THE
HOSPITAL
IN
MODERN
SOCIETY

Edited by

Eliot Freidson

The Free Press of Glencoe

COLLIER-MACMILLAN LIMITED, LONDON

THE

HOSPITAL

IN

MODERN

SOCIETY

FOR
MARION

Preface

In the most general sense, the hospital is a place in which ailing people sleep and receive care. Because ailing people live in it, the hospital will always have some attributes of the hotel or dormitory: some of its personnel will play domestic roles and others will supervise them. Because ailing people receive some sort of care while they are living there, the hospital will always have some of the attributes of the school or prison: some of its personnel will assume responsibility for the inmates. Provision of hospital care thus implies a profound division of people into those who assume responsibility, those for whom responsibility is assumed, and those who keep house. The nature of that division has varied with prevailing notions of what ails people and what must be done to help them. In all, the word "hospital" has been applied to institutions that have on one occasion or another resembled a Skid Row hostel, a religious retreat, a school, a prison, a hotel, an elephant's graveyard, and a hospital. Such variation is not entirely historical. In the United States there are gross and important differences among proprietary hospitals, rural community hospitals, religious-administered hospitals, public hospitals, and university hospitals, not to speak of differences between general hospitals and those devoted to specific diseases like mental disorder and tuberculosis.

The Study of Hospitals and the Social Sciences

Its very variation makes the hospital a particularly useful object for study by social science. Social science has been handicapped continually by the problem of controlling the variables it studies, and has in only narrowly limited areas been able to perform the laboratory experiments common to disciplines concerned with the physical world. More commonly, it has used the survey method to gather a large enough mass of material to allow sorting out the influence of a number of variables by statistical means; but studies in which control of organizational variables can be central to analysis have been rare. This deficiency is partly a technical problem, but at least as much a problem of access to an adequate range of organizational variation. American factories were the first organizations to be studied in any great detail by a fairly wide range of modern social scientists, but access to them has been limited, and even the clear-cut variable of technology has lacked systematic control. The hospital has unique and valuable virtues that can overcome this persistent problem. The virtues of the hospital are that it is an ubiquitous institution, that its character varies both widely and significantly, and that it is more likely than most organizations to be accessible.

That the hospital is more ubiquitous than most organizations, with the possible exception of schools, is self-evident enough to require no discussion. Similarly, its range of variation is obvious. Although the primary aim of hospital work is application of therapy to persons rather than the production of goods, many other significant elements vary. Some hospitals are run for profit from client fees, like a factory or a hotel; others subsist on fees supplemented by donations and volunteer staffing; others subsist on private or public donations alone. Technology varies: that of a mental hospital is considerably different from that of a physical-rehabilitation hospital. Clientele vary: legally committed patients in a mental or tuberculosis hospital are in a considerably different position from that of patients in a swank lying-in or proprietary hospital. And as more than one of the papers of this volume makes clear, there are also profound differences in staff organization to be found among hospitals that probably exceed those to be found in any other institution of modern society. Therefore, hospitals provide a number of "natural experiments" in human organization.

Finally, they are more accessible than most organizations. Even when they are run privately for a profit, hospitals tend to be responsible to the state. Morally, they tend to be part of the public domain. Since they are generally identified with the universalism of science, they cannot easily excuse themselves from study by reference to competitive trade secrets. And, since they are supposed to have ameliorative aims, they may be positively eager to be studied in the hope that they may be able to improve themselves.

One purpose of this collection of papers is to indicate the range of possibilities for study the hospital provides for the social scientist. While the collection is not completely representative of all present research on the hospital, it does represent the scope of present work—from large-scale institutional studies to the very particular studies of the experiences of patients. Furthermore, by virtue of the fact that the papers suggest more than they actually demonstrate (which is what good papers should do), many possibilities for further research are indicated. In this, then, it is hoped that the collection will be provocative for social scientists.

Social Science Methods and the Hospital

For those concerned with the practical affairs of the hospital, this collection will be of somewhat different interest. Many hospitals have been opening their doors to social scientists recently, and others will no doubt be doing so in the near future. The inclination of most in so doing is likely to be practical in origin, guided by the desire to answer such questions as: How can we obtain more donations from the community? Why do so many patients leave against medical advice? Why is there such high staff turnover? Why is there persistent grumbling among the house staff and how justified is it? Why do patients seem to be so unhappy on one floor and so satisfied on another? Some of the papers in this collection actually address themselves to such questions, but they do so in a way that may not seem justified to the practical reader. Nonetheless, there is justification.

It is perfectly clear that, in so far as practical questions do not require description so much as explanation, they are not so straightforward as they look. Any halfway good answers will have ramifications in a variety of areas, so one becomes involved in an enormous clutter of particularistic facts and variables. Perhaps merely in self-defense, more likely because it is aesthetically gratifying and practically necessary, the social scientist is likely to sort out the clutter by the use of concepts and an assumption that he can proceed as if all else outside his concepts were held constant. Inevitably he is led to a degree of abstraction from the concrete problem he studies, even if his study was not guided by any elaborate conceptualization in the first place. The consequence very often is that, although the results of the study may be "interesting" to those involved, they do not tell the host institution in detail what to do about the problem that led it to invite the study in the first place. Sometimes the findings are such that the institution studied is presented in a grotesque, almost unrecognizable light. Aside from problems requiring only description of the distribution of attributes in a given situation (for which social science has fairly routine tools of some precision), this result is partly inevitable and in fact quite desirable.

The aim of social science is the aim of all science—understanding through the development of empirically testable, universal propositions. Social science is thus trying to penetrate the unchanging core of a diffuse contemporaneousness. It follows that its task requires seizing upon the apparently strategic and exploiting it while deemphasizing the apparently trivial and tangential. It further follows that the quality of the task it performs is no better than the quality of its guide to what is chosen as strategic. The particular virtue of the guides used by social science is their systematic and self-conscious character—a character that, in the long if not the short run, far surpasses the uncontrolled selectivity of common sense. The source of this systematic approach varies. Sometimes it is a limited theory that has been worked out on empirical grounds, sometimes a logically derived taxonomy, sometimes the insight of the individual researcher. The strategy of this systematic approach also varies. Sometimes it is based on a closely argued view of the interrelations of a number of variables, sometimes rotation of a number of variables to sort out relative influence of each, sometimes the use of an analogy to order the data, sometimes the pursuit of the diverse ramifications of a single important theme or fact. It is only the approach itself—not its source, its strategy, or its content—that may be considered typical of social science. In so far as this collection reflects some of that unity of approach and diversity of style, it may serve both to expand and to temper the views of social science held by those preoccupied with the practical affairs of health institutions.

Summary of the Papers

Briefly summarized, the papers have been arranged to move from the widest possible historical and cross-national scope to progressively more detailed views of the hospital. In the first paper, Rosen presents a sociologically oriented history of the hospital that shows the rich potentialities of the topic for comparative historical study. In the second, Glaser presents a systematic review of the strategic differences between hospitals as they exist today in the world, suggesting a variety of ways in which those differences influence hospital operations. Elling, focusing on the place of the hospital in the local community, presents a case study of the way in which attempts to plan hospital facilities rationally in an American city became transformed by political forces mobilized by individual hospitals seeking to preserve their own interests.

Focusing on control *within* the hospital, Perrow presents a case study of how the balance of policy-making power in an American hospital has shifted from one to another agent as institutional goals have changed—shifts fairly representative of those taking place in American voluntary hospitals in general. Looking at the hospital as a whole, Strauss and his associates argue that the most appropriate model for the analysis of the hospital (and other organizations that, like the hospital, typically bring together a variety of professions) should not stress organizational structure so much as the continuous negotiation and renegotiation of order among the participants. Goss, restricting herself to analysis of the medical staff in a teaching hospital, seeks to determine how the presumed incompatibility between formal bureaucratic organization and professional autonomy are reconciled without excessively dysfunctional conflict. She suggests a new analytical model that she labels "advisory bureaucracy."

Kendall presents survey material indicating something of the range of variation among hospitals in the learning environment provided for interns and residents, suggesting how elements of hospital organization vary and the significance of such variation to medical education. Coser seeks to explain differences in alienation from work among nurses in two units of a hospital by analyzing how staff organization stimulates and maintains a strong sense of occupational identity. Rosengren and DeVault explore the implications of the temporal and spatial organization of an obstetrical unit for staff behavior and definitions of patient behavior. Roth analyzes the transmission of information between staff and patient, and among the staff, emphasizing the inadequacy of the process and the inevitability of conflict in the process. And, finally, Sommer and Dewar discuss the psychological significance of the physical environment of the ward to the patient.

The Theme of Environment

Taken as a whole, it would be folly to assert that any single theme dominates this collection. There is one, however, that seems to serve as a focus for many of the papers. The relation of the hospital to its environment enters into the papers of this collection in more than one way.

Consonant with the expanse of time covered, Rosen's paper

indicates very clearly how the environment forms the organization. We can follow the founding, governing, reform, or decline of hospitals, not as something mysteriously proceeding from within organizations themselves (which is the view we are most prone to get from empirical studies of the hospital from the inside), but as something reflecting the demands made on them by the political and economic forces of the community. Indeed, in Elling's paper we see how hospitals dependent on the support of the local community struggle to capture for themselves the loyalty of influential community elements—how, in fact, hospitals in such circumstances are likely in part to make themselves into the image they believe is attractive to the community and, in part, to persuade the community that what they are is good and worthy of support. Both Glaser and Perrow comment on how this immediate dependence on local public support on the part of the American voluntary hospital shapes so many of the services it provides. These papers all imply that one quite important task, as yet unperformed in the study of hospitals, is to distinguish clearly what is effectively internal to organization and what may be better examined as a function of the external environment. That something goes on within the walls of a building does not mean it is sociologically internal.

Another side of the problem of defining the relation of organization to its environment complicates matters considerably. It is raised when we address ourselves to the question of the best kind of model for the analysis of staff relations in the hospital. As Goss points out, the classic model of bureaucratic organization is far enough removed from American hospital organization to raise the question of adopting another model entirely, or at least of elaborating variant submodels. Her own suggestion of "advisory bureaucracy" is eminently appropriate for the situation she discusses and, in conjunction with the variants suggested by other students, goes pretty far toward creating an adequate range of subtypes by which we may classify analytically significant aspects of organizational variation. Explaining why these variations occur, however, is another thing.

From what Glaser tells us about European hospitals, something very much like the classic model of bureaucratic organization exists there, with neither the markedly dual line of authority mentioned by observers of American hospitals, nor the advisory pattern of control of medical staff described by Goss. Indeed, Glaser's description resembles Victor Thompson's discussion of "monocratic" organizations. But what varies in the comparison? Medicine is practiced in each locale; professionals practice it; why should there be such marked differences? I suspect that explanation lies in one of the major variables uncontrolled by gross European-American comparisons—the career environment outside the hospital for the staff working inside.

An organization can be treated as a thing in itself, its staff arranged in the positions by which we delineate formal structure. This method of treatment usually ignores staff turnover largely because it is the position, not its incumbent, that is the focus. Another way of looking at the organization, however, treats the staff position as a stage of an occupational career, so that turnover becomes very much the focus, and the organization is seen as a place where people may come together momentarily while on their way somewhere else. Considering the hospital as a focus for occupational careers, the alternative jobs offered outside the hospital are a critical element in assessing positions inside the hospital. Under the proper circumstances, the organization of staff positions and privileges within the hospital may be seen as in part something continuously negotiated in the light of the opportunities available to the staff in the outside environment. This, of course, is a crude example of the negotiations discussed by Strauss and his associates.

As Glaser notes, one gross difference between European and American hospitals is the sharp segregation of opportunities in the hospital from those in the community. Specialty- and hospital-oriented physicians in the United States have considerably greater flexibility of choice among career alternatives than is the case for their opposite number in Europe; it is the exception in America who is wholly dependent on a hospital staff appointment and hospital-dispensed patronage (though this situation may be changing). All this means, to put it bluntly, that some of the difference in organization of European and American hospitals can be ascribed plausibly to the fact that the American attending staff doctor is in a better position to bargain. As a "guest" he can avoid much of the administrative "dirty work," and in turn escape the exercise of much administrative and advisory influence. Thus, career alternatives outside the organization constitute an independent variable that qualifies the position of a worker within the organization. The exact influence of this factor on formal organization remains to be demonstrated, but should it be done for hospitals (in which the profession is held constant but staff organization varied) we may find we have been ascribing too much influence on organization to professionalism and too little to the professional market place.

Aside from the organization and its environment, another theme runs through many of the papers of this collection that joins together many superficially disparate topics. I refer to the concept of observability, attention to which has been drawn by Merton, and in this volume emphasized by Coser. As a concept it is intimately attached to the physical and technological world, for some kinds of work are by their nature more observable physically than others. But it is just as intimately connected with social structure and even, as Coser suggests, with self-identity. It may turn out to be a crucial concept for the analysis of the central problem of organizational studies—the character of supervision and control of work. However, it cannot be discussed at length here, any more than can others. The papers must be left for the reader to explore for himself in the following pages.

ELIOT FREIDSON

CONTRIBUTORS

Rue Bucher is Research Associate at the Department of Psychiatry, University of Illinois.

Rose Laub Coser is Associate Sociologist in the Social Science Department of McLean Hospital, and Research Associate at Harvard Medical School.

Spencer DeVault is Staff Psychologist at Emma Pendleton Bradley Hospital, and Assistant Professor of Psychology at Rhode Island College.

Robert Dewar is on the staff of University Hospital, Saskatoon, Saskatchewan.

Danuta Ehrlich is on the staff of the Psychiatric Institute, Michael Reese Hospital, Chicago.

Ray H. Elling is Assistant Professor at Sloan Institute of Hospital Administration, Cornell University.

Eliot Freidson is Associate Professor of Sociology at New York University.

William A. Glaser is Research Associate at the Bureau of Applied Social Research, Columbia University.

Mary E. W. Goss is Research Associate at New York Hospital-Cornell Medical Center.

Patricia L. Kendall is Research Associate at the Bureau of Applied Social Research, Columbia University.

Charles Perrow is Assistant Professor of Sociology at University of Michigan.

George Rosen is Professor of Health Education at Columbia University School of Public Health and Administrative Medicine.

WILLIAM R. ROSENGREN is Assistant Professor of Sociology at Brown University.

JULIUS A. ROTH is Research Scientist at New York School of Social Work, Columbia University.

MELVIN SABSHIN is Chairman of the Department of Psychiatry, University of Illinois Medical School.

LEONARD SCHATZMAN is Research Sociologist on the Staff of the San Francisco Medical Center, University of California.

ROBERT SOMMER is Assistant Professor of Psychology at University of Alberta.

ANSELM STRAUSS is Professor of Sociology in the School of Nursing, San Francisco Medical Center, University of California.

Contents

(**xix**)

THE
HOSPITAL
IN
MODERN
SOCIETY

1

The Hospital

HISTORICAL SOCIOLOGY OF A

COMMUNITY INSTITUTION

GEORGE ROSEN

Introduction

Illness creates dependency. The sick need not only medical treatment but also personal care and shelter. Throughout history societies have accepted such need as a responsibility of community life, and have created various institutions to provide the necessary services. One of these institutions, the hospital, is today a cornerstone of any modern system of health care.

Arrangements to provide for the needs of the sick have always been intimately linked with the varying economic, political,

This study was financed by a grant (M-3171) from the National Institute of Mental Health, U. S. Public Health Service. The paper is an expansion of one read at the 1960 meetings of the American Sociological Association.

(1)

social, and cultural conditions that govern the life of man.
Whether man lived in a city or on the land, whether he suffered
scarcity or enjoyed abundance, how he saw his fellow men and
how they looked upon him, the religion he practiced and the
values he prized, the learning, arts, and sciences that gave
shape to his society—all have affected the development of the
hospital, the form it has achieved, and the services it offered. To
be understood, the hospital has to be seen, therefore, as an organ
of society, sharing its characteristics, changing as the society of
which it is a part is transformed, and carrying into the future
evidence of its past.

A historical sociology of the hospital in this sense requires a
delineation of political and economic conditions, social structure,
value systems, cultural organization, and social change in relation
to the health conditions and needs of populations at various
historical periods. However, a task of this kind far exceeds the
limits of this chapter, and will not be undertaken here. Instead,
I have selected a number of hospital types that can be distinguished in different historical periods, and in each case described and discussed how the hospital was conceived, organized,
financed, and operated, how it was related to its societal context, and how it changed or gave way to other kinds of
institutions.

The Medieval Hospital

The concept of a need for social assistance in case of sickness
or other misfortune was highly developed during the Middle
Ages. This was as true of the Moslems and Jews as of the
Christians, and was most evident in the creation of hospitals.
Religious and social considerations were pre-eminent in the
development of these facilities.

To be sure, separate institutions for the care of the sick existed
even earlier. Temples were probably the earliest institutions
concerned with such care, as in the case of the cult of Asclepius.
Separate medical institutions for the care and shelter of the sick
first appear in Rome,[1] but the guiding motives in their develop-

ment were clearly military or economic for the most part, and obviously related to the structure and purposes of Roman society. Other values underlie the creation of hospitals by Christian communities during the later Empire and the medieval period. The teaching of Paul, "and now abideth faith, hope and charity, these three; but the greatest of these is charity," sets forth one of the basic values that motivated the rise of such institutions. The Christian had a duty to his sick and suffering fellows, and the practical expression of this charitable idea became evident after Constantine accepted Christianity and recognized it as a state religion. Bishops had an obligation to receive strangers or the needy into their homes, or to see that they were cared for by the community in other ways. The Council of Nicaea (A.D. 325) instructed the bishops to establish a hospital in every city that had a cathedral, and at the end of the fourth century the Council of Carthage (A.D. 398) urged them to maintain a hospice (*hospitiolum*) not far from the church. The model for these Christian institutions was very probably the Jewish hospice, which already existed in the Talmudic and pre-Christian period.

The motive of charity was reinforced by another Christian value—that Grace and salvation might be achieved by giving alms. Thus, the so-called second letter of St. Clement, which dates from the second or third century, informed the congregation of Corinth that "almsgiving relieves the burden of sin." [2] Moreover, through sickness and suffering man became a participant in the Grace of God. To care for the sick was not only a Christian duty but also beneficial for the salvation of the soul. Through association with the sick, and by providing for them, the healthy could participate in their grace. Had not Christ said: "I was sick and you visited me. Whatever you have done unto one of these, the least of my brethren, you have done it unto me"? This motive is found throughout the entire medieval period.

From the fourth century on, institutions were founded to care for the sick and those in need. An early example is the hospital established by St. Basil at Caesarea in Cappadocia (369–372). [3] This institution comprised several sections, and cared for travelers, the indigent, the infirm, and the sick. Even those suffering from contagious ailments such as leprosy were admitted. The entire staff, including physicians, resided in the hospital. The land with which the Emperor Valens had endowed the church of Caesarea was its principal source of revenue. The example provided by St. Basil was followed in 398 by St. John Chrysostom when he became Patriarch of Constantinople. A number of similar hospitals were constructed in the capital. The administration of each of these establishments was entrusted to two priests. Institutions of the same kind also came into being at Alexandria and elsewhere in the Eastern Empire.

While these early institutions combined social and medical functions, hostels, hospitals, and other charitable establishments were set up separately. Fabiola, a Roman matron who had aided in founding a hospice at Ostia, also created an infirmary (*nosocomium*) in Rome, and according to St. Jerome "gathered into it sufferers from the streets, giving their poor bodies worn with sickness and hunger all a nurse's care." An awareness of the distinction between the hospital in a strict sense and other facilities designed for the care of groups with different needs is evidenced by the various terms used to designate them.[4] *Xenodochia* were hostels or hospices for pilgrims, travelers, and all those who needed a lodging when in a strange town. *Nosocomia* designated hospitals, that is, institutions for the care of the sick. *Gerocomia* were establishments for the aged; *lobotrophia* provided asylum for the disabled or for lepers; *orphanotrophia* were orphanages, and *brephotrophia* designated foundling homes.

A number of different officials administered these institutions. In imperial decrees, the director of such a facility is designated as *administrator, antistes, or praepositus*. When referring to the chief administrator of a specific type of institution, terms such as *nosocomos* or *xenodochos* were employed. Such titles as *oeconomos* or *circuitor* designated the superintendent of an institution.

The degree to which the hospital in the East Roman or Byzantine Empire tended to achieve a clear-cut institutional character is most sharply revealed by the organization of the important hospital attached to the Monastery of the Savior Pantocrator at Constantinople, Our knowledge of this and similar institutions is derived from their *typica*, or charters of foundation. The monastery and its associated welfare facilities were established by John II Comnenos in 1112, and seem to have been completed by 1136.[5]

The hospital had an outpatient department and five sections, each for a different class of ailments. A surgical ward of ten beds was provided for patients with fractures and wounds. A second ward of eight beds was assigned to patients with acute infectious diseases, particularly ailments of the eyes and the intestinal tract. Twelve beds in another ward were reserved for women. Then there were two wards of ten beds each for simpler cases. Furthermore, each ward had an extra bed for emergency cases. However, in addition to these there were six more beds, each with a mattress that had a central hole, for patients so seriously ill that they could not move.

The medical staff was quite large. Each ward had no less than two physicians, three assistants, and several orderlies. The women's ward had a woman physician in addition to the two male physicians. These women physicians probably developed from midwives, and it is quite likely that obstetrics was practiced on the women's ward.[6] Two chief surgeons headed the surgical service of the hospital, and provided care for female patients when required. In addition, the surgical service included a specialist for hernia operations. Furthermore two physicians, two surgeons, and eight assistants provided care for ambulatory patients in the dispensary. In difficult cases the chief physicians were called upon for consultation. The entire medical staff was divided into two groups, each serving alternately for a period of a month. Physicians on service were expected to visit patients at least once daily and twice a day in summer. Physicians also had night duty. The hospital was administered by two physicians, the *primmikerioi*. Under their direction two chief physicians supervised the medical staff.

Both the Moslems who overran large parts of the Eastern Empire and the Europeans who came into contact with it for religious, commercial, or political reasons were impressed and influenced by its hospitals and other welfare institutions. At first the Moslems used existing institutions; then they built new ones. In the ninth century, during the reign of the Caliph Harun al-Rashid, a hospital was founded at Baghdad. Another hospital was built there in the next century by the Caliph al-Muktadir. A third hospital founded at Baghdad in 970 had a staff of twenty-five physicians and was used for the teaching of medical students. All in all, there are records of some thirty-four hospitals in countries under Islamic rule. These hospitals were generally well organized, and reflect the high state of development attained by medicine in Moslem lands. At Cairo, for example, the hospital founded in 1283 had separate sections for patients with febrile illnesses, for the wounded, and for those with eye diseases, as well as special rooms for women. Medical care was provided by a staff of physicians under a director, and three male and female nurses or aides. The similarity to the type of institution exemplified by the Pantocrator is unmistakable.

The hospital as concept and as institution developed much more slowly in the West. In view of the close linkage to the Church, it is not surprising that the most significant early contribution to the establishment of hospitals came from medieval monasticism. The manner in which the monks cared for their own sick became a model for the laity. The monasteries had an *infirmitorium*, where the sick monks were taken for treatment, a pharmacy, and frequently also a garden with medicinal plants. In addition to caring for members of the monastic community, the monasteries also provided for pilgrims and travelers. The beginnings of this practice cannot be precisely established, but it is quite likely that they go back to the early Middle Ages.

Benedict of Nursia, the founder of Western monasticism, dealt with these matters explicitly in the code of religious life that he created on Monte Cassino about A.D. 535. In Chapter 36 of his *Rule,* Benedict specified that "a cell be set apart by itself for the sick brethren, and one who is God-fearing, diligent and careful, be appointed to serve them." Another chapter deals with guests who are to be received like Christ Himself. Moreover, special care should be "taken in the reception of the poor and of strangers." For this purpose a guesthouse is to be established.[7] Other monastic orders had similar rules. The Franciscans were told to care for the sick in the same manner that they themselves would wish to be treated in case of illness.

As monastic houses were established, these injunctions were carried out, and the simple cell set aside for a sick monk in many instances became a large institution. Thus, an architectural plan of the Abbey of St. Gall, in Switzerland, in 820 contains a hospital, with rooms for seriously ill patients (*cubiculum valde infirmorum*), for a chief physician (*mansio medici ipsius*), and for other physicians (*domus medicorum*). Nearby is the pharmacy (*armarium pigmentorium*), and behind the physician's quarters lies the herb garden with sixteen plots for various plants.[8]

The visitor to Tintern Abbey, in Monmouthshire, founded in 1131 for monks of the Cistercian order, will find a similar establishment. The infirmary of the abbey housed both the sick and the aged monks, and comprised a large hall, a cloister, and a kitchen. Attached to the hall at one end is a room with a drain that was probably the latrine. A passage connects the infirmary hall with the church.[9] Similar arrangements can be found in various parts of Europe.

Further important impulses toward the creation of hospitals came from ecclesiastical as well as secular sources. At the Council of Aachen, in 816, it was decided that a refuge for the poor (*receptaculum, hospitale pauperum*) would be established by bishops and abbots.[10] In the course of the following two to three hundred years, establishments for the poor, the sick, and for strangers were founded at bishops' sees and in connection with cathedral chapters and religious communities. Meffert has clearly demonstrated this development for Bavaria.[11] In Germany, hospitals were first founded in the seventh century in the Rhineland-Westphalia area, and not earlier than the ninth century in the northern section.[12]

The hospital also spread because it became a central institution around which great hospital and nursing orders established themselves. Thus, hospitals were founded along the routes taken by the Crusaders, and several knightly orders organized during the holy wars assumed the mission of establishing and maintaining hospitals. The best known of these orders, the Knights of St. John or the Hospitalers, for example, founded hospitals as far apart as Malta and Germany. Another trend developed with the founding of the Holy Ghost Hospital at Montpellier by Guido, a pious layman. Sanctioned in 1198 by Pope Innocent III, the Order of the Holy Ghost established and maintained similar hospitals throughout Europe.

As time went on, many different kinds of benefactors founded hospitals. Kings, queens, high ecclesiastics, noble lords, wealthy merchants, guilds, fraternities, and municipalities—all endowed houses for the care of the sick, the poor, the infirm, the aged, and for numerous other purposes. The first hospital in England was founded in 937 by Athelstan, favorite grandson of Alfred the Great, at York, and was dedicated to St. Peter. Later, in 1155, after a great and destructive fire, it was reestablished by King Stephen and dedicated to St. Leonard. It became a vast establishment which in 1370 maintained over two hundred sick and otherwise infirm inmates. Still surviving today is the vaulted undercroft that was the basement story of a large infirmary hall.[13]

Another extant relic in York is the undercroft or hospital in the Merchant Adventurers' Hall. Built between 1357–1368, the hall housed the guild of York mercers and merchants. The guild was a dual organization comprising (1) a fraternity concerned with religious and social matters and (2) a mystery concerned with trade and commercial affairs. In 1371 the fraternity created a hospital. Two years later, the Archbishop of York undertook the reorganization of the hospital, and Johannes de Roncliff, a benefactor of the guild, became its patron. Thirteen poor and feeble people, apparently impoverished mercers, under the charge of a resident master, were to inhabit the hospital. Attached to the hospital was a chapel in charge of a chaplain. The hospital was called the Hospital of the Blessed Mary and the Holy Trinity. With the Reformation, the religious aspects of the hospital disappeared, but the pensioners remained. Indeed, pensioners continued to live in the accommodations on the street floor of the hall until the end of 1900. Thereafter they were boarded out with relatives or others.[14]

York simply illustrates a significant trend. The guilds took an important and active part in founding hospitals as well as other establishments for medical care and social assistance. Funds were created for the relief of their sick and disabled members. Wealthy guilds built their own hospitals; others paid regular fees to a cloister hospital that assumed responsibility for the accommodation and care of their members.

By the end of the fifteenth century, as a result of the developments described above, Europe was covered with a network of hospitals. For example, in England alone, by the middle of the fourteenth century, there were more than six hundred institutions of this kind, ranging in size from numerous small foundations caring for a dozen or so persons to the great establishments like St. Peter's and St. Leonard's of York.[15] Developments on the Continent were similar. According to the chronicler Giovanni Villani, Florence in 1300, with a population of some ninety thousand inhabitants, had thirty hospitals and welfare establishments capable of providing medical aid and shelter to more than a thousand sick and needy people. They were staffed by more than three hundred monks or other nursing personnel. During the later fifteenth century, under Lorenzo the Magnificent, there were some forty hospitals of various kinds. Paris at the beginning of the fourteenth century is reported to have had about forty hospitals and as many leper houses.

The hospitals varied considerably in purpose, and there were variations in the way they functioned. The medieval hospital was not only a center for medical care but a philanthropic and spiritual institution as well. Provision was made at various times and in different places for lepers, orphans, pregnant women, the aged and invalid, and strangers, as well as for those suffering from illness. Smaller establishments frequently dealt with a limited group or specific problem, while large institutions handled a wide range of health and welfare problems. Actually, this was a logical consequence of the premises on which the whole system developed, namely, the religious obligation to provide care and support for the sick, the poor, and the disabled. Those admitted to a hospital were to be received and cared for in a spirit of Christian charity. Tierney in discussing medieval poor law notes that the church lawyers of the period seldom discussed in detail the kind of administrative problems that have most perplexed writers on institutional poor relief in more recent times. There is very little, for instance, on criteria of admission to hospitals, or on the relative values of outdoor relief and institutional care in different types of cases. There was certainly no idea of a "workhouse test." [16]

While the hospital was created as a philanthropic institution and an agency of poor relief, it was simultaneously also a religious and spiritual institution. Spiritual care, prayer, and religious provision for the dying were predominant in every Christian hospital. Even when hospitals were taken over from the ecclesiastical authorities by municipalities in the later Middle Ages, they were not secularized.[17] Essentially, the hospital was a religious house in which the nursing personnel had united as a vocational community under a religious rule.[18] Spenser in *The Faerie Queene* sums up succinctly this side of the institution:

> Eftsoones unto an holy Hospitall
> That was foreby the way, she did him bring:
> In which seven Bead-men, that had vowed all
> Their life to service of high heavens King,
> Did spend their daies in doing godly thing.
> Their gates to all were open evermore,
> That by the wearie way were traveiling;
> And one sate wayting ever them before,
> To call in commers-by that needy were and pore.[19]

The medieval hospital generally had clergy attached to it; frequently it was also a church, and religious services were conducted in it for the edification of the faithful. In short, the hospital was a *locus religiosus* from an ecclesiastical viewpoint, and legally a *pia causa*. As such it enjoyed certain privileges and rights. Most frequently the hospital was tax-exempt; thus, the Hôtel-Dieu of Angers was able to sell its wine to taverns without paying any taxes to the government. The right of burial (*jus funerandi*) was also granted to hospitals, as was the right of asylum.

The financing of the medieval hospital reflected its origins and purpose. Medieval charity was a consequence of one of the strongest and most widespread feelings of the period, the desire for salvation and sanctification. An effective means for the achievement of this aim and to avoid suffering and pain in the next world was the performance of good works, including charity toward the poor and needy. Countless endowments, almshouses, hospitals, and other charitable institutions bear witness to the strength of this religio-social principle. Endowment, legacies, donations, offerings, lands and buildings provided the financial basis for the medieval hospital. The revenues of the Hôtel-Dieu of Beauvais in 1450 may serve as an example (Table 1).

Table 1

Revenues of Hotel-Dieu of Beauvais, 1450

Revenues (in specie)	Livres
Quitrents, leases, farms	144
Legacies, donations, offerings, and so forth (including 11 livres from the sale of beds, clothes, and the like)	27
Seigneurial rights	2
	173
Revenues (in kind)	
Quitrents, tithes, and so forth	33
Direct exploitation	
Wine	297
Wheat	170
Grains	56
Animals	35
Wood	2
	593
Grand Total	766

A number of hospitals at the death of a member of the parish took the bed and linen of the deceased. Judicial fines were sometimes given to hospitals by royal or seigneurial order. In 1395, for example, the Parlement of Paris laid a fine of 10,000 livres on the Jews living there, of which 500 livres were to go to the Hôtel-Dieu of Paris, the remainder for the construction of a bridge that would essentially serve the needs of the same institution.

The concept of good works as a means to salvation tends to emphasize the role of the donor in giving charity. It is the giving that is important—this is the essential good work. However, the founder, sponsor, or patron of a charitable institution had certain rights in it that were determined by law. All such institutions operated under a constitution granted by the local diocesan bishop. By 1414, the Archbishop of Canterbury had formulated a general framework for this purpose, namely, "The Statutes of St. James, according to the use of the Church of England." [20] Founders or patrons could determine what kinds of persons were to be admitted to the institution; they appointed the administrator (warden, master, keeper) and had a right to make a visitation whenever they desired to inspect the premises, the observance of the rule, the accounts, and other aspects of the operation of the institution. Moreover, they could set rules of behavior and punish those who broke them.[21] Indeed, even when municipal or national governments took over the administration of hospitals and other charitable institutions, the rights and intentions of the original founders were taken into account.[22] As Tierney points out, canonistic writers on hospital law were largely concerned with the regulation of the property rights of the institution and the definition of its legal status in relation to the local parish and diocesan authorities.[23]

But while a bishop could act to prevent maladministration of charitable bequests in his diocese, before the fourteenth century there was no general regulation of hospitals and related institutions. The individualistic, private characters of these caritative foundations made possible the appearance of various abuses, especially during the later Middle Ages. Hospital funds were misappropriated; in various instances hospitals were turned into ecclesiastical benefices to provide an income for some cleric; and toward the end of the Middle Ages hospitals frequently became boarding homes for the aged or for able-bodied individuals. In 1321, for example, Bishop Johann von Strassburg ordered the master of the Andreasspital at Offenburg to receive only the infirm and invalid poor and not to admit any idle, healthy individuals who could support themselves outside the institution. Excepted were persons who had sufficient means to support themselves and would therefore not disadvantage the sick.[24] Similarly, in 1414, an English statute for the institution of hospital reforms is justified on the basis that "many hospitals . . . be now for the most part decayed, and the goods and profits of the same, by divers persons, spiritual and temporal, withdrawn and spent to the use of others, whereby many men and women have died in great misery for default of aid, livelihood and succor." [25]

Ecclesiastical authorities were aware of various abuses that had become notorious, and in 1311 Pope Clement V promulgated the decretal *Quia contingit,* later incorporated in the *Extravagantes Joannis XXII.*[26] This decretal required all administrators of hospitals to swear to administer honestly property entrusted to them, and to prepare for the bishop an annual statement of hospital accounts. Moreover, the administrator did not have to be a cleric; that is, the hospital was not to be considered an ecclesiastical benefice, and its resources were to be devoted wholly to the charitable end for which it was created. Bishops were required to look into the administration of all hospitals in their dioceses, and to correct abuses.

The Medieval Hospital in Transition

Despite such efforts, however, the decline in the medieval hospital system continued. The authorities, both ecclesiastical and civil, neglected to take action where abuses existed and to enforce reforms; founders or their descendants failed to curb the malfeasance of administrators; and a number of other influences and elements, economic, social, and political, came into play to create a new situation.[27] For one thing, from the thirteenth century on, the hospital came increasingly under secular jurisdiction.

As cities in Europe prospered and the bourgeoisie grew wealthy and powerful, municipal authorities tended to take over or to supplement the activities of the Church. In part, this was politically motivated, a desire of the civil authorities to be independent of clerical domination or to render the ecclesiastical power subordinate. Yet, this does not mean that the clergy were entirely eliminated. Monks and nuns continued to provide nursing care as they had done before. Administratively, the municipal authorities were responsible for the hospital facilities, but the Church might participate in some way. At Amiens, in the fifteenth century, for example, the master of the Hôtel-Dieu was elected by the municipality, but installed in his office by the bishop. At Louvain from 1473 to 1476, the ecclesiastical authorities played a part in removing two unsatisfactory administrators from the town hospital.[28]

Second, the hospitals and related establishments were increasingly inadequate to deal with new situations, in which problems of health and welfare were considered from a new viewpoint. From the medieval standpoint, the poor, the sick, and the infirm might almost be considered necessary for the salvation of the donor of charity. They did the almsgiver a service, and had they not been present they might have had to be created. However, such an attitude tended to encourage begging and the acceptance of the beggar as a necessary part of human society. Little or no consideration was given to bettering the condition of the poor and the sick. During the late Middle Ages, and especially following the Reformation, the whole approach to this problem changed.[29]

Though the causes of poverty changed but little from the thirteenth century to the sixteenth, economic and social circumstances altered their significance and intensified their impact. As a result, the condition of the poor, which was bad in the earlier period, had become increasingly severe by the early sixteenth century. Increased unemployment, higher prices, enclosure of peasant lands and related factors brought into being the problem of vagrancy, which was constant throughout the fourteenth and fifteenth centuries. Vagrancy appeared in the Netherlands and Germany even earlier than in England, and then assumed increasingly large proportions. In their endeavors to piece out a livelihood, many vagrants pretended to be crippled or diseased, so as to be able to beg with impunity and to obtain admission to a hospital. There is little doubt that the large number of poor and sick wanderers overtaxed the facilities available in various countries. Whether these vagrants were sick or not, there was a great deal of economic and social distress by the sixteenth century, and the problem was what to do about it. As Simon Fish put the case in 1529 in his famous *Supplicacyon for the Beggers*: "But whate remedy to releve us your poore sike lame and sore bedemen? To make many hospitals for the relief of the poore people? Nay truely. The moo the worse, for ever the fatte of the hole foundacion hangeth on the prestes berdes." [30] Fish proposed a solution: that the clergy be expropriated and the hospitals and related facilities be taken in hand by the king.

In fact, this was the course followed, a course influenced essentially by the Reformation and the rise of the absolutist state. While the intervention of the civil authorities in matters of welfare and health before the sixteenth century has been noted, the notion that poor relief, including medical care, was a community and not a church responsibility was definitely established during the Reformation period. Those who wished to bring some order into the area of welfare and health, whether Vives in Bruges or Zwingli in Zürich, were guided by the same principles and were oriented to the same goals: elimination of all beggary, organization of effective agencies of public assistance, and unification of all facilities and resources (hospitals, domiciliary relief, and the like) in the hands of municipal or national authorities.

However, throughout the period the hospital changed little in its character. It remained a combination of an institution for the care of the sick, an old-age home, an almshouse, and an orphanage, possibly a guesthouse. Many aspects of medieval hospital administration were retained. For example, religious services continued to be held in many places, not only in Catholic countries. Sweden's first general legislation on hospital administration of 1571 laid down specific instructions that at least once a day, at a given time, prayers were to be said collectively for peace on earth, for the welfare of the authorities, and for all concerned with the management of the hospital.[31]

Hospital administration of the period is clearly described in an account of the organization of the London hospitals in the middle of the sixteenth century.[32] Over-all administration was in the hands of a board of governors comprising sixty-six members. Of these, fourteen were aldermen and fifty-two "grave commoners, citizens and freemen of the said citie." Furthermore, the latter group included at least four scriveners, or notaries. The board of governors was headed by two aldermen termed governors general; the other twelve aldermen and the fifty-two commoners were divided into four subcommittees, each of which supervised one of the four London hospitals. Each subcommittee had at least sixteen members; one of these, an alderman, acted as president, and another, a commoner, served as treasurer. Members of the board of governors were elected at an annual meeting held on St. Matthew's day at Christ's Hospital or one of the others. A majority of the board was required, and each new member was elected for a two-year term. In a special situation a longer term was permitted.

The administration of each hospital was in the hands of a staff consisting of two groups. Officials concerned with the business management and administration of the institution were called governors, and comprised the following: a controller general and a surveyor general who were responsible for all the affairs of the hospital and represented it at meetings of the governors of the London hospitals; a president who was the actual director or administrator of the hospital; a treasurer who looked after the financial affairs and internal property; three almoners who supervised the inmates, their diet, activities, hygiene, as well as the personnel who looked after such matters (matron, nurses, steward, and others); two "scruteners" who were responsible for gifts, legacies, and bequests given to the hospital, and in general for fund raising in our terms; a renter who collected rents on all properties and holdings of the hospital; and two surveyors who were responsible for managing the real and other property of the hospital.

In addition to the above officials, or governors, the hospital staff, or officers, consisted of the following personnel, whose titles essentially describe their jobs. The clerk acted as secretary and bookkeeper. Those concerned with housekeeping functions included the matron, the steward, the cook, the butler, the porter, and the beadle. The matron was responsible for all women and children in the institution, as well as for the nurses and keepers of the wards. In addition, she was a housekeeper who looked after laundry, bedding, and the like. Food supply and maintenance were the major responsibilities of the steward, while the butler dealt with the baker and the brewer who supplied the hospital with bread and beer. A separate official maintained liaison with the churchwardens and the local parish collectors who had to bring in money to the hospital and with the poor who needed care and assistance. A surgeon and a barber were connected with the hospital and provided the necessary professional and technical attention.[33]

The medical staff and its activities are essential to the hospital as we conceive it today. As has already been indicated, this was not the case in the medieval hospital in Europe. During the early Middle Ages the presence of monastic physicians in religious houses makes it probable that the sick received some medical care.[34] From the fourteenth century on, however, physicians were increasingly associated with hospitals to provide care for patients. Thus, in Frankfurt am Main the municipal surgeon appointed in 1377 was required to treat surgical patients at the Holy Ghost Hospital. Similarly, the municipal physician appointed in 1381 agreed to attend gratis all persons employed by the municipality and to care for patients in the hospital.[35]

In Nürnberg a specific hospital physician was first appointed in 1486 at the new Holy Ghost Hospital with private funds.[36] By the beginning of the sixteenth century, this example began to be followed by other communities. This was done in Strassburg around 1515 on the ground that medical attention might help some patients and would eventually cost less than if no medical care was provided. It had been noted that patients who received no medical care remained longer in the hospital, and even though some died, the expenses to the institution were higher.[37]

Karl Sudhoff suggested that the association of the physician with the hospital and the provision of medical care in it became permanent when the inunction cure of syphilitics required public funds and when results showed that this treatment was successful.[38] As we have indicated, however, this trend began earlier, and was influenced by other factors as well. The so-called "Reformation of the Emperor Sigmund" (*Reformatio Sigismundi*), a work prepared in or about 1439, which contains proposals for the reform of medical care in the German cities, indicates that this was a problem that caused considerable concern.[39] The author insisted on the need for a municipal physician in every town, and emphasized that the medical profession should attend the poor gratis. This work was widely circulated during the fifteenth century and may have influenced governments to provide care by physicians on a more regular basis.

As it emerged from the medieval period the hospital was essentially an instrument of society to ameliorate suffering, to diminish poverty, to eradicate mendicity, and to help maintain public order. It had also come under different management in many places, under the jurisdiction of the royal power, of a municipality, or of some voluntary charitable organization. The same period also saw the beginning of an association with the medical profession, but the physician was not yet a part of the hospital, and remained independent. However, this association did provide the basis for another trend that from the seventeenth century on would lead the medical profession increasingly to use the hospital for the study of disease and for its own practical education. The view that hospitals should be places for the treatment of the sick and at the same time centers for the study and teaching of medicine was to have extraordinarily fruitful consequences in succeeding centuries. Holland led the way in this development; bedside teaching was established at Leyden in 1626. The same idea was also advanced in England by Francis Bacon, Samuel Hartlib, William Petty, and John Bellers.[40] Later, in the eighteenth century under the leadership of Hermann Boerhave, this idea was developed at Leyden and put into practice so that other medical centers were influenced, notably Edinburgh.

New Conditions Produce New Hospitals

The eighteenth and early nineteenth centuries saw a growth of hospitals in Great Britain, on the European continent, and in America that exemplified and was formed by major political and social currents, especially mercantilism and enlightened despotism, private initiative and cooperative action, and the concept of a national health policy. Taking as a point of departure the mercantilist position in relation to health, a few far-seeing men had been led in the seventeenth century to adumbrate the idea of health as a significant element of national policy. Problems of health were considered chiefly in connection with the aim of maintaining and augmenting a healthy population, and thus in terms of their significance for the political and economic strength of the state. On a theoretical plane, this idea had been developed in varying degree in different countries. However, owing to the lack of knowledge and administrative machinery, it had nowhere been possible to develop and to implement a health policy on a national basis. While this goal was not actually achieved until the later nineteenth century, significant changes occurred during the eighteenth and earlier nineteenth centuries that did affect the hospital.

During the period under consideration, health problems in Great Britain were handled overwhelmingly by local authorities. Local government was carried on by the counties and the parishes into which the counties were divided. These administrative units provided the frame of reference for thought and action in matters of community health. Furthermore, the Elizabethan Poor Law (1601) had laid upon the parish the duty of providing relief for the indigent, and in time this came to include medical care. Each parish was responsible for the maintenance of its own poor, and consequently was concerned to reduce this burden as far as possible. It was believed that this could be accomplished by arranging to employ the poor in workhouses. While the enthusiastic belief in the efficacy of workhouses to deal with poverty was never realized, many of the plans and programs developed for this purpose also turned attention to health problems. As a result there was an increasing recognition in Great Britain of the need for medical assistance to certain groups of the population.[41]

It was this period, particularly the years from 1714 to 1760, that witnessed the creation in London and the provinces of dispensaries and general hospitals, as well as hospitals for special groups. The hospital and dispensary movement found its impetus chiefly in private initiative and contributions, although there was some governmental assistance in the form of legislative action. To be sure, private benefactions had never been absent in the support of the older London hospitals. In fact, as Jordan has recently shown, the sums contributed by private persons between 1480 and 1660 were large.[42] Moreover, fund-raising appeals to the public and the establishment of charities were not unknown before the eighteenth century.[43] The development of private initiative coupled with cooperative action, which is so characteristic of Britain in the eighteenth century, is to a very considerable degree related to the character of activity by local government. While the parish officers had to assume considerable responsibilities, generally they had neither the training nor desire to perform their functions. In many ways, this very aspect of the governmental system gave increasingly greater scope to private initiative, making it necessary and possible to deal pragmatically with new problems as they presented themselves. Indeed, throughout this period parliamentary action was generally undertaken on the basis of previously initiated local programs and projects.

The first institutions to provide medical care for the sick poor appeared in London. The metropolis was growing, wages were high, and workers were attracted to the city. Many of them, however, unable to establish the needed residence requirement, were ineligible for parochial relief when sick. The Act of Settlement of 1662 gave the parish authorities the right to remove within forty days any newcomer unable to rent a dwelling worth £10 if they believed that such a person was likely to be a burden to the parish.[44] Furthermore, the two older hospitals, St. Bartholomew's and St. Thomas's, were overcrowded and unable to care for all those in need. Recognizing the problem, a group of London laymen and physicians in 1719 organized the Charitable Society in Westminster to provide for such sick persons as were unable to obtain proper care. This was the beginning of the Westminster Hospital, which was soon followed by the establishment of other institutions: Guy's (1724), St. George's (1733)) London Hospital (1740). About the middle of the century special hospitals were created. The Middlesex Hospital was founded in 1746 for smallpox patients and to encourage inoculation. The same year also saw the establishment of the Lock Hospital for patients with venereal diseases. St. Luke's, for the reception of mentally ill persons, was established in 1751.

From 1760 to 1800 the growth of hospitals in London slowed down, but thereafter the process of development was resumed. During the first four decades of the nineteenth century, fourteen hospitals were founded in London. While some were general hospitals, it is noteworthy that most of them were special hospitals. Thus, the London Fever Hospital was founded in 1802, the Royal London Ophthalmic Hospital in 1804, the Royal Chest Hospital in 1814, the Royal Ear Hospital in 1816, and the Royal National Orthopedic Hospital in 1838.

The influence of these trends was soon felt and paralleled outside London. The movement began to spread rapidly to Bristol (1737), York (1740), Exeter (1741), and Liverpool (1745). By 1760 there were 16 provincial hospitals of which 14 were general in character. There were 38 by 1780, and 114 by 1840. Similar forces were at work in Scotland and Ireland, and by the end of the eighteenth century hospitals were to be found in most of the cities and larger towns of Great Britain.[45]

But even while hospitals were being founded, it was realized that these institutions would have to be supplemented by some other kind of establishment. To fill this need the dispensary was developed. The dispensary idea may be traced to the seventeenth century, but it was not until 1769 that a more permanent establishment of this type came into being. This was the Dispensary for the Infant Poor, opened by Dr. George Armstrong at a house in Red Lion Square, Holborn, London. The opening of Armstrong's dispensary was followed in 1770 by the founding of the General Dispensary by John Coakley Lettsom, a Quaker physician, and a group of associates. Following the example set by Lettsom, dispensaries sprang up in London and the provinces. From 1770 through 1792, fifteen were founded in London, and from 1775 through 1798, thirteen in the provinces.[46]

The causes of this expansive growth were varied, but they may be considered in two major categories: medical and scientific, and socioeconomic. The great scientific outburst of the sixteenth and seventeenth centuries laid the foundation for the application of science to medical care, and increasingly knowledge of the structure of the human body was provided through dissection and observation by Vesalius, his contemporaries, and his successors. Obstetrics and surgery were already able to benefit from this knowledge in the eighteenth century. Equally basic, though on a more complex level, was Harvey's discovery of the circulation of the blood, which provided a firm basis for consideration of the body as a functional system. Observation and classification also made possible the more precise recognition of diseases. In creating institutions where it was possible to apply this knowledge, the hospital and dispensary movement gave a concrete form to the social philosophy of Bacon, Petty, and others who saw in science a means for improving human health and welfare.

However, the mere accretion of medical ideas and knowledge cannot of itself assure application. Social environment and intellectual milieu must provide favorable conditions and patterns of behavior in terms of which knowledge can be put to use. Precisely this, however, characterized England during the eighteenth century, particularly during the latter part of the period. The tempo and character of economic life had been changing in England before the middle of the eighteenth century, but by comparison the industrial and agricultural changes during the latter half of the century were both rapid and radical. These profound alterations in the economic life of the country necessarily disturbed its social structure and gave rise to a new attitude of mind toward problems of community life. Representing essentially the views of the middle classes, this distinctive ethos was characterized by two dominant facets: an insistence on order, efficiency, and social discipline, and a concern with the conditions of men. Appreciation of the social factors and consequences of ill health led merchants, physicians, clergymen, and other public-spirited citizens to undertake ameliorative efforts. It is significant that the hospital and dispensary movement, the infant-welfare movement, and other similar activities originated in urban centers, first in London, then in other cities and towns. Wealth, commerce, and industry were largely centered there, and at the same time it was much easier for the middle class, many of whose members were Dissenters, to make themselves felt. They fostered the growing social conscience, but it was a humanitarianism coupled with a firm belief in the sober and practical virtues of efficiency, simplicity, and cheapness.[47]

The English colonies in America followed the general pattern set by the mother country, but with a considerable lag. The first successful effort to establish a general hospital occurred in Philadelphia, in the middle of the eighteenth century, with the opening of the Pennsylvania Hospital in 1751. The causes that led to its founding were well stated by Benjamin Franklin in 1754:

About the end of the year 1750 [he wrote] some persons, who had frequent opportunities of observing the distress of such distemper'd poor as from time to time came to Philadelphia, for the advice and assistance of the physicians and surgeons of that city; how difficult it was for them to procure suitable lodgings, and other conveniences proper for their respective cases, and how expensive the providing good and careful nurses, and other attendants for want whereof, many must suffer greatly, and some probably perish that might other wise have been restored to health and comfort, and become useful to themselves, their families, and the publick for many years after; and considering moreover, that even the poor inhabitants of this city, tho' they had homes, yet were therein but badly accommodated in sickness, and could not be so well and so easily taken care of in their separate habitations, as they might be in one convenient house, under one inspection, and in the hands of the skilful practitioners; and several of the inhabitants of the province, who unhappily became disordered in their senses, wander'd about, to the terror of their neighbours, there being no place (except the House of Correction) in which they might be confined, and subjected to proper management for their recovery, and that House was by no means fitted for such purposes; did charitably consult together, and confer with their friends and acquaintances, on the best means of relieving the distressed, under those circumstances; and an Infirmary, or hospital, in the manner of several lately established in Great Britain [was proposed and approved].[48]

Franklin also pointed out that the hospital could serve an educational purpose by training physicians. Moreover, the idea that in terms of social economy it may be cheaper to provide medical care in an efficient and accessible way so that sick persons can be restored, if possible, to a useful place in society, which had been noted in the early sixteenth century, now appears as an integral motivating value of the eighteenth-century hospital movement.

The hospitals founded in Great Britain and in America during the eighteenth century and the early nineteenth century were not governmental undertakings. They were the outcome of voluntary efforts by private citizens, and were financed by subscription and bequest. It is clear that the voluntary hospital was not an outgrowth of experience with the social and economic changes brought about by the Industrial Revolution in the nineteenth century, but preceded them. Moreover, the voluntary hospital had a purpose that was primarily social rather than medical. It was intended to serve the sick poor "whose home conditions were deficient in the accommodation their distress needed." [49] However, the sick poor who had to go to a hospital because they could not obtain care at home were faced with two possibilities: they might be admitted by a voluntary general hospital; if not, the almshouse or the workhouse was their lot. The choice was determined by hospital policy. Patients with chronic, incurable, or terminal conditions were not accepted by the voluntary hospitals. For example, in 1808 attention was drawn to the circumstance that certain medical practitioners tended to refer to the Dundee Royal Infirmary patients far advanced in illness who had no prospect of recovery. These people were not regarded as "proper objects" of the infirmary, which was "never intended as an almshouse or poorhouse." Furthermore, with a limited number of beds such a practice would tend to exclude those who might truly benefit from the care provided by the institution. Finally, "what opinion would the public form of the skill of the medical attendants in the house, if upon looking at the annual reports it should appear that the cases of death were to those of recovery as three to one?" [50] This situation continued to exist throughout the nineteenth century. Louisa Twining commented some seventy years later that there were "a large number of persons afflicted with incurable disease who are not proper objects for admission into general hospitals." Furthermore, the workhouses were "hospitals for those who are incurable, and who are turned out of our best London hospitals." [51]

On this basis there developed in Great Britain, and in a modified form in the United States and Canada, a pattern of hospital services that persisted until well into the twentieth century and whose influence is still evident in hospital organization in the United States. Hospitals were simply institutions maintained through public funds or private charity, where the indigent poor could be cared for more economically than in their own homes. Voluntary hospitals tended to take acute cases, the short-stay patients, while the chronic cases, the incurable, the insane, and those suffering from communicable diseases went to public institutions.

This pattern explains in part the number of hospitals, hospital beds, and hospital patients in the United States and Britain in the nineteenth century. As late as 1873 there were only 149 hospitals and related institutions in the United States, and of those one-third were for the mentally ill. Fifty years later there were 6,762. During the same period the number of beds increased from 35,453 to 770,375. Similarly, in 1851, in all of

England and Wales the census enumerators recorded only
7,619 patients as resident in hospitals. In 1871 there were 19,585
patients in general and special voluntary hospitals, but over
50,000 patients in workhouse infirmaries.[52]

The public hospitals of this period, and to a lesser extent
the voluntary general institutions, left much to be desired.
Owing to prevailing concepts of administrative economy, wards
were overcrowded, hygienic conditions were poor, and nursing
was primitive. Small wonder when as late as 1877, W. Gill Wylie,
a prominent physician, asserted that hospitals did more harm
than good by removing the "healthful stimulus of necessity"
that was essential to recovery. In his opinion, hospitals should
be limited "to those who have no homes and to those who
cannot be assisted at their homes." [53] However, Wylie did emphasize the importance of hospitals for medical education, a
view that was stated even more strongly by John Green, another
physician concerned with hospital construction and operation.
Hospitals, he said, "are essentially charitable institutions, and
the welfare of the patients must ever hold the first place in the
minds of their founders. Nevertheless, we must not lose sight of
the fact that they are also our great schools of clinical observation and instruction; and have thus, perhaps, rendered their most
important service to mankind." [54]

Hospital organization and staffing of the nineteenth century
were simple. The Charity Hospital in New Orleans was jointly
administered at first by the state and the city through a board
of administrators, and later by a state board. The operating
personnel of the hospital consisted in 1823 of an attending
physician, an apothecary who also served for a time as a house
surgeon and purveyor, an assistant apothecary, a ward master,
a porter, and ten nurses, including slaves belonging to the
institution. Later, the board annually elected four physicians,
one visiting surgeon, and a house surgeon to provide professional
attendance. In 1843 the number of attending physicians was
increased to eight, the surgeons to two, and elections to these
posts were made semiannual. About six medical students served
as interns and performed tasks ordered by the attending
physicians.[55]

The Modern Hospital Appears

Application of the knowledge derived from bacteriology and laboratory studies in clinical medicine led in the twentieth century to an increase in the number of medical and technical personnel required by the hospital. A striking illustration of this development was offered in 1938 by Alphonse R. Dochez in a comparative picture of the complex changes in hospital medical practice during the first three decades of this century. He did this by contrasting the histories of two patients with similar types of heart disease; one was recorded in 1908, the other at the same hospital in 1938. The total written record of the first patient occupies two and one-half pages, and the observations represent the combined efforts of two physicians, the attending and the house officer, and of one specialist, a pathologist-bacteriologist. The record of the second patient, who was still in the hospital when Dochez made this comparison, comprised twenty-nine pages and represented the combined observations of three visiting physicians, two residents, three house officers, ten specialists, and fourteen technicians, a total of thirty-two individuals.[56] Naturally, such an elaborate study as that of the latter patient is not made of everyone admitted to a hospital, but the organization necessary for such studies is continuously maintained, not only for patients with heart disease but also for others.

Obviously the change described by Dochez could not have occurred without specific alterations in the hospitals and in the communities they served. Thus, it had long been recognized that different categories of patients should be separated. In 1865, for instance, a report to the administration of the Paris hospitals advised a reorganization of the maternity service, that patients be separated into appropriate groups, and the building of special pavilions for those with communicable diseases.[57] However, this reorganization was not undertaken until 1880. This was also the period in which operating rooms were constructed that took account of the principles of asepsis and were specifically designed for the purpose. Hospital laboratories were also introduced in the eighties and nineties. The first laboratory in a municipal hospital in Paris was created in 1893.[58] Lankenau Hospital in Philadelphia established the first bacteriological and chemical laboratory in that city in 1889, and the first hospital X-ray laboratory in 1896.[59]

It was also during this period that nursing was reformed and training schools for nurses were introduced. This along with the increasing recognition of the medical value of bedside care led to changes in hospital administration. The introduction of trained nurses involved conflicts with the physicians, the older nurses, and the administration. As Abel-Smith has so succinctly put it: "If the new matron was to undertake what she considered to be her duties, she had to carve out an empire of her own. She had to take over some of the responsibilities of the medical staff and some of the responsibilities of the lay administration. In addition she had to centralize the administration of nursing affairs," thereby lowering the status of the other nurses.[60] Moreover, not only for the matron but also for the nurses under her direction there existed the problems of role definition, status, and the other sociological elements involved in such innovations. Doctors were afraid that nurses would undermine their authority, and no one had yet drawn a line between general nursing that was a responsibility of the matron and her staff and medical treatment for which the physicians were responsible. Eventually, of course, a *modus vivendi* was developed, and, especially in the English voluntary hospitals, nursing became essentially an independent department, of which the head had a position of authority between the medical staff and the lay administration. Similar changes in the English workhouse infirmaries occurred much more slowly, essentially because of the deterrent philosophy that was the basis of the whole system of poor-law administration.[61]

The suspicion and hostility encountered by the trained nurses when they first entered the hospital were not peculiar to this group. Such attitudes and the conflicts they engender have been the fate of other new groups also. This happened to the first social workers in hospitals and for the same reasons. Richard C. Cabot found such a situation at the Massachusetts General Hospital. In 1909 he wrote:

Unless there is at least one doctor who really knows what the social worker is trying to do, the scheme fails. If he thinks of her merely as a nurse and asks of her only such help as a nurse can render, she will either fall short of his expectations . . . or finally she will exceed his expectations and his horizon—which will make him think her "uppish" or interfering or visionary. Unless a doctor has already acquired the "social point of view" to the extent of seeing that his treatment of dispensary patients is slovenly, without some knowledge of their homes, their finances, their thoughts and worries,—he will think that the social worker is teaching him how to do his work whenever she does what he didn't and couldn't do before. Naturally he will resent this indignantly . . . he will not care to be advised by any "woman charity worker." [62]

In this manner the hospital in the more developed countries of the world was taking unto itself the various elements that were eventually to create the institution that we know today as the workshop of the physician and the eventual community health center. At the same time other factors also made their impact felt. One of these was urbanization; the other was population growth. During the later nineteenth century more and more hospitals were constructed.

In New York City twelve hospitals came into existence from 1850 to 1860, at a time when Brooklyn was not yet a part of the greater city. The decades of the seventies and eighties were prolific in the creation of new hospitals. Many of the special hospitals were created during this period. This growth of special institutions was due in part to the development of specialism, but even more so to the limitations of the voluntary general hospital. The latter had no facilities for the new specialties as they appeared, nor could they undertake any pioneering initiative because of financial limitations.

Furthermore, public attitudes toward hospitals changed. As early as 1802, the municipal authorities of Paris converted the Hospice de Jésus into a hospital known as the Maison Dubois to which paying patients were admitted,[63] and in New York City, St. Vincent's Hospital, built in 1850, was the first to provide private accommodations. None the less, the rich for a long time continued to receive medical care, including surgery, at home, and the poor feared admission to the hospital as a death sentence, a way station to a pauper funeral. By the middle of the second decade of the twentieth century, the situation had changed completely. Around the turn of the century the adoption of asepsis had so lowered operative mortality that the public began to accept hospitals as agencies of social good. It was realized that various forms of ill-health could be treated more effectively in the hospital than in the home. This trend was further strengthened and intensified by the development of roentgenology, of laboratory techniques for diagnosis, and of a variety of costly therapeutic modalities. At the same time the value of the hospital as an educational institution for physicians, students, and nurses was increasingly recognized. As a result, by the beginning of the twentieth century hospitals were admitting increasing numbers of paying patients in private rooms and other accommodations set apart from those for the indigent.[64]

With increasing complexity of medical care and increased acceptance of hospital service, there developed a need for adjunct services in addition to the usual medical and nursing care. These have involved social work, nutrition, and more complex record and business procedures. As hospitals had to accommodate more complex functions, additional personnel, facilities and equipment, their organization has also grown increasingly complex and their operation more costly. These consequences, interacting with or affected by developments outside the hospital, have in turn led to new phenomena and situations, namely, the appearance of hospital administration as a profession, the growth of voluntary prepayment plans for hospital expenses, an increased awareness and greater attention to the quality of hospital service and medical care, and a more prominent role of government, at all levels, in the hospital field, especially in the financing and construction of hospitals.[65]

The consequence of these developments has been to give the hospital a central role in modern medical care, to make it responsible for complex and wide-ranging tasks, but at the same time to produce painful tensions and conflicts most evident in the voluntary general hospital.

The source of this situation is to be found in the characteristic administrative structure the voluntary hospital inherited from its eighteenth century origins in Great Britain and the United

States.[66] Each voluntary hospital was an independent institution managed by its own trustees or governors, and staffed by physicians and surgeons who donated their services gratis. In return the medical staff were enabled to use suitable and interesting cases for teaching and research. Later, as the public began to accept the advantages of hospitalization, physicians began to use the hospital for their private patients. At the same time, the physician had no administrative or financial responsibility to the hospital. Moreover, as scientific medicine emerged and became institutionalized in the hospital, the physician became essential for its operation, while the institution became more and more indispensable for the practice of good medicine. This administrative duality was possible as long as most of the patients were indigent, as long as the hospital tended to remain a self-contained, relatively simple organization, and as long as the physician could use the hospital and still retain his position as an independent entrepreneur.

However, as the hospital increased in size and complexity, as the development of medicine required the use of costly equipment, as changing social and economic conditions altered the financing of medical care and created new patterns of hospital utilization, the organizational relationships within the hospital have been disturbed and have become unstable. It is no longer a question of trustees, administrator, and medical staff alone. Another set of people, the organized consumers, have to be considered and satisfied if possible. In short, having become a large-scale organization, the hospital requires a more explicit organizational division of labor and more efficient, responsible management. For the physician this means accommodation to institutionalized teamwork, a prospect that is highly distasteful to many. The degree of control will vary with the hospital, but the prospect is that increased administrative rationality will characterize the developing hospital and that the practice of the physician will be under the continuing scrutiny of others, not only his professional colleagues, who will appraise his activities. Indeed, the very nature of large-scale organization raises problems of administrative efficiency and rationality, productivity, and accountability of all personnel, including physicians.

Conclusion

At various periods in history the need to care for the sick and the disabled, the needy and the dependent has crystallized sufficiently in terms of attitude and practice that one may speak of institutional models characteristic of certain societies. In this sense, the history of the hospital may be seen in terms of certain types that have predominated in given historical periods. The medieval hospital in all its varied forms was essentially an ecclesiastical institution, not primarily concerned with medical care. This institutional type was eventually replaced in the sixteenth century by another kind of hospital whose goals were not religious, but primarily social. To achieve this, the medieval hospital was to a large extent secularized, placed under governmental control, and its activities accepted as a community responsibility. In its organization and operation, however, the early modern hospital still retained various features of its predecessor, one being that medical care was not its primary function. That is, the hospital as it existed from the sixteenth century into the nineteenth century was intended primarily to help in the maintenance of social order while providing for the sick and the needy. During this period, however, various forces and developments external to the hospital eventually transformed it into what is now characteristic of economically developed countries. This hospital, the product of the industrial and scientific revolutions, may be called the health-workshop or medical-factory type. Here medical care is the primary goal of the institution, and its provision is governed chiefly by scientific-technological norms and the requirements of organizational rationality and economy. Yet this hospital type still has features derived from its past that are not always congruent with its ostensible goals and norms. For this reason, the better we understand how "within living memory an age-old institution has been transformed from a hostel for sick-poor into a medical center for everyone," [67] the clearer will we as scientists be able to see the hospital, and the more effectively can we as practitioners contribute to its evolution.

NOTES

1. Cyril Bailey, ed., *The Legacy of Rome* (London: Oxford University Press, 1951), pp. 292-296.

2. "The So-called Second Letter of St. Clement," trans. Francis X. Glimm, *The Apostolic Fathers*, The Fathers of the Church Series (New York: Cima Publishing Co., 1947), p. 76.

3. E. Jeanselme and L. Oeconomos, "Les Oeuvres d'Assistance et les Hôpitaux Byzantins au siècle des Comnènes," *1er Congrès de l'Histoire de l'Art de Guérir (août, 1920)* (1921), pp. 239-256.

4. *Ibid.*, p. 240.

5. Georg Schreiber, *Gemeinschaften des Mittelalters. Recht und Verfassung. Kult und Frömmigkeit*, Gesammelte Abhandlungen, Bd. I (Regensberg Münster, 1948), pp. 3-80 (p. 10); Steven Runciman, *Byzantine Civilization* (New York: Meridian Books, 1956), p. 190.

6. Schreiber, *op. cit.*, pp. 45-46.

7. *The Rule of St. Benedict*, ed., with an English translation and explanatory notes by D. Oswald Hunter Blair, 3rd ed. (Fort Augustus, Scotland, Abbey Press, 1914), pp. 101-103, 133-137.

8. F. Keller, *Bauriss des Klosters St. Gallen vom Jahre 820, im Faksimile herausgegeben und erläutert* (Zurich, 1844). Cited by Alfons Fischer, *Geschichte des deutschen Gesundheitswesens*, 2 vols. (Berlin: F. A. Herbig, 1933), Vol. I, p. 49.

9. These comments are based on a personal inspection of the site in 1960. See also O. E. Craster, *Tintern Abbey, Monmouthshire*, Ministry of Works Official Guide-Book (London: H.M.S.O., 1956), pp. 17-19; also plan between pp. 11-12.

10. Wilhelm Liese, *Geschichte der Caritas*, 2 Bde. (Freiburg im Breisgau, 1922), Vol. I, p. 143.

11. Franz Meffert, *Caritas und Krankenwesen* (Freiburg, 1927), p. 147.

12. Liese, *op. cit.*, Vol. II, p. 118; E. A. Meinert, *Die Hospitäler Holsteins im Mittelalter*, Kiel Dissertation (1949).

13. J. M. Hobson, *Some Early and Later Houses of Pity* (London: George Routledge and Sons, 1926), pp. 14-15.

14. Maud Sellers, *The Merchant Adventurers of York*, Printed for the Company of Merchant Adventurers of the City of York (Ben Johnson & Co., Ltd., 1946, reprinted 1956). Comments based also on visit to building in 1960.

15. For a list of the English hospitals, see D. Knowles and R. N. Hadcock, *Medieval Religious Houses* (London: Longmans, Green & Co., Ltd., 1953), pp. 250-324.

16. Brian Tierney, *Medieval Poor Law: A Sketch of Canonical Theory and Its Application in England* (Berkeley: University of California Press, 1959), p. 87.

17. Siegfried Reicke, *Das deutsche Spital und sein Recht im Mittelalter*, Kirchenrechtliche Abhandlungen (Stuttgart, 1932), p. 198.

18. For different religious rules of various French hospitals in the twelfth, thirteenth, and fourteenth centuries, see Léon Le Grand, *Statuts d'Hôtels-Dieu et de Léproseries. Recueil de textes du XIIe au XIVe Siècle*

(Paris: Alphonse Picard et Fils, 1901); also Dorothy-Louise Mackay, *Les Hôpitaux et la Charité à Paris au XIIIᵉ Siècle* (Paris: Honoré Champion, 1932), pp. 34-50.

19. *The Faerie Queene*, Book I, Canto X, 36.

20. Rotha Mary Clay, *The Medieval Hospitals in England* (London: Methuen & Co., 1909), pp. 120-126.

21. *Ibid.*, p. 138; Liese, *op. cit.*, Vol. 1, p. 173.

22. F. R. Salter, ed., *Some Early Tracts on Poor Relief* (London: Methuen & Co., 1926), pp. 10-11, 117.

23. Tierney, *op. cit.*, p. 87.

24. W. Haid: "Über den kirchlichen Charakter der Spitäler, besonders in der Erzdiözese Freiburg," *Freiburger Diozesanarchiv*, Bd. 2 (1866), p. 136, 2.2, p. 305, Document No. 7; cited by Fischer, *op. cit.*, Vol. I, p. 137.

25. Clay, *op. cit.*, p. 212.

26. Tierney, *op. cit.*, p. 86.

27. W. J. Ashley, *An Introduction to English Economic History and Theory*, 2 vols. (New York: G. P. Putnam's Sons, 1893), Vol. II, p. 319.

28. Martha Goldberg, *Das Armen- und Krankenwesen des mittelalterlichen Strassburg, Freiburg Dissertation* (Strassburg, 1909), p. 2; E. Becker, "Geschichte der Medizin in Hildesheim," *Archiv für klinische Medizin*, 38 (1899), p. 317; Reicke, *op. cit.*, pp. 93-97; Liese, *op. cit.*, Vol. I, pp. 231 ff.; A. de Calonne, *La Vie municipale au XVᵉ siècle dans le nord de France* (Paris: Didier et Cie, 1880), p. 126.

29. Charlotte Koch, *Wandlungen der Wohlfahrtspflege im Zeitalter der Aufklärung*, Erlangen Dissertation (Erlangen, 1933), pp. 11-29.

30. Simon Fish, "A Supplicacyon for the Beggers" (1529), in *A Miscellany of Tracts and Pamphlets*, ed. A. C. Ward (London: Oxford University Press, 1927), pp. 1-17 (p. 16).

31. Claude Lillingston, "Sweden's Hospital Administration in the Sixteenth Century," *British Medical Journal* (December 10, 1955), p. 1445.

32. *The Order of the Hospitals of K. Henry the VIII and K. Edward the I, viz. St. Bartholomew's. Christ's. Bridewell. St. Thomas's.* By the Maior, Cominaltie, and Citizens of London, Governours of the Possessions, Revenues and Goods of the sayd Hospitalls, 1557.

33. The organization as described in the preceding reference lists a surgeon and a barber, but does not discuss their duties or their specific position as members of the hospital staff.

34. E. A. Hammond, "Physicians in Medieval English Religious Houses," *Bulletin of the History of Medicine* 32 (1958), pp. 105-120.

35. G. L. Kriegk, *Deutsches Bürgertum im Mittelalter*, 2 vols. (Frankfurt am Main, 1868-1871, Vol. I, pp. 8, 53, 524.

36. Ernst Mummenhoff, "Die öffentliche Gesundheits- und Krankenpflege im alten Nürnberg," in *Festschrift zur Eröffnung des neuen Krankenhauses der Stadt Nürnberg*, herausgegeben von den Städtischen Collegien (Nürnberg, 1898), p. 53.

37. O. Winckelmann, *Das Fürsorgewesen der Stadt Strassburg vor und nach der Reformation bis zum Ausgang des 16. Jahrhunderts*, Quellen und Forschungen zur Reformationsgeschichte (Leipzig, 1922), Vol. V, p. 25; Fischer, *op. cit.*, Vol. I, p. 140.

38. K. Sudhoff, "Ein Wendepunkt im Spitalwesen des Mittelalters," Bericht über einen am 24 Sept., 1913, gehaltenen Vortrag, *Münchener medizinische Wochenschrift* (1913), p. 2482.

39. *Die Reformation Kaiser Sigmunds, Eine Schrift des 15. Jahrhunderts zur Kirchen und Reichsreform,* herausgegeben von Karl Beer, Beiheft zu den Deutschen Reichstagsakten herausgegeben durch die Historische Kommission bei der Bayerischen Akademie der Wissenschaften (Stuttgart, 1933), pp. 124-126; Karl Beer; "Was ein deutscher Reformer vor einem halben Jahrtausend vom Ärztestand erwartete," *Gesnerus,* 11 (1954), pp. 24-36; Lothar Graf zu Dohna, *Reformatio Sigismundi. Beiträge zum Verständnis einer Reformschrift des fünfzehnten Jahrhunderts* (Göttingen, 1960).

40. George Rosen, "Medical Care and Social Policy in Seventeenth Century England," *Bulletin of the New York Academy of Medicine,* 29 (1953), pp. 420-437.

41. Dorothy Marshall, *The English Poor in the 18th Century* (London: George Routledge & Sons, 1926), pp. 127-128; Karl de Schweinitz, *England's Road to Social Security* (Philadelphia: University of Pennsylvania Press, 1943), pp. 53-55; H. R. Fox Bourne, *The Life of John Locke,* 2 vols. (New York: Harper & Brothers, 1876), Vol. II, pp. 376-392; A. Ruth Fry, *John Bellers, 1654-1725: Quaker, Economist and Social Reformer* (London: Cassell & Co., 1935), pp. 5-28; George Rosen, "An Eighteenth Century Plan for a National Health Service," *Bulletin of the History of Medicine,* 16. (1944) pp. 429-436; Bernard Mandeville, *The Fable of the Bees: or Private vices, publick benefits. With an essay on charity and charity schools . . . ,* 5th ed. (London: J. Tonson, 1728), pp. 341-366.

42. W. K. Jordan, *The Charities of London, 1480-1660: The Aspirations and the Achievements of the Urban Society* (London: George Allen and Unwin, 1960), pp. 186-196.

43. *Bute Broadsides* (Houghton Library, Harvard University), Vol. 1, pp. 44, 53, 65, 76-77, 164-166.

44. Dorothy Marshall, *English People in the Eighteenth Century* (London: Longmans, Green & Co., 1956), pp. 186 ff.

45. B. Kirkman Gray, *A History of English Philanthropy* (London: P. S. King & Son, 1905), pp. 126-131; S. Wilks and G. T. Bettany, *A Biographical History of Guy's Hospital* (London, 1892), pp. 52-53, 56-73; Thomas Ferguson, *The Dawn of Scottish Social Welfare* (Edinburgh: Thomas Nelson & Sons, 1948), pp. 255-284; K. H. Connell, *The Population of Ireland 1750-1845* (Oxford: Clarendon Press, 1950), pp. 198-207; M. C. Buer, *Health, Wealth and Population in the Early Days of the Industrial Revolution* (London: George Routledge & Sons, 1926), pp. 257-258.

46. Ernest Caulfield, *The Infant Welfare Movement in the Eighteenth Century* (New York: Paul B. Hoeber, 1931), pp. 55-58, 146-176; Gray, *op. cit.,* pp. 132-134; A. M. Carr-Saunders and P. A. Wilson, *The Professions* (Oxford: Clarendon Press, 1933), pp. 72-73; Harvey Cushing, "Dr. Garth. The Kit-Kat Poet," *Bulletin Johns Hopkins Hospital* 17 (1906), pp. 1-17; G. F. Still, *The History of Pediatrics* (London: Oxford University Press, 1931), pp. 417-421; J. J. Abraham, *Lettsom, His Life, Times, Friends and Descendants* (London: William Heinemann, Ltd., 1933), pp. 109-110; T. J. Pettigrew, *Memoirs of the life and writings of the late John Coakley Lettsom . . . ,* 3 vols. (London, 1817), Vol. I, pp. 36-38; J. C. Trent, "John Coakley Lettsom," *Bulletin of the History of Medicine,* 22 (1948), pp. 528-542.

47. *Reports of the Society for Bettering the Conditions and Increasing the Comforts of the Poor* (London, 1802), Vol. III, p. 2; Dorothy Marshall,

English People in the Eighteenth Century (New York: Longmans & Co., 1956), pp. 147-157.

48. Benjamin Franklin, *Some Account of the Pennsylvania Hospital,* ed. I. Bernard Cohen (Baltimore: Johns Hopkins Press, 1954), p. 3; see also p. 19-22.

49. Henry J. C. Gibson, *Dundee Royal Infirmary with a Short Account of More Recent Years* (Dundee: William Kidd & Sons, 1948), p. 11.

50. *Ibid.,* pp. 12-13.

51. Louisa Twining, *Recollections of Workhouse Visiting and Management during Twenty five Years* (London, 1880), p. 37; *idem, A Letter to the President of the Poor Law Board on Workhouse Infirmaries* (London, 1866), pp. 26-27.

52. Michael M. Davis, *Clinics, Hospitals and Health Centers* (New York: Harper & Brothers, 1927), pp. 4-5; Brian Abel-Smith, *A History of the Nursing Profession* (New York: W. Heineman, 1960), pp. 2, 4.

53. W. Gill Wylie, *Hospitals: Their History, Organization, and Construction* (New York: D. Appleton & Co., 1877), pp. 60, 67.

54. John Green, *City Hospitals* (Boston: Little Brown & Co., 1861), p. 14.

55. Elizabeth Wisner, *Public Welfare Administration in Louisiana* (Chicago: University of Chicago Press, 1930), pp. 37-38.

56. Alphonse R. Dochez, "President's Address," *Transactions of the American Clinical and Climatological Association,* 54 (1939), pp. 19-23.

57. Pierre Vallery-Radot, *Un Siècle d'Histoire hospitalière de Louis-Philippe jusqu'à nos jours (1837–1949)* (Paris, 1948), pp. 27-28.

58. *Ibid.,* pp. 31-32.

59. Herman M. Somers and Anne R. Somers, *Doctors, Patients and Health Insurance* (Washington, D.C.: Brookings Institution, 1961), p. 63.

60. Abel-Smith, *op. cit.,* p. 25.

61. *Idem,* Chaps. 2–3.

62. Richard C. Cabot, *Social Service and the Art of Healing* (New York: Dodd, Mead & Co., 1931), pp. 180-182; see also E. Moberly Bell, *The Story of Hospital Almoners: The Birth of a Profession* (1961), pp. 27-30.

63. René Sand, *The Advance to Social Medicine* (New York: John de Graff, Inc., 1952), p. 86.

64. Davis, *op. cit.,* pp. 13-14; Somers and Somers, *op. cit.,* pp. 64-65.

65. George Rosen, "Hospital," *Encyclopedia Americana* (1959), Vol. XIV, pp. 432-433.

66. George Bugbee, "The Physician in the Hospital Organization," *New England Journal of Medicine* (1959), pp. 896-901.

67. Michael M. Davis, *Medical Care for Tomorrow* (New York: Harper & Brothers, 1955), p. 111.

2

American and Foreign Hospitals

SOME SOCIOLOGICAL COMPARISONS

WILLIAM A. GLASER

Nearly all sociological research about hospitals has been performed in America. A comparison of hospitals in America and in foreign societies would make valuable contributions to sociological analysis. First, we can see what propositions about American hospitals are true only of them, and what propositions are generally true of hospitals in different contexts. Such universally true propositions would reveal certain functional prerequisites inherent in hospital organizations and in modern medical care; such structural elements would clearly be so

This article may be identified as Publication No. A-339 of the Bureau of Applied Social Research, Columbia University. This investigation was supported by Research Grant, RG-7934, awarded by the National Institute of Health, Public Health Service. For helpful comments on an earlier draft, I am indebted to Simon Btesh, Lyle Creelman, Milton Roemer, Marjorie Duvillard, and Ray Elling.

important that they can resist cross-national variations in the social environment. Second, cross-national comparisons could identify how specific variations in the social context correlate with variations in hospital organizations. Therefore, we could pass beyond sociological descriptions of American hospitals and begin sociological explanations of *why* particular characteristics are true of American hospitals while other characteristics are true elsewhere.

For convenience in exposition, this chapter will contain many simplifications. I shall contrast American and "foreign" hospitals, but of course the reader must never forget that the word "foreign" embraces a great variety of forms. International variations in government structure, economic prosperity, skilled manpower, styles of medical practice, and other factors produce a great range of hospital types in the world.[1] Highly developed countries with social and medical structures much like America's, such as Canada and Australia, have hospitals that are sociologically similar.[2] Northern and Western Europe resemble America in some ways and differ in others; hospitals in the underdeveloped countries of Asia and Africa are yet more different. For the most part I shall be comparing the kinds of large general hospitals that American sociologists have usually studied, but occasionally I shall mention the smaller private and rural hospitals.

This chapter can be considered as no more than an introduction to a complex problem. My conclusions are little more than impressions and informed hypotheses based on personal observations in American and foreign hospitals, interviews with informants, and a review of the literature. Carefully designed and thorough comparative studies would be necessary before we can state final conclusions about how and why American and foreign hospitals differ in some ways and are alike in others.

Administration and Administrative-Therapeutic Conflicts

When a sociological participant-observer enters an American hospital, he is immediately struck by the large number of administrative offices near the front entrance and by the numerous administrative employees, such as full-time or nearly full-time executives, purchasing officers, bookkeepers, personnel officers, secretaries, file clerks, receptionists, messengers, and others. Many of these tasks and personnel are concentrated in central offices; others are parts of the separate medical services of the hospital. Some social scientists have made intensive studies of the administrative personnel themselves.[3] A principal theme in many sociological studies of hospitals has been conflicts between the administrative and therapeutic personnel, arising from their different conceptions of the hospital's goals and priorities.[4]

But if the same sociological participant-observer entered a hospital in nearly any foreign country he would notice fewer administrative offices, fewer administrative personnel, and a smaller volume of administrative work. There may be fewer conflicts between the administrative and therapeutic needs of hospitals, and thus between administrators and therapists.[5] These fundamental differences have numerous causes. In many countries the nature of medical care, simpler payment methods, the expectations of patients, and the character of the society require fewer administrative tasks. In nearly all other countries certain administrative tasks performed inside the American hospital are performed on a higher level of the society. In many countries certain tasks performed in America by central administrators for the entire hospital are performed by the separate medical services within the organization. In nearly all other countries administrative work is more clearly subordinated to clinical work; it may be delegated to lay employees who clearly possess less education, lower prestige, and fewer rewards.[6]

DIFFERENT AMOUNTS OF MEDICAL ADMINISTRATION

Many characteristics of American medical care produce a larger volume of administrative work. For example, compared to most countries, American hospitals use larger amounts of new equipment and new drugs, and they perform more diagnostic tests.[7] Many administrative tasks result. Proposed equipment and drugs must be inspected and evaluated, the money raised by someone, sales and delivery negotiated and checked, special parts of the hospital building planned and adapted for the location of equipment in use or for the storage of materials and drugs, the orderly movement of materials and drugs throughout the hospital arranged, timetables prepared and checked for use of facilities, for the personnel who man the facilities, and for the patients who are diagnosed or treated by the equipment or drugs. Reports about patients' tests or treatments must be prepared and sent to the physicians who requested them, capital costs amortized in some way, and so on. Countries whose medical care is less technical—and this includes most of the world—have a smaller volume of such tasks in their hospitals and thus a smaller need for administrative specialists.

America integrates hospital practice and clinical medical research more than most other countries, and this too creates more administrative tasks than appear abroad. Since considerable prestige, professional advancement, and money are conferred upon the scientist in American medicine, more American than foreign hospital doctors perform research on their patients and write reports or journal articles. To a greater extent than in corresponding types of foreign hospitals, house staffs in larger American institutions conduct in-service educational programs that emphasize scientific lessons from the hospital's practice.[8] Even when American clinicians or administrators are not making original investigations of their own patients, more often than their foreign counterparts they may read the medical literature and check in their own hospitals whether certain new scientific findings are true. For such reasons, American hospitals have more specialized clerical personnel to file records, get information from files, aggregate facts about separate patients, type manuscripts, manage hospital libraries, and search the published literature.

Even the numerous American hospitals performing no research and no in-service staff education keep more voluminous records than their foreign counterparts. One reason is the need to protect the hospital and doctor in case of malpractice lawsuits. Such suits—very rare except in the Anglo-Saxon countries— must be defended by the hospital and doctor themselves with the aid of written evidence. Another reason for voluminous records is that they facilitate continuity of care over several hospital visits and American medicine practices such continuity more than most other countries. In a few other nations where continuity of care is attempted, such as England, the Soviet Union, and Israel, efficient patient files are kept in record rooms much like America's. Therefore, for a variety of reasons—research, in-service education, protection of the hospital, continuity of care, and American cultural habit—American hospitals keep more detailed, more voluminous, and more typewritten patient records than most foreign hospitals. American hospitals tend to keep these patient records in central and efficient files, a system that adds additional administrative tasks to the hospital.

Much of American hospital care is performed by private practitioners who visit the hospital for short periods either to treat their personal patients or to do voluntary work in clinics or on wards. In nearly every other country, hospital care is given only by permanent staff members, many of them full-time; if outside practitioners enter the hospital, they only give or receive information, and rarely do they participate in patient care. Since the "attending doctor" system produces larger and more mobile medical staffs, American hospitals have more administrative tasks. A larger number of doctors tends to work on each case than is true abroad, and the arrival of one doctor may not coincide with the time schedules of the other doctors and nurses. Thus the American doctor is more likely to communicate with other doctors and nurses by writing his findings and orders in the patient's charts and in the ward's order book; in most other countries the stable and small medical staff can more often communicate by face-to-face conversations.[9] Since a large number of private practitioners are continually entering, circulating in, and leaving American hospitals, the establishments must administer elaborate systems for taking messages, paging doctors, and sending information to private offices outside. In addition, the hospital must maintain and continually revise appointment calendars for the attending physicians' clinical work and case conferences. Finally, since the busy American private practitioner often views the hospital as a device for conserving his time and enabling him to increase the size of his practice, he may expect the hospital to perform tasks that many foreign counterparts would do themselves, such as filling out charts, making appointments, sending messages, doing diagnostic tests, and so on. Some of these delegations involve transferring administrative chores from private office practice to the hospital, and in addition the very fact of delegation itself creates tasks of communication, record-keeping, and double-checking that most foreign hospitals avoid.

American hospitals must perform other administrative tasks because American patients expect more than patients in foreign public hospitals, or because American hospital executives try to please them more. In part, these tasks are designed to promote recovery, in part to maintain the favorable public images that are necessary to avoid losing public subsidies and fee-paying customers, in part to be consistent with the American cultural tradition that no products or services should displease the user. For example, many American public and voluntary hospitals—but few of their foreign counterparts—have reception staffs to give advice and specially prepared pamphlets to new patients. Many American hospitals—but few foreign ones—have elaborate catering services, often with specially trained dietitians and complex delivery services, so that patients can make choices of palatable food from varied menus. Many American—but few foreign hospitals—have special shops for ambulatory patients, such as beauty parlors, newsstands, and post offices. American hospitals usually have more elaborate libraries and recreational services. They also have more extensive public relations programs designed in part to relieve the anxieties and puzzlement of past and future patients, and to cushion the shock of admission.[10] Competition among American public and voluntary hospitals for funds and for paying patients steadily increases these public relations functions,[11] but such competition among foreign public hospitals usually takes a different form, such as political pressures within the government rather than the more laborious and expensive appeals to local constituencies and to patient clienteles. Practically the only foreign hospitals that have such comforts and public relations techniques are those with similar problems of winning patients and funds under competitive conditions, namely the small profit-making hospitals owned by doctors in the cities of Europe, Asia, and Africa.

Finally, the American hospital has a number of administrative tasks found less frequently abroad because of the administrative propensities of American society itself. More than foreigners, Americans are likely to conceive of a hospital as an organization like any other, and thus to install in the hospital administrative practices and types of administrative personnel that have established their usefulness in business or in other lay bureaucracies. For example, although the cross-national differences have recently begun to diminish, American hospitals are still more likely to employ lay administrative procedures in their financial departments, in purchasing, and in intrahospital communications. Such more sophisticated and efficient procedures require more administrative effort and a larger staff that thinks in lay rather than in clinical terms. In addition, Americans generally are more likely to think of the hiring, screening, and assignment of personnel as a specialized administrative problem requiring files and a staff. Just as American organizations are more likely than their foreign counterparts to have special personnel staffs, so American hospitals have more personnel officers and more personnel procedures. Practical needs as well as cultural fashion underlie the greater American attention to personnel management; American hospitals may have higher personnel turnover than any other country's, and thus the hospital must always cope with the screening and placement of new employees and the discontent and departures of old ones.

MEDICAL ADMINISTRATION INSIDE OR ABOVE THE HOSPITAL

American hospitals have more administration because they are more autonomous than hospitals in most foreign countries, and they must make many decisions, or perform many functions that are more often conducted on a "higher" level of the society abroad. Many such differences are financial. In most countries hospitals are owned and managed by a "higher" authority, such as local or national governments, religious orders, national trade unions, or other larger-scale organizations. Even when foreign hospitals are theoretically autonomous, they may actually be the agency of a more powerful authority that governs the hospital through regulations and subsidies. Since each voluntary and religious hospital in America must raise its own money for large capital expenses or for covering deficits, its executive (sometimes including special fund raisers) must devote time to seeking and administering charitable gifts or special grants. The greater the number of competitors for the donors' money, the greater the number of donations received by the hospital, and the more varied the sources of its funds, then the more complex the administrative task and the greater the number of specialized fund raisers and financial administrators the American hospital must employ.

American hospitals have much administrative work because most decide their own fees, many patients pay entirely from personal funds, and fees may exceed the sums guaranteed by insurance funds. Much administrative attention and many persons are involved in calculating operating costs, setting over-all fee policies, investigating each patient's ability to pay, determining each patient's daily fee, sending and collecting bills, and hearing complaints from the patient and from the patient's personal physician. But in most foreign hospitals large business offices need not exist, since the hospitals do not make their own fee decisions and since collection is simpler. Most fees are standardized on a regional or national basis according to type of treatment or according to type of patient, and fees are not determined by individual hospitals or by individual physicians. In many such countries, billing and payment are simple matters of correspondence involving long lists of patients between the hospital on the one hand and either the government treasury or insurance funds on the other. Of course, there remain some countries (although a decreasing number) where the fees of large public and voluntary hospitals are discretionary and are paid in whole or in part by the patient. One expects such hospitals to have administrative functions and administrative roles much like America's, but no comparative social research has yet been done.

American hospitals usually make their own personnel decisions. Therefore administrators must hire personnel and negotiate wages and hours according to the needs and bargaining power of the hospital. But in many countries wages and hours of nurses, auxiliaries, and sometimes even doctors are decided by higher authority—either by government statutes or by collective bargaining agreements between unions and regional or national hospital boards. In some countries the hospital directors have little voice in hiring or assigning doctors. In some, hiring is decided by competition according to statutory rules, and the hospital itself is not represented on the panel of judges. In a few countries, both the hospitals and doctors are parts of a governmental medical service, and doctors are assigned or transferred according to judgments made in the Ministry of Health, with only limited participation by the hospital.

Much of American hospital administration is devoted to planning and constructing new buildings, acquiring land, and adapting and installing new equipment. Here, too, some countries differ. In a few with government health services, the decision to build a new structure or to adapt an old one will be made by regional hospital boards or by the health ministry of the locality, region, or nation. The hospital director will participate in the new planning and decisions, but much of the administrative work will be done by the personnel of the higher agency. In a few countries new building styles and new equipment are not the subjects of extensive administrative investigation and judgment as in America, but certain standard patterns are followed throughout the hospital service.

CENTRALIZED AND DECENTRALIZED SYSTEMS

Administrative tasks and personnel are less prominent in the hospitals of most foreign countries because these establishments are usually more internally decentralized than the American. Tasks are spread out among the powerful chiefs of service and need not be performed by any central administrators. For example, in the large hospitals in a few countries the chiefs hire and direct the other doctors; in some they hire and direct the nurses and auxiliaries; in many countries each service has its own laboratories, x-ray equipment, catering service, and rehabilitation service; in some countries, each surgeon has his own operating room and recovery room. There is less decentralization in the small than in the large hospitals abroad and the trend everywhere is toward more central services, but decentralization probably is greater in each type of foreign hospital than in its corresponding type in America. Throughout the United States today labs, x-ray departments, catering, rehabilitation, operating rooms, recovery rooms, and many similar facilities are financed, staffed, and managed by the central administration for the hospital as a whole. Since many of these American central services are more elaborate than the facilities scattered through foreign hospitals, they require more money and administrative effort.

ADMINISTRATION AS A RIVAL TO THERAPY

Administrative-therapeutic conflicts seem to occur less frequently and with lower intensity in foreign hospitals. In previous pages I have suggested why administrative personnel are less important and less numerous in the hospitals of most foreign countries. In addition, the specialized administrators who exist abroad are less likely to be rivals of therapists.

In America, particularly in the large general or mental hospitals that sociologists have studied, there is an increasing tendency for administrators and clinicians to be different people. The administrators might be laymen or doctors in full-time administration. Occupying high positions in the organization and committed to the structural and financial order of the hospital, they may disagree with clinicians over the application of existing policies or the creation of new ones.

Such administrative challenges to clinical primacy are much more rare abroad. First, in most countries the administrative tasks of hospitals are usually performed by clinicians whose primary commitment is to clinical medicine. This combination of administrative and clinical tasks is possible because both are less burdensome; foreign administrative work is simpler and less time-consuming, and foreign hospital doctors may see fewer patients than their American counterparts. Foreign chiefs of service may be more willing than Americans to accept administrative duties as part of their leadership responsibilities and may be more accustomed to using their administrative positions to wield authority over younger doctors, nurses, and other personnel. (If the service chief delegates this work to anyone, he gives it not to a lay administrator but to his clinical assistant, namely, the chief resident of his service). In contrast, the American hospital doctor may more often seek to acquire respect and power in the organization through recognized clinical skill, through research findings, and through a large and lucrative patient load.

A second reason for the possible rarity of administrative-therapeutic conflicts is that, until recently when lay administrators were incorporated into foreign hospitals, they were almost always placed in unambiguously subordinate positions. They were called "secretaries," "business managers," or "engineers," but rarely anything like "directors." Their span of control was always much narrower than that of American lay administrators. They were usually subordinate to hospital directors who were clinicians.[12] Lay hospital administrators directly responsible to governing boards are now arising in England, France, Italy, Switzerland, and some other countries. Because their positions are so new, rivalry with the clinicians has not yet become general, although the visitor notices some of the beginnings of the American-type conflict. But whether they are officially subordinate to or independent of medical directors, foreign lay administrators may be more deferential to the doctors than are their American counterparts. Usually they come from class backgrounds and from educational curricula (such as commercial high schools and the business schools of universities) that give them considerably less prestige than the doctors in the eyes of both the hospital and of the larger society. In America, class consciousness is generally lower, doctors and lay administrators spring from less dissimilar class origins, lay administrators like doctors get a university education and a university degree, and administration is a job that attracts more public respect.

THERAPY'S DEMANDS UPON ADMINISTRATION

Just as foreign administrative structures and administrators may pose fewer challenges to the therapists, so therapists may do fewer things upsetting to the hospital organization. For example, American doctors are often eager to use laboratory tests and the newest equipment. Such routine orders given by many physicians, each with only slight thoughts about costs, are one reason why American hospital administrators must cope with mounting deficits and rising patient fees. In many (and perhaps most) foreign countries, doctors routinely request fewer tests, use less diagnostic and therapeutic equipment, and may be slower in asking the hospital to employ the newest techniques. As a result, they make fewer costly demands, hospital costs rise at a slower rate than in America, and fewer administrator-therapist disputes may arise over new and excessive expenses.

Compared to the American physician, the hospital doctor in most countries seems less hurried. Few are trying to combine more than one task at the same time, such as private and hospital practices or research and hospital practice. The minority of doctors with both hospital and private practices usually are supposed to separate the two by reserving fixed morning hours for the hospital and seeing private patients elsewhere during the rest of the day. During comparable time spans spent in the hospital, the foreign doctor may see fewer patients than the American. For all these reasons, he may be less peremptory in giving administrative orders than his American counterpart, he may be present to guide the implementation and repercussions of his orders, and he is available for questions. Many of the tensions between administrators and clinicians in the American hospital are due to the fact that the American doctor is often hurried, peremptory, unaware of the results of his orders, and difficult to find. The administrator and nurse in the American hospital have the added irritant of knowing that many of the doctor's demands are designed to assist his lucrative private practice, rather than to assist the hospital.

ADMINISTRATIVE-THERAPEUTIC CONFLICTS

Thus, for many reasons, administrative and therapeutic structures are probably less distinct in foreign than in American hospitals, and conflicts between administrative and therapeutic roles may be less frequent and less acute. But the differences must everywhere be matters of degree, since no organization can ever be without certain functional needs that may compete with therapeutic ends. For example, every hospital in the world needs to budget its resources, and such budgeting usually conflicts with therapeutic ideals about giving maximum care to all potential patients; auxiliary personnel in every hospital in the world seem to prefer predictable work schedules, but such routine may conflict with therapists' demands for emergency action.

Certain types of administrator-therapist conflicts are different abroad, because of the different organization of public and voluntary hospitals. In many countries conflicts arise over the therapist's allocations of time between the hospital and his private practice. In theory this conflict is avoided where the senior hospital doctors are supposed to devote their mornings— usually from 8 A.M. to 2 P.M.—exclusively to the public hospital. But since these doctors earn three-quarters or more of their incomes from practice in their private offices or in their private hospitals, they often reduce their time in the public hospital by arriving late, leaving early, using some of their public hospital time for lunch, and often arranging not to be called for emergencies in their public hospital departments during afternoons or evenings. Since most countries lack the funds for salaries high enough to compensate service chiefs for loss of private practice, usually hospitals are powerless to enforce work hours on the part-time senior men. Where the system of part-time service chiefs operates in this way, there result strains for the hospital management and considerable irritation among the low-salaried full-time house staff.

Furthermore, conflicts somewhat different in character and scope from the American-style incompatibilities between organizational stability and therapeutic success within each separate hospital are likely to be found in countries where a lay public policy governs a subordinate system of hospitals. Hospital administrators implementing governmental or church orders might collide with doctors concerned only with the welfare of individual patients. For example, the Soviet Ministry of Health under Stalin obeyed the government's policy of keeping workers at their job, and hospital administrators and local party representatives responsible to the Ministry placed pressure on doctors to limit hospital admissions and accelerate discharges.[13]

Medical Staff

STRUCTURE OF AUTHORITY

American sociologists have studied authority and work relations among hospital doctors. In some of the studies, superior-subordinate relations have been examined—for example, between fully qualified physicians and students, between the influential leaders of the local medical community and aspiring hospital doctors, and between the heads and members of surgical teams.[14] But one gets the impression from these studies that authority is considerably diffused within American medical staffs, and in fact some social scientists have suggested that clinicians cannot be said to have any definite organizational structure at all.[15] Medical staffs have been studied by medical sociologists much less than some other aspects of the hospital, and one reason may be the absence of the kind of structural clarity that facilitates sociological analysis elsewhere in the hospital and in other bureaucratic organizations.

But if one examines medical staffs in many foreign countries, one finds clear-cut hierarchies of the type that characteristically attracts the interest of sociologists. A number of reasons may make American medical staffs more egalitarian and more diffuse structurally.

One reason is the combination of leadership roles in certain strategic statuses, particularly the chiefs of service in the foreign hospital. These men are multifunctional experts, performing a set of roles that are often spread among many senior persons in the American hospital. The foreign "patron" or "kliniksdirektor" may be at the same time chief clinician in his service, chief administrator, and chief educator. In each role, he may share his authority less than the American counterpart. For example, the foreign chief clinician may exercise ultimate responsibility over a larger proportion of the patients in his service; he may seek other doctors' advice less and insist more on the enforcement of his own medical judgments. As chief administrator of his service, the patron does not try to delegate the managerial and clerical chores that American doctors often avoid, since it is recognized that being a patron includes the continued exercise of organizational authority. The patron's administrative resources often exceed the American service chief's since many foreign hospitals give him control over budget, nurses, equipment, and other personnel and facilities that would often be centralized in an American hospital. As chief educator of his service (if he is a service chief in a teaching hospital), the patron would give the principal lectures in his specialty and conduct the most important and best-attended teaching rounds. Such educational duties are more widely spread in America among hospital doctors and among clinicians who are medical-school faculty members rather than hospital doctors.[16]

The clinical hierarchy is more clear-cut and authoritarian in many foreign countries because, compared to young Americans, the young hospital doctor is usually more dependent on his superiors for career advancement. At an earlier age than the American, he may be committed to a single career. By entering the hospital hierarchy he makes a lifetime commitment to specialty practice in hospitals; he would prefer not to switch into general office practice, since it is much less rewarding than a hospital career, and usually he cannot switch into a research career, since research opportunities are few and may not exist outside the hospital. Young American hospital doctors can and do find many other jobs throughout their large country; but the young foreign doctor, either because geographical mobility is unusual in his country or because good hospital jobs are few, is far more likely to stay in one hospital in the metropolis or in his home locality, if he can. Since challenging a patron may damage one's career while his favor might yield great prizes—even including designation as his successor—only a foolhardy doctor would risk displaying imprudent independence. Instead, the more important the patron, the larger the number of students at his lectures and rounds, the more numerous the applicants for his service, and the greater the deference to him.

Certain national variations in medical practice help account for the lower amount of deference by subordinates toward higher hospital doctors in America. Compared to many other countries, American medicine makes greater use of scientific and technical knowledge, and its content changes more rapidly. Among a group of doctors knowledge is more widespread, and decisions can better be made by questioning and by many contributions from among members of teams. Knowledge and skill may not always correlate with official rank, and therefore American service chiefs may be demonstrably surpassed on specific problems or in general ability by doctors junior in both rank and age. American medical culture, to a greater extent than those of many foreign countries, emphasizes the uncertainty of knowledge and judgment. Consequently decisions are often preceded by group discussions, by the critical questioning of senior men, and by citing clinical evidence, and a senior doctor addicted to *ex cathedra* assertions is suspect.

Certain national cultural differences underlie the less deferential habits of American clinical subordinates. In general, American leader-follower relations include less social distance and permit more free-and-easy fellowship than is true in most other societies.[17] Compared to most other countries, American premedical and medical education provide less rote memorization and encourage more independent critical thinking, and these habits of questioning and discussion are retained by both superiors and subordinates in clinical staffs. Possibly more than foreign patrons, American senior physicians may admire and reward the junior colleague who is an independent thinker and skilled critic.[18]

Finally, not only do the attendings in American hospitals represent a large element of instability and limited commitment, but even the regular hospital staff may not be full-time participants in their own clinical services. In most countries, doctors spend most of their hospital duty hours close to their own departments. But in American hospitals, and particularly in the large medical centers, a doctor not only sees patients in his own service but often is called for consultation about any patient elsewhere in the hospital who might present a problem in his specialty. For such consultations, the American hospital doctor may go to see the patient instead of waiting for him to be brought. Most foreign hospitals have considerably less movement of doctors through the corridors and across the thresholds; as a result, each clinical service is a more stable social structure.[19]

FUNCTIONS OF THE HOSPITAL FOR THE PROFESSIONAL COMMUNITY

As sociologists and others have long realized, American hospitals perform crucial functions in the community of private practitioners. The right to hospitalize and care for one's own patients in a good hospital is essential for a successful private practice. The hospital staff becomes a "club" of professional allies who provide advice and patient referrals. In most American communities there is a stratification among hospitals, so that the better one's hospital, the higher one's income and repute. The granting of hospital privileges and internal reviewing mechanisms such as Tissue Committees and rounds become methods by which the professional community regulates the clinical and personal behavior of its members.[20]

Participation by all doctors in hospitals is nearly unique to America. In most countries general practitioners cannot work in hospitals, even when their own patients are hospitalized. The separation of most private practitioners from the public and voluntary hospitals abroad results in a professional community much different from the American. Paradoxically, the integration of private and hospital practices in America produces a more diffuse medical staff structure inside the hospital and a more orderly structure in the community of private practitioners. Since the majority of doctors in most countries practice outside the public and voluntary hospitals, rank in these institutions cannot be used to arrange a hierarchy in the medical profession generally. Granting or withdrawing hospitalization privileges cannot be used to regulate professional and personal behavior; in fact, this use of hospitalization privileges makes America one of the few countries with any controls over the quality of private practice.

Abroad, the hospital reinforces the position of the leaders of the foreign professional community, but does little more. To become a professor in the medical school and service chief in the teaching hospital seems to ensure a doctor's power and prosperity in the local medical community in all countries, and usually also in the nationwide medical profession. Since foreign cultures glorify the university professor more than America, such an appointment results in even greater rewards and power abroad. Becoming a service chief in a nonteaching hospital abroad often will make a doctor one of the recognized leaders of his specialty in the locality. The appointment is a kind of free advertising and is public certification of his competence, but his position in the medical community will also depend on the success of his private practice, either in his office or in his private hospital. The hospital staff and the leadership structure of the medical community are not always articulated; in some countries, such as parts of Greece, it is not generally assumed that leading specialists must be service chiefs in public or voluntary hospitals. Doctors can build reputations and high incomes through their own private hospitals, and they may even avoid the time-consuming and unremunerative obligations of the public hospital. However, a few countries integrate the hospital and the local medical community, sometimes going even farther than the United States. For example, in the Soviet Union the outpatient polyclinics that give all ambulatory and home care to Soviet citizens are attached to the hospital. All specialists and general practitioners in the locality hold ranks in the same medical organization, belong to the same chapter of the Medical Workers Union, and sometimes rotate between the hospital and the polyclinic. The sociological functions performed by the hospital in the medical community of such a highly integrated system would merit future research.

Morale of Nonmedical Staff

One theme that recurs in American medical sociology is the low morale of nurses and auxiliary workers. Many sociological studies were initiated because hospitals needed to learn the causes and remedies for high personnel turnover and widespread discontent. The malaise has been attributed to various causes—the peremptory behavior of doctors, insufficient pay, blocked mobility, frustration of humanitarian motives, and so on.[21] As in many other sociological findings about hospitals, the American facts and reasons have been stated as if they were inherent in hospital organizations.

Here too, there may be considerable cross-national variation, with America having an unusual degree or unusual forms of employee discontent. First, hospital employees in most countries are probably more satisfied than Americans. The absence of comparative research about morale makes such estimates precarious, but turnover seems smaller abroad. One set of reasons arises from the economy. America has many competing, better paid, and more glamorous jobs in white-collar work and in industry. In many countries, hospital work is considered a better job than it is in America because other good jobs are scarcer, and the discrepancies in pay and pensions between hospital and other jobs is smaller. In many underdeveloped countries, unlike America, hospital work is quite prestigeful, since it provides steadier employment than other proletarian jobs and since it makes the employee a participant in modern urban activities.

Discontent may also be lower in some foreign countries because the average doctor irritates the nurses and auxiliaries less. Since his patient load is lower, he is less hurried and peremptory, less pressed to delegate work to already overworked subordinates, and more able to provide continuous supervision. Because the great majority of foreign hospital doctors have no private practice while most of the others conduct it outside the public and voluntary hospitals, other hospital employees may not feel they are helping the doctors become rich. Where service chiefs acquire the reputation of neglecting their hospital duties for longer hours in private practice, I have sometimes noticed an increased solidarity between the house staff and the nurses; they are united by common responsibilities and by a common irritant. In America, the nonmedical staff may bear a more generalized grievance against all doctors.

Discontent may be lower abroad for cultural reasons. American norms about individual competitive striving toward success and wealth cause considerable frustration among the unsuccessful throughout American society, and this seems true of many hospital employees. In many other countries, proletarians such as hospital employees seem more resigned and less overtly bitter. In America chain reactions of rebellion and conflict often develop between workers and employers or co-workers, because of the cultural habit of speaking frankly. A discontented hospital employee abroad may more often keep his grievances to himself or confide them to his peers, thus avoiding the vicious circle of rejection by a superior and increasing bitterness.

Employee discontent exists abroad, of course, but often it is directed at targets other than the doctors or hospital administrators.[22] For example, in the numerous countries where wages and working conditions are set by law or by collective bargaining agreements, discontented nurses and auxiliaries blame the government or regional hospital boards rather than their own hospital. In both the informal conversations of foreign nurses and in the official announcements of nursing groups, the grievances that seem most salient are higher pay, shorter and more convenient hours, and better living conditions in the hospital; action consists of regional or national organized appeals to public opinion, to the government, or to other high-level authorities.[23] In contrast, American nurses and auxiliaries usually concentrate all their discontent against the doctors and administrators in their own hospital.

National or regional standardization of wages and working conditions in many foreign countries has the additional effect of reducing personnel shifts as a solution of discontent. If all hospitals have similar wages and conditions, the discontented employee will gain little from transferring, and may lose the seniority rights and informal social statuses he had at his first hospital. In comparison, invidious contrasts among hospitals and job shifts among them cause considerable discontent and weak job commitment in America.

Nurses

Much social research has been done about the recent changes and present characteristics of American hospital nursing. Foreign nursing in many respects is quite unlike America's. In some ways, widely standard foreign patterns exist that are altogether different from those in America. In other ways, a great variety of forms exist abroad, each being different from those in America. Sometimes one can find trends in the American direction, but large differences of degree remain.

ASPIRATIONS FOR PROFESSIONAL STATUS

Women in America have achieved a higher economic and social status than in most other societies. And compared to most countries, America's nurses have higher aspirations relative to doctors. The leaders of American nursing and apparently the bulk of the practitioners seek considerably more prestige, autonomy, responsibility, and rewards than heretofore—in short, recognition as the doctor's colleague rather than as his helper. Although the beginnings of such lay professional aspirations can be seen in some European and Anglo-Saxon countries, nursing leaders and practitioners in these and the other parts of the world generally have different self-images, job conceptions, and aspirations.[24] In many countries, particularly where women still have only limited educational and economic opportunities, nurses may perceive themselves as skilled employees performing socially useful, interesting, but subordinate work. In countries where Catholicism and evangelical Protestantism are strong, many nurses may perceive their work as a divinely blessed vocation.

As a result of the greater social opportunities of American women and as a result of their more professional aspirations, American hospital nurses differ from their foreign counterparts in many ways. They have more years of education, in many cases even including a few years of college, and their schooling includes more liberal arts and science. They may be more eager to take on technical and administrative work, and to delegate housekeeping work. They seem to be more resentful of subordination to doctors and hospital administrators, particularly when they are not consulted or notified in advance about decisions or changes in plans. Compared to most foreign hospital nurses, the individual American staff nurse may be more accustomed to exercising her own discretion and may prefer more autonomy from her own superiors in the nursing service. American nurses probably receive and read more professional literature.

The professionalizing tendencies in American nursing have certain effects upon hospitals that occur rarely or never in foreign countries. Because nursing leaders emphasize that improved education is essential to achieve full professionalization, there is a rapidly spreading trend for all undergraduate students to be taught by specialized clinical nursing instructors in place of the ordinary clinical nurses. Thus every American hospital with a nursing school is acquiring two nursing hierarchies—clinical and educational—with the resultant drawbacks of occasional conflicts and many additional salaries. In foreign countries, clinical care and teaching are combined in the same persons, with lower overhead costs and with fewer opportunities for structural conflict. Because of the American emphasis on good professional nursing education—including much reading and didactic instruction—and because students are not yet considered sufficiently skilled for membership in a professional clinical complement, American hospitals no longer rely upon students as much as foreign hospitals for the provision of ordinary nursing services. There is an increasing tendency to accord American students the typical rights of all students in American professional schools, such as considerable free time, living and eating outside the hospital, marrying, and so on. Such changes have just begun abroad, and in some countries the daily lives of students and sometimes even of staff nurses are still closely supervised by the hospital.

Some of the policies of American organized nursing have had fundamental consequences for hospitals. For example, an increasing number of hospitals have agreed to the nursing associations' recommendations that postgraduate education be a prerequisite for promotions in the hierarchies of clinical administration and student education. As a result, a nurse often cannot be promoted simply by virtue of seniority or experience, as she would in most foreign countries,[25] but she would need to take the time and bear the expense of graduate education. Some observers believe that blocked mobility for nurses without appropriate educational preparation is a principal reason for the very high and costly turnover on American nursing staffs. American hospitals must adapt their work schedules to an often substantial number of nurses who are taking courses during the evenings, weekends, or summers. American hospitals have the further complication—also rare or non-existent abroad—that the university instructors who are teaching these nurses may be teaching professionally ideal doctrines and techniques that contradict hospital practice.

In a few countries nurses, and particularly the matron, exercise even more authority in the hospital than do Americans. But their role is that of skilled organizational managers, and they are not trying to become professional colleagues of the doctor in the sense of applying their own scientific knowledge to the patient's problems, developing programs of patient care in collaboration with doctors, making decisions by agreement among equal and autonomous individuals, and so on. For example, the hospitals of England and of many Commonwealth countries are ruled by vigorous matrons and disciplined nursing hierarchies, whose managerial prerogatives are scrupulously respected by the doctors. In parts of Western Europe there are hospitals owned and managed by Lutheran deaconesses and Catholic nuns; doctors usually think of themselves as guests of the order and are carefully deferential to the sisters in personal and administrative matters. All these arrangements seem to be maintained by a combination of separate functions, elaborate personal etiquette, and strict time schedules. Doctors concentrate on patient care, and the matron and her nurses are the hospital administrators; the nurses act as assistants rather than as equal colleagues of the doctor in patient care, and they accept the doctor's judgments about medical needs. If an experienced nurse believes an inexperienced doctor is making a mistake in caring for a patient whose conditions she well understands, she may volunteer information and advice, but with a degree of subtlety and formal etiquette that is rare in America.

DIVISION OF LABOR

It is difficult to make cross-national comparisons of nursing work for many reasons. Scientific job analyses have been conducted only in a few countries.[26] International comparisons are complicated by the fact that the distribution of tasks varies considerably within certain countries; this is true of the United States, as a result of its system of many local independent hospitals. A further complication is that the nursing corps is not the same everywhere; most countries have few graduate nurses and many practical nurses with limited formal training, while a few European countries have many graduate nurses and few practical nurses.

A few very tentative comparisons may be hazarded. Since

American hospitals keep more records than foreign hospitals, American nursing complements may devote a larger number of man-hours to records. Since American hospitals use more equipment and more complex diagnostic and therapeutic methods than most foreign hospitals, American nursing complements may devote a larger number of man-hours to work with equipment on wards and to complex calculations concerning metabolic balances, fluid intake-output balances, and so forth. In many American hospitals, but less frequently abroad, central services relieve the nursing complements of some domestic tasks, such as collecting and distributing laundry, collecting and distributing dishes and food, cleaning floors, and sometimes even making beds. Throughout the world administrative and technical work is considered more skilled and prestigeful than housekeeping work, and as a result American nursing seems to have a more technical and skilled image.

The distribution of tasks within the nursing complement is different in some ways. To simplify very drastically, American graduate nurses may give less bedside patient care than European graduate nurses, but more than the graduate nurses in underdeveloped countries. Because of the shortage of graduate nurses in underdeveloped countries—often none, one, or two in hospitals of up to three hundred beds—practical nurses have more administrative and clinical responsibility than American practical nurses, and far more such responsibility than the Western European auxiliaries. Student nurses in America, however, give considerably less administrative, clinical, and domestic work to the hospital than do students in any other country; in much of the world, a third-year student in a graduate nursing curriculum is performing all the tasks and has all the responsibility of any staff nurse, including the charge of wards and even of the entire hospital at night.

One might expect that their longer periods of technical education and their more professional aspirations would lead American nurses to acquire more medical tasks from doctors than do foreign nurses. Certainly in recent years busy American doctors have delegated a number of routine but responsible medical chores to graduate nurses and even to staff nurses, such as starting and refilling blood transfusions, doing diagnostic tests, and so on. But throughout the world, particularly in hospitals without large numbers of undergraduate and postgraduate medical students, graduate nurses and practical nurses do the same tasks, sometimes with even less close medical supervision than in America. Possibly local custom and shortages of doctors in rural areas give nurses in many countries even more medical responsibility than American nurses, such as performing normal deliveries and giving all types of anesthetics. Possibly the only cross-national difference concerning such medical delegations to nurses is whether it is cause for worry. American and British hospitals have become anxious over the location of legal responsibility in such delegations, because of the danger of the malpractice lawsuits peculiar to the Anglo-Saxon countries.[27] But in my visits I have detected little more than regret elsewhere, accompanied by the hope that an increased number of doctors and graduate nurses might make such delegations less frequent or less risky, in the future.

Volunteers

One of the reasons why American hospitals seem to have more diffuse and less disciplined organizational structures is the presence of many volunteers. Some are men and women who raise funds and serve on management committees. Others are adult women or teen-age girls who work inside the hospitals at various tasks, such as running the library for patients, helping patients in many personal matters, managing canteens, or running errands.[28] The volunteering spirit and the provision of volunteers for hospital work occur in America for various reasons. The American class structure can supply a large number of middle-class men and women whose ideology emphasizes public service and whose economic security enables them to devote much time to unpaid work. Business firms and other organizations believe that such voluntary service by their employees and by the wives of employees will be valuable for public relations. Churches, clubs, and other groups encourage beliefs in charitable service. American hospitals benefit from all these circumstances, because most are closely integrated into their localities and are favorite objects of local pride.

Hospital volunteers are nearly unique to America, because different social conditions exist abroad. Ideologies about voluntary "good works" by the ordinary citizen exist in few cultures. Many countries are split between a self-centered elite and a mass of employees and farmers, and no social source can provide numerous lay volunteers. In many countries hospitals cater only to one special clientele—that is, public hospitals for the poor and private commercialized hospitals for paying patients—and there may be no community-wide hospitals that might attract a potential volunteer desiring to serve the entire community. In most countries hospitals are managed by professionals designated by the national organization that owns the hospital, and the employees are confined to salaried workers belonging to trade unions that seek to protect jobs and wages, and for these reasons the hospital organization has no place for volunteers. In most countries the hospital is viewed as a facility provided by some absentee organization such as the national government or the church, and local citizens do not feel they have a responsibility to provide support. Only in a few countries are the American social conditions reproduced and are the countervailing conditions weak, and therefore only a few other countries have hospital volunteers.[29]

Patients

Since the behavior of patients throughout the world is a function of cultural norms and social roles generally, considerable cross-national variations have been discovered in the anthropological research so far completed. A few studies have been done of hospital inpatients in America, and we may make a few preliminary guesses about hospital patients abroad. American patient roles may differ slightly from those in Western Europe and other Anglo-Saxon countries, but they may diverge greatly from hospital patients in underdeveloped countries.

American hospital patients may be more active both physically and mentally than foreign patients, although the contrast is smaller as one makes comparisons with the more developed countries. One reason for the greater physical activity is that American patients become hospitalized at an earlier stage of disease and for less handicapping diseases than do patients abroad, particularly in agricultural societies; among the reasons are the greater self-insight, the greater lay knowledge about medical symptoms, the lower tolerance of sick persons by homes and work sites, the higher ability to pay for hospitalization, and the more effective referral network between private practitioners and hospitals. Physical and mental activity may be higher among American patients because of the cross-national differences in the hospitals themselves; in America there are earlier ambulation, shorter stays, a faster turnover, more numerous and more frequent diagnostic and therapeutic procedures, and possibly more questioning of patients by doctors and nurses.

The greater physical and mental activity of American patients may create certain cross-national sociological differences in patient-staff relations and in the patient community, but at present we can do no more than speculate. The greater medical understanding and worldly sophistication of some American patients may induce them to question and criticize the medical staff more, suggest treatments themselves, and have less confidence in folk remedies. The greater ambulation may cause more interaction and possibly greater solidarity in the patient communities on American wards.

The American patient communities studied by medical sociologists consist of nothing but patients. But in some countries patient communities would include other family members, who live in the patients' rooms or who visit for long periods each day. In Greece, Japan, and a few other countries, these family members give much of the nursing care.[30] Obviously their presence, often in very large numbers, creates a much different social environment from America's, but as yet we have little sociological knowledge about their roles. In some of the underdeveloped countries, family members provide powerful competition with medical authority by secretly bringing in their own folk remedies and food or by privately ridiculing some of the doctors' decisions. In some of the more gregarious societies, such as rural Greece or Cyprus, the separate families of various patients acquire considerable solidarity among themselves and develop a kind of "public opinion" that the medical and nursing staffs must appease; meetings among families in the hospital sometimes become opportunities for the exchange of nonmedical news among separate villages. On the other hand, a few countries, such as the Soviet Union and China, afford even less participation by healthy family members in ward life by providing even shorter visiting hours than do American hospitals.

Some American sociologists have emphasized the evolutionary character of the American patient role. The patient is expected to adjust completely to the hospital's demands for passivity at first, but as his medical condition improves, he is expected to aspire increasingly to resume his normal family and occupational responsibilities.[31] Probably the same evolution is expected to occur in other societies emphasizing personal achievement in the family and at work. There may be some societies, however, where interruption of normal family obligations is considered so wrong that patients may not assume patient roles as readily as Americans; they may be more reluctant to enter hospitals and more uncooperative and more unhappy after they enter. On the other hand, in many societies with underemployed labor forces, weaker achievement and autonomy norms, and inferior housing, patients may be less eager to abandon their passive hospital roles and return to work. There are many specific stimuli in the American hospital that motivate the patient's desire to go home and resume work—frequent visiting hours have the latent function of reminding him of the outside world; the fact that family members cannot stay with him around the clock prevents him from making the hospital a second home; opportunities to send and receive telephone calls and mail remind him of his outside obligations; and hospitalization and disability insurance benefits cannot reproduce the normal way of life of Americans as well as they can abroad.

Some as yet unexplored sociological differences must result

from the sizes of wards. American medical sociologists have studied small groups, since American hospitals have small wards, often split into a series of small rooms. In the public hospitals of much of the world, large rooms with fifteen or more beds are still common; in some of the ancient hospital buildings of France and Italy, occasionally one can still see large rooms with as many as fifty beds. The large number of small rooms in the newest American and foreign hospitals permits the separation of patients according to stage of illness; American sociologists consequently have studied patient groups that are approximately homogeneous in level of activity. But in many countries the lack of private rooms and of portable screens often results in the presence of unconscious and seriously ill patients on the open wards; perhaps one reason that foreign patient groups seem quieter than the American is the inhibiting effects of such critically ill patients upon the others.

Types of Hospitals

From the standpoint of the internal social structure customarily studied by American medical sociologists, American public and voluntary general hospitals differ from those abroad. But since foreign medical and social systems vary considerably, no single type of "foreign" hospital can be contrasted with an equally misleading simplification called the "American hospital." Instead, a range of types can be found abroad, just as within America. It is possible that some of the criteria may correlate, so that a few principal social types might ultimately be identified after rigorous research and theorizing. Following are a few types that I have noticed in different countries. I present them only as the kinds of preliminary impressions and guidelines that are essential at the earliest stage of research and that soon become obsolete simplifications.

In one type of hospital, a cross section of the entire community becomes patients, as the result of either comprehensive insurance or socialized medicine. Hospital jobs become a prized asset in a doctor's career, hospital work is rewarding both medically and financially, and therefore the community's better doctors work in the hospital for all or much of their time. Since such hospitals are usually found in the developed countries, they have a substantial number of competent nurses and technicians. Medical and administrative regulations are obeyed.

Another type of hospital is perceived as a charitable institution for the poor. It is a very common type in both Europe and the underedeveloped countries. Patients are drawn from the urban proletariat or from the peasants; they tend to be quiet, elderly, poorly nourished, very ill, and docile. The medical staff is headed by a small number of service chiefs who devote most of their time and attention to private practice outside the hospital; the bulk of the doctors are younger full-time house staff members, many of whom are ill-paid or discontented, all of whom are putting in a prescribed number of years in hospital service until they can establish their own specialty practice or emigrate to richer countries. The nursing staffs are very young on the average, obedient both to medical orders and to hospital regulations, and divided into a small number of professionally trained supervisors and a large number of persons without formal training.

In the most underdeveloped countries, the foregoing type of hospital exists, with certain modifications. Immense numbers of patients come to outpatient clinics, and therefore staff time and resources must be diverted away from inpatient care. Many hospital employees are poorly paid male "sweepers" who lack any technical or administrative skills, who work slowly and inefficiently, and who spend much of the day idly waiting for the assignment of some task. Unfamiliarity with Western scientific knowledge and with administrative norms results in frequent violations of sterile technique, medical orders, and administrative obligations by the nursing and administrative staffs. Where the culture emphasizes duties to one's own family rather than charitable service to humanity at large, nurses and other employees may give to patients only the minimum services ordered by doctors and by supervisors. In some—but not all— impoverished countries, economic necessity may induce the nurses, employees, and even some doctors to pilfer hospital property and to solicit tips from patients. In short, there may be considerable order when superiors are present, but much less in their absence.

Another widespread type of hospital is the private clinic. It is owned and managed nearly full-time by one doctor. The need to attract paying patients results in heavy investment in private rooms, furnishings, diet, and other amenities resembling nearby hotels. The need to earn net profits results in employment of very young and medically untrained domestics who are called "nurses" and who do all the nursing care. Also, for reasons of economy, there may be no other doctors. Unless the owner lives on the premises, there is no doctor present at night. Since they are most profitable and have the high recovery rate essential to protect the reputation of the clinic, patients are accepted who have mild disorders and who stay for short periods. Visiting hours are unlimited and family members sometimes live with the patient; consequently patients interact more with outsiders than with fellow patients.

Here, then, are some of the differences between American and foreign hospitals. Although some differences stem from cultural and social traditions, others result from economic necessity. As other countries became richer, they will acquire the facilities and the better trained hospital staffs that will lead to organizational changes in an American direction. Meanwhile, certain social changes in American medicine, particularly the spread of nation-wide prepaid systems for paying for medical care, may change American hospitals in a more "foreign" direction. Besides these unconscious tendencies toward greater similarity, much conscious emulation will have the same effect. Each country's best medical achievements have always spread abroad, and at present hospital administrators from all countries are traveling and learning from one another. Currently the visitor can find foreign hospitals that are partially organized according to American principles and that are expected to become the models for the hospitals of entire countries when more money becomes available; meanwhile, some critics and reformers in American hospitals are advocating changes that will follow certain foreign patterns, particularly those of Scandinavia. Perhaps in the future the hospitals of the world will somehow manage to combine both unity and diversity, and thereby gratify two contradictory aims; namely, to provide the same high-level services demanded by patients throughout the world, while retaining enough cross-cultural variations to interest the medical sociologist!

NOTES

1. For a discussion of international variations in hospitals and for a description of the research methods that yielded the present article, see my forthcoming book tentatively titled *Social Contexts and Health Institutions*. Many other administrative differences among foreign medical services are reported in the numerous writings of Milton Roemer and Franz Goldmann.

2. Oswald Hall presents some sociological generalizations common to both American and Canadian hospitals in "Some Problems in the Provision of Medical Services," *Canadian Journal of Economics and Political Science*, 20 (November, 1954), pp. 456–466.

3. For example, Edith Lentz, "Morale in a Hospital Business Office," *Human Organization*, 9 (Fall, 1950), pp. 17-21.

4. See the many sources listed in George Reader and Mary Goss, "Medical Sociology with Particular Reference to the Study of Hospitals," *Transactions of the Fourth World Congress of Sociology* (London: International Sociological Association, 1959), Vol. II, p. 46.

5. This is generally but not universally true. In some Asian cultures, complex administrative procedure is a cultural norm and clerical jobs are very prestigeful. Therefore, the hospitals of such countries may have more administration and more administrators than a Western sociologist might consider functional for medical and organizational success. Certainly they have more bureaucrats and more red tape than the doctors think necessary! Administrative-therapeutic conflicts may result. For example, see R. E. Rewell, "Medicine in the New India," *The Lancet* (September 13, 1958), pp. 575, 577.

6. These differences have been noticed by other travelers, such as Frederic C. Le Rocker, "Hospitals without Administrators," *Hospitals*, 35 (January 1, 1961), pp. 47-49; and Milton I. Roemer, "General Hospitals in Europe," in J. K. Owen, ed., *Modern Concepts of Hospital Administration* (Philadelphia: W. B. Saunders Company, 1961). Detailed cross-national comparisons of administrative practice are still rare, but some exist. For an able comparison of hospital organization and procedure in America and in a developing country with typical problems, see Ahmed Kamel Mazen, "Development of the Medical Care Program of the Egyptian Region of the United Arab Republic," Stanford, Calif.: Stanford University, unpublished dissertation for the Ph.D. in Medical Care Administration, 1961. For a good comparison of American and English hospitals, see B. H. Chubb and A. Ashworth, *A Study of Staff Organization in Relation to Design of Selected Hospitals in the United States of America* (Sheffield: Sheffield Regional Hospital Board, 1962).

7. Foreign visitors are invariably struck by the higher technical level of American facilities and the greater use of the laboratory. For example, International Hospital Federation, *Report of Study Tour of Hospitals in the United States of America* (London: International Hospital Federation, 1961), pp. 42-59 *passim,* and the unpublished reports by individual tour participants; Claude Huriez, "Les Hôpitaux Américains," *Techniques Hospitalières,* 12 (October, 1956), pp. 4-7.

8. International Hospital Federation, *op. cit.,* pp. 2, 56-57, Urs Peter Haemmerli, "Principes d'organisation dans un hôpital d'enseignement Américain," *Médecine et Hygiène,* 17 (January 30, 1959), p. 39.

9. Paul A. Lembcke, "Hospital Efficiency—A Lesson from Sweden," *Hospitals,* 33 (April 1, 1959), p. 38; Roemer, *op. cit.*

10. These public relations services are very striking to foreign visitors. International Hospital Federation, *op. cit.,* pp. 43, 56; and unpublished reports by individual participants on the Federation's study tour.

11. Ray Elling, "The Hospital-Support Game in Urban Center," Chap. 3 in this volume, and his other writings cited therein.

12. Le Rocker, *op. cit.;* Roemer, *op. cit.*

13. Mark G. Field, *Doctor and Patient in Soviet Russia* (Cambridge, Mass.: Harvard University Press, 1957), Chaps. 9 and 11.

14. For example, Temple Burling, Edith Lentz, and Robert Wilson, *The Give and Take in Hospitals* (New York: G. P. Putnam's Sons, 1956), Chaps. 6, 15, 16, 17, and 18; Patricia Kendall, "The Learning Environments of Hospitals," Chap. 7 in this volume, and her other publications cited therein.

15. Amitai Etzioni, "Authority Structure and Organizational Effectiveness," *Administrative Science Quarterly,* 4 (June, 1959), pp. 52-66.

16. This comprehensive role-set is true of all patrons, regardless of the amount of time they spend in the hospital. Apparently the more time the patron actually spends in the hospital, the more of this work he personally performs. Part-time service chiefs abroad delegate some paper work, the supervision of nurses, and routine care of charity patients to their full-time chief residents. But almost everywhere the chief resident thus acts as the service chief's representative and assistant, and the tasks have not been formally transferred and have not become his own autonomous responsibility. An exception is teaching in foreign university hospitals; younger staff members have their own lecture courses and their own bed-side teaching rounds, on the basis of an appointment legally made by the entire faculty and by the Ministry of Education. In practice, however, most patrons dominate the teaching of their juniors, since they really decide who shall receive the junior appointments and what teaching facilities will be available for each instructor.

17. This is obvious to any traveler. For a sociological comparison in a nonmedical field, see Stephen Richardson, "Organizational Contrasts on British and American Ships," *Administrative Science Quarterly,* 1 (September, 1956), pp. 204-207.

18. Foreign doctors who have spent their residencies in American teaching hospitals are repeatedly struck by these intellectual and personal differences. For some typical comments, see Haemmerli, *op. cit.,* pp. 38-39; Huriez, *op. cit.,* pp. 10-11; J. F. Stokes, "A British View of an American Hospital," *New England Journal of Medicine,* 260 (January, 8, 1959), p. 69. Americans studying abroad quickly notice the same difference. For

example, Frances and Donald Widmann, "London Clerkship," *Western Reserve University School of Medicine Alumni Bulletin*, 24 (First Quarter, 1960), p. 8.

19. Some important exceptions exist. Some English and Scandinavian teaching hospitals have long traditions of interdepartmental case conferences. In an increasing number of countries there are hospitals recently reorganized on American lines and staffed by American-trained doctors; such hospitals have more case conferences and more traffic through the corridors than the other more typical hospitals of those countries.

20. Oswald Hall, "The Informal Organization of the Medical Profession," *Canadian Journal of Economics and Political Science*, 12 (February, 1946), pp. 30-44; Hall, "The Stages of a Medical Career," *American Journal of Sociology*, 53 (March, 1948), pp. 327-337; Hall, "Types of Medical Careers," *American Journal of Sociology*, 55 (November, 1949), pp. 243-253.

21. For example, Everett C. Hughes, *et al.*, *Twenty Thousand Nurses Tell Their Story* (Philadelphia: J. B. Lippincott Company, 1958), especially Chaps. 7 and 9, and sources cited therein.

22. The text says that the incidence of discontent against one's own doctors and hospital may be higher in America, but of course discontent is not absent abroad. I have heard many complaints about doctors and hospital officials who were allegedly arbitrary and unwilling to listen to the employee's viewpoint. Such complaints have been spreading among nurses in Europe as the status of women and of nursing increasingly resemble the American pattern. Quite significantly, I have heard many of these complaints from European and Asian nurses who received graduate education in America.

23. For example, *Denkschrift zur Lage des Krankenpflegeberufes in der Bundesrepublik Deutschland* (Hannover: Agnes Karll-Verband, 1950). Many such appeals to public opinion and to governments have been issued by European and Asian nursing associations in recent years.

24. The differences in viewpoint between English and American nursing are described by a leader of English nursing, in B. A. Bennett, "We Have Been Warned! By 20,000 Nurses Telling Their Story," *Nursing Mirror*, 108 (May 29, 1959), p. xiii. Other foreign nurses who have worked in or have been educated in America have noted many of the same differences between their own countrywomen and Americans.

25. The new trend abroad is to follow in the American direction. An increasing number of countries are now adopting civil service and other regulations reserving supervisory jobs for graduates of three-year nursing curricula, and in practice nurses who return from postgraduate courses abroad get very high posts.

26. The principal American studies are summarized in Hughes, *op. cit.*, Chap. 6. Some comparable English studies have been done by H. A. Goddard, particularly *The Work of Nurses in Hospital Wards* (London: Nuffield Provincial Hospitals Trust, 1954); and *The Work of Student Nurses and Pupil Assistant Nurses* (London: South-East Metropolitan Area Nurse-Training Committee, 1957).

27. For example, "When Should Nurses Give I.V. Medications?" *Hospitals* (Chicago), 32 (October 1, 1958), pp. 68, 70; "Nursing or Medicine?" *Hospital* (London), 54 (November, 1958), pp. 779-781.

28. Visitors to America are often struck by the number and importance

of volunteers. See International Hospital Federation, *op. cit.*, p. 56, and unpublished reports by tour participants; also Chubb and Ashworth, *op. cit.*, pp. 32-35.

29. England has always had strong traditions of "good works," its hospitals have always had close ties to the community, and volunteers continue to serve as management committee members and as hospital workers. See John Trevelyan, *et al.*, *Voluntary Service and The State* (London: George Barber & Son, 1952). Volunteers work inside some Israeli hospitals. Local leaders serve on management councils of Greek government hospitals.

30. Ernestine Friedl, "Hospital Care in Provincial Greece," *Human Organization*, 16 (1958), pp. 25-26; Edwin Crosby, "Observations on Japanese Hospitals," *Hospitals*, 31 (August 1, 1957), p. 35; Eugene Schoenfeld, "A Summer at Dr. Schweitzer's Hospital," *Journal of Medical Education*, 36 (March, 1961), pp. 224, 226. A common sight in many underdeveloped countries is large numbers of visitors submerging the hospital after the guards unlock the front gates at the start of visiting hours. Maurice Orbach, "Visit to Egyptian Hospitals," *Hospital*, 51 (November, 1955), p. 741.

31. Talcott Parsons and Renée Fox, "Illness, Therapy, and the Modern Urban American Family," *Journal of Social Issues*, 8 (August, 1952), pp. 31-44.

3

The Hospital-Support Game
in Urban Center

RAY H. ELLING

Introduction

It is important to recognize the extent to which "rational planning" on a community-wide or regional basis has gained currency as a watchword in the hospital field.[1] The goal of planning efforts in this field is to bring the best health facilities and care to the most people for the least cost. The emphasis is on conscious, rational choice as regards expansion of facilities, extension of services, and support of programs. Coordination and cooperation among health organizations and personnel are core ideas. Yet the proliferation of organizations in the health

---

This research is supported by National Institute of Health grant, W-127. The assistance and encouragement of my colleagues at the Sloan Institute is gratefully acknowledged, particularly that of Dr. Milton Roemer and Rodney White. Others have also been of great help. These include my sociological colleagues in Urban Center, some of whose writings would be cited in the relevant places were it not for a danger of unduly identifying the locale of this game to the possible displeasure of some other citizens who also have been of great assistance.

and welfare fields and the lack of coordination and cooperation among them have been noted many times.[2] In short, there has been little realization of planning ideals. How is this the case? What are some of the important sociological considerations that inhibit, or if taken into account may facilitate, a greater actualization of coordinating plans? The present study, in examining the game of obtaining hospital support from the point of view of each organization, hopes to achieve a better understanding of the fundamental dialectic existing between the organization and its environment such that planning based on the community as a whole is frequently undermined by lesser units such as the hospital.

This is the story of the hospital struggle in a medium-sized metropolitan center. Our story covers ten long years during which no new hospital beds were put in place in Urban Center. With an acute hospital-bed shortage recognized at the beginning of the period, one citizen's committee after another was formed to decide on the raising of funds and distribution of them among the competing hospitals. The third and last committee succeeded in devising a plan and raising the requisite funds. The implications of this plan for existing hospitals and the distribution of resources among them over the ten-year period can be analyzed in terms of winners and losers of support. This is a study of the social relationships and conditions associated with winners and losers.

The game metaphor is used for several reasons. For one thing, it allows us to keep our sense of humor. As one leader in Urban Center put it, "This hospital business is no joke. Some people got bloody noses out of it; in fact, a few leading citizens still aren't speaking to one another many years after." Second, as Long suggests in the article from which this orientation is taken,[3] the game framework directs our attention to the process of interaction as well as to its products. In part, at least, each person plays for the play itself, as a part of a game larger than himself and his own behavior.

The Game

Urban Center is located along a major thoroughfare. It early served as a way station and source of supply. In the period of industrialization, with water supplies and raw materials at hand, and a trade artery passing through, native industry raised some old families to prominent positions. It has grown to include about a half-million people in its metropolitan area.

Only in the last quarter-century has national industry moved in and begun to create a community in transition. The wife of one of the vice presidents of a national organization described the move of her husband's firm into Urban Center: " 'The trek' was funny in a way. Here we were the newcomers. All the old dowagers of Urban Center were expecting great things from this new company. They took their slightly yellowing kid gloves out of moth balls to welcome the women at a few social gatherings." [4] At present, the original members of the 100 Club are still involved in downtown development and in cultural and artistic affairs. The club itself still stands on George Street, but it has been invaded by the managers and is surrounded by agencies and bureaus. The financial and legal elite, composed in part of members of the old families and in part of bright new-comers, provide a bridge between the periods, and integrate but also depend upon the new managerial elite. The latter have become dominant in the philanthropic and board activity of the community.[5] It is against this background that part of the hospital game in Urban Center is to be understood, for certain hospital boards, having ties to the past through their old family members, are reluctant to see the role of the board shift, as it has, from *noblesse oblige* toward "the working board."

With the increased complexity of each type of community service—whether it be in social work, hospital administration, or some other sphere—and with the growing number of special services, the professional has begun to have a voice in the councils of the great. But if the professional is heard in Urban Center, he does not direct. As one professional who serves on several boards put it, "I can be the technical expert, give advice and all, but if I start acting like a power person, I'm dead." Or, as an executive of a large health insurance agency put it, after naming several "real movers" of community projects, "I didn't include myself with those boys; I'm not quite in that league." This part of the setting also aids our understanding of the game, for the struggle of professionals to maintain their hospital teams in spite of the wishes of the managerial, financial, legal, and religious elite of the community is a central part of the contest. In spontaneously commenting on the claims of professionals and those of the old order, the head of the last, and successful, Citizens' Hospital Planning Committee stated: "The business point of view has to predominate in hospitals. Tradition and patient care and all are fine, but the business sense has to be upheld. Why have three or four laundries, pharmacies, and so on, if you could have a central one?"

Still another background theme of considerable importance is the growth in authority of the Medical School. It has become the "keeper of the keys" to the temple of medical learning to a vastly greater degree than in the preceptor days that preceded the Flexner Report. In a way, the Medical School can be seen as umpire or referee, and the resource providers and resource channelers among the elite public as the fans who must accept the standards and judgments passed down by the Medical School.[6] Thus the proximity of each team to the main stream of medical care (the main stream being that which the Medical School evaluates highly and which in turn is evaluated highly by important resource channelers in the community) is an important part of the apparatus that is given careful consideration in planning strategy.

THE FIRST PERIOD

In 1950 all four of the hospital teams we are discussing, plus two others, made a play for community support. The war years had held construction back. The Hill-Burton Act (Hospital Survey and Construction Act) was passed by the United States Congress in 1946. It provided for federal funds to match those raised by local communities in areas with high priorities as to hospital bed needs. By 1948 it was ready to operate in Urban Center. Priorities had been estimated, and local hospitals became aware of the eligibility of their community and were anxious to make up for lost time. The administration of the Act pro- vided, in the case of this state, for one-third federal funds to be matched by two-thirds local funds. St. John's, with a head start it gained by a fund drive in 1947–1948 yielding $1,500,000, received $450,000 in Hill-Burton aid in 1949. Then in 1950, the community still remaining in the high-priority category, all six hospitals submitted applications to the Urban Center Regional Hospital Planning Council, a cooperating agency of the Joint Hospital Survey and Planning Commission of the state. At a special executive committee meeting of the Planning Council held in April, 1950, the following resolution was passed:

Whereas six Indian County applicants wish Federal aid under Public Law 725, and whereas it would be difficult for the Council to pass judgment on the merits of these applications without consider- able study and investigation, now, therefore, be it resolved that it is the sense and judgment of this Executive Committee that a survey of hospital facilities, including teaching bed facilities be sponsored by the Council.

After this, the Regional Hospital Council requested the Council of Social Agencies of Urban Center to appoint "a representative Citizen's Committee to study the medical care facilities in Urban Center, and the hospital needs of Urban Center and Indian County."

As already noted, these moves of the various hospital teams were preceded by "the Catholic Hospital," St. John's, having just completed a fund drive (held largely among Catholics) for a new south wing. St. John's appeared in good repair in spite of being the oldest hospital in Urban Center, for it had kept apace. It had adequate parking space, and its connection with the Medical School (even though located across town) was rela- tively secure because of the large Catholic population and the consequent numbers of patients it could supply to the teaching program. Its addition of 100 beds in 1950 brought St. John's up to 300 beds, the largest voluntary hospital in Urban Center.

At the same time as St. John's applied, an application was submitted jointly by Crestview Hospital and the Medical School Hospital, requesting support for new facilities to be shared by the two. Crestview is located right in the Medical Center along with the Medical School Hospital, Doctors' Memorial Hospital, and other health organizations. This makes parking tight. (It can be noted, however, that Crestview has a larger lot than Doctors'.) In spite of the crowding, a joint proposal as a strategy is bound to have a certain attraction for citizen planners. Besides, there was an integral relationship existing between Crestview and the Medical School in the form of shared medical staffs. Its physical plant was in good repair and presented a good appearance. With 280 beds, it had been the largest hospital prior to St. John's expansion in 1950. Crestview long enjoyed a prestigeful, even if sometimes cold and lofty, place among the hospitals of Urban Center; it became known by some as "the address." Its plan was to be carefully weighed.

As far back as 1937, Doctors' Hospital had called in consultants to develop building plans. Throughout the war period, particularly in 1944–1945, it had been "laying plans for expansion," as an annual report puts it. In 1948, Doctors' Memorial got in touch with the Community Chest and received what the administrator later described as "tacit approval to go ahead with our plans." Although of fair size, 220 beds, Doctors' occupancy was generally high. In terms of physical condition and crowding, it was clearly in the sorest need. According to a present-day Medical School official, it was started by "two rebellious doctors who had a falling out with the Medical School." One of these men had many strong admirers among his patients and others in the community, and was able to obtain enough funds to convert a large apartment building located next to the Medical School complex into a private hospital. This was converted, a short time after founding, into a voluntary community hospital regulated by a board in trust for the community. Thus with the narrow corridors of an old apartment building, years of postponed plans, and a heavy patient census, Doctors' felt thoroughly justified in making its move for support.

Central, a somewhat smaller hospital than the others (with 130 beds in 1950 as compared with St. John's 300, Crestview's 280, and Doctors' 220), not to be outdone, also submitted an application. Central began before the turn of the century as a homeopathic hospital and only in 1921 changed its name, substituting "Central" for "Homeopathic," thereby making a move to join the main stream of medical care. Its physical plant was in almost as much need of attention as was Doctors'. The hospital had grown like Topsy over the years, with a yellow-brick wing here, a gray-brick section around the corner, and a red-and-gray section farther down the block. Small sections were built in 1904, 1922, 1926, 1928, 1943, and 1949. The last segment, a small portion built on top of what was otherwise a three-floor structure, was a matter of immediate pressure and not a large enough development to exclude Central from the competition for Hill-Burton funds and general community support.

These first moves hold several lessons as to strategy. It is important, first of all, to give the appearance of upholding the values of important publics. Having submitted a "solo" plan, but recognizing the attractiveness to community leaders and planners of the "joint" proposal submitted by Crestview and the Medical School Hospital, the president of the board of Doctors' Memorial called publicly in the papers for "joint planning for all hospital facilities." It was a move to identify with "the community good" and an attempt to overcome any initial advantage of a competing team by seeking common evaluation. Reflecting back on this decision, ten years later, the administrator of Doctors' said: "Maybe that's where we made our first mistake. Maybe we should have stood and fought them from the beginning." Later this team followed such a strategy. But at the outset, at any rate, a cooperative course was followed. Perhaps the really shrewd thing would have been to cooperate in common, community planning throughout. With such a course, the outcome could not have been a great deal worse for Doctors', and it may have been a great deal better.

Another tactic of apparent importance in the over-all strategy of this game is for a team to seek legitimation of its plans. In time of threat, it is good to be close to the ideals if they themselves are not threatened. In this connection, the role of the

Medical School is important and the closeness of Crestview to it significant. Crestview was in the best position of all the teams to form such an alliance with the Medical School. Like Doctors', Crestview was located in the Medical Center; but, unlike Doctors', it had no history of estrangement from the Medical School; unlike Central, it had never operated outside accepted medical tradition as a homeopathic hospital; and, unlike St. John's, it was not across town from the Medical School.

Reaching out to establish connections with community power figures is also important. Early in the game, before any of the proposals were actually submitted in 1950, some of the teams began recruiting top-level people onto their boards. Crestview already had powerful elements of the community represented on its women's board. But it began to involve its councilors (largely the husbands of the women on the board) to a greater extent. St. John's, with the help of a very able monseigneur from the bishop's office, recruited a very powerful board of advisers. Several of these persons were also on Crestview's Board of Councilors. Central had had a large board, but added a few significant community figures. It was not until after the game was under way and proposals submitted to the Planning Council that Doctors' made similar moves. Whereas Crestview had had real power on its board in 1950, both old-family members and managers of national firms, Doctors' had had a relatively in-grown board of local business people and physicians who had served possessively for many years. Recognizing this weakness, when it became clear that there would be a contest for community acceptance of the several expansion programs, this team began recruiting new players to its board from among managers of national industrial firms. The board was increased from seven to eighteen inside a six-month period! According to a lawyer for the manufacturer's association, "All of the additions were executives of national firms or representatives of 'downtown' [that is, banking and legal] interests."

Another essential of strategy, of course, is to get in the game. St. John's, having the money in hand from a drive it conducted in 1948 and having already received some Hill-Burton aid, might have felt that its needs were met, at least for the time being. But this team had nothing to lose and a fair chance of gaining, for there may be an advantage to having one's foot in the door. Central, realizing that an impasse would be reached, decided to enter the game with an application and thereby have at least a claim to be evaluated along with the others. An additional small hospital following the same philosophy also entered an application. In this respect, the hospital game is like poker: as the saying goes, "You can't win staying out."

The First Citizens' Committee, headed by a partner of the most important law firm in town, held its first meeting in February, 1951. It went thoroughly into the needs and facilities available in Urban Center and Indian County. An outside hospital consulting firm was brought in to aid with what the committee eventually took to be its task—the piecing together of "a master plan to provide for the development of health and hospital facilities and services in the next several decades." Such a task takes time and exhaustive evaluation. Consultations were held with Medical School personnel and representatives of the county medical society. The latter body, it should be noted, had the job throughout the game of representing the interests of its members who had appointments on one team or another. Three years later, there emerged a 105-page official report and a 90-page staff report containing detailed statistical tables.

While this First Committee was at work, the teams in this game were not idle. Perhaps the busiest of all was Doctors' Memorial. First of all, it continued the purchases it had begun years before of old buildings and land in its immediate vicinity. Second, it expended (the reported amounts vary according to informant; therefore, no exact figure is given) several thousand dollars on the development of a specific construction plan and presented it to the committee. As matters of strategy, perhaps the investment in land can be seen as a move to improve the team's apparatus; the investment in plans as demonstration of confidence and determination. Attention could later be called to both of these investments as resources that would be lost if the community "let Doctors' go down the drain." But the First Committee's report was very favorable to Doctors', concluding:

It now owns in a solid block sufficient land so that without disturbing its present hospital building it can erect a new hospital and also have sufficient parking areas. Its existing hospital building can, therefore, be retained and converted for auxiliary uses. It would seem, therefore that a new hospital of at least 300 beds should be constructed on these Doctors' Memorial Hospital lands.

Central had done nothing more than to present its needs to the committee and otherwise cooperate with it. The conclusion was:

With the exception of a possible addition of a nursing unit over the wing of the nurses' home, future expansion does not seem feasible.
The sub-committee agreed that the beds in the present Central Hospital are suitable for long-term use for inpatient care.

Thus, while not too well favored by this first report, Central was not left out. In fact, a newspaper report of March, 1957, states that a fifty-bed addition was recommended, though only the above recommendation can be located in the official report.

Crestview was in the process of preparing specific plans for the addition of a wing as the report was issued. The report recommended that some part of a total of 400 new beds for the community could be placed in such a wing. The news report cited above stated that 100 beds were recommended.

St. John's, with one of its two main buildings completed in 1951 from the money raised in 1948, was still considered favorably by the committee, which concluded that "the funds to be raised should provide for the construction of new facilities for the nurses and nursing education at St. John's."

Each team would have got something. The news report already cited stated: "The hospital people were happy with this one. The money raisers weren't." As one of the major money givers put it when referring to the First Committee's report, in an interview held in 1961: "It turned out to be a thick, vague thing with no very specific recommendations and no price tag. It kissed the ass of every hospital in town and would have cost $13,000,000." The recommendations were not adopted.

But something had to be done. The hospital needs left over

from the war years were still unmet when the First Citizens'
Committee began, and in the three years of committee work
nothing in the way of new construction had been put in place.

THE SECOND PERIOD

The grand old man of Urban Center (referred to by many as
"Mr. Urban Center"), a lawyer whose father had been a Cabinet
member of the United States and whose firm served the manufacturers and their "association," stepped into the picture at this
point. In his capacity as chairman of the finance committee of
the Community Chest and council, he went with a number of
associates to one of the major industrialists and suggested, "John,
it's your turn."

The meaning was clear. It was "Mr. Industrialist's" turn, according to "the voluntary way," to serve the community by
helping solve the hospital crisis. The chosen man was, as he
himself put it in an interview, "new" to the community; he and
his wife had been there almost ten years at the time, but he
was not so rooted as the man who came to call. This industrialist,
although new and without the power that goes with acceptance
and knowledge of local culture and people, was one of the
largest employers in the community and could give, or not, as
he put it, "10 per cent of any fund drive you want to have in
this town." He agreed to take the job. His one condition for
serving was that he be able to select his own committee. "Not
one picked by the Community Chest that I couldn't get to
work at it." [7] It is worth noting how members were picked, the
connections each had to the teams involved in the game, and
the rationale offered by "Mr. Industrialist" for their selection.

A meeting was held at the 100 Club, and a nominating committee of three was appointed by "Mr. Industrialist." These three,
with his approval, selected a committee of five, including himself
as chairman. The dean of the Medical School and the chairman
of the First Citizens' Committee were also brought on. Later
on, two more members were added; finally, two additional persons were asked to serve.

The primary members, "Mr. Industrialist" and "Mr. Urban

Center," had both had connections through their wives (and in the case of the law-firm head, also through his daughter) to the women's board of Crestview and were themselves members of Crestview's Board of Councilors. The lawyer, "Mr. Urban Center," also had a connection with St. John's through serving on its advisory board. Others among the first group were picked "to represent the various hospitals." Curiously enough, although he had no connection with any hospital board, an officer of one of the local industries that had become one of the largest firms of its kind in the country through supplying equipment to Catholic churches was selected as "a prominent Catholic layman" to represent St. John's. The treasurer of the committee was a banker who was on Central's board. One person from the board of Doctors' Memorial was asked to serve. He was one of the industrialists added to the board of Doctors' at the beginning of this period of the game. He was a large employer representing a national firm. Significantly enough, none of the more indigenous members of this board were chosen.[8] The chairman of the First Committee was asked, "to lend continuity to our work." He was, as noted earlier, a partner in "Mr. Urban Center's" firm. The dean of the Medical School represented the Medical School Hospital and among other things had the significant task of helping to hold off on building plans of the Medical School Hospital so as to keep the community from losing its Hill-Burton priority before it could carry out some plan of its own.

The later additions to the committee were chosen to "represent particular segments of the community." As if the business, financial and industrial interests were not already taken care of, the president of a department store who was also the president of the Chamber of Commerce was added. He was connected with Crestview through membership on its Board of Councilors. The president of another large department store was added "because he comes in contact with the general public and knows many people." He had no direct hospital connections. The head of a large real-estate firm' was added as "another prominent Catholic." The last person mentioned in the interviews was, as the law-firm head put it, "a prominent Jew" added because "there was no Jewish member on the committee." He was the president of an automotive and engineering supply house and served on the Board of Councilors of Crestview. A public relations man was retained as assistant to the chairman, to "backstop me," as the chairman put it. He was a member of the advisory board of St. John's. Thus the hospitals had the following number of official board–Citizens' Committee connections: Crestview, 4; St. John's, 2 (with an additional person seen as representing St. John's because he was Catholic although he was not on its board); Central, 1; Doctors', 1.

It is worth considering the chairman of this Second Citizens' Committee. Although "rules of irrelevancy" may apply to personal qualities in some games, in this one the qualities of this man were important for the outcome of the game. Personality may not be an important variable for every player, but it would seem to have an effect in the case of a member of the elite public who had the potential of channeling major resources one way or another among the teams. Clearly, there is an interweaving here. The position of power may draw a man who has characteristics that match such a position. Nevertheless, there are variations in style.

"Forceful" is the word for the chairman of the Second Committee. He is tall and commanding. Just inside the entrance to the central building of "his" company, one sees a quotation from the man himself. Written in eight-inch-high silver letters on a black wall, it states, "Being Big Will Not Replace Being Great." One filters through three waves of receptionist-secretaries before entering his expansive office. On the floor is a rich carpet, and along the walls are lighted alcoves containing hand-carved jade and ivory figures. His mahogany desk with built-in clock facing him (he can control the situation rather than the visitor) has on it three phones, each of a different color. His interests, in so far as this game is concerned, are in rationality and saving money. In the community from which he came, as chairman of the finance committee of the Community Chest, he put the Boy Scouts on a paying, even profit-making basis! He also succeeded in closing down the social evenings of two organizations that drew some of the same crowd as those of a third. His summary of his activities in that position was, "I saved the community $30,000 in one year." If allowed 50 per cent of whatever he could save the Chest in Urban Center, this man believes he would come out well ahead of the $125,000 a year he makes as chairman of the board of his firm. Having this forceful chairman, with these interests, the hand-picked Second Citizens' Committee went to work.

The first thing it did was, as the chairman put it, "determine the size of the piece of cloth." A fund-raising firm was brought in, and reported that they could raise $6,000,000. Then the chairman canvassed friends and experts all over the country as to whom to get as a consultant. The First Committee's reports were examined, and conversations were held with various people in the community. But on this point, it is important to note that the teams themselves felt slighted. As one administrator put it: "He [the chairman] picked his men and wrote his own report. The report is his report. He never talked to anybody over here." One of the older board members of Doctors' Memorial noted: "We had absolutely no representation on the committee he set up. [This statement was made, it should be noted, even though one of the newer members of the board, a manager of a national firm was on the committee.] Nor were we ever contacted during the hearings and discussions this committee had. Well, the first thing we knew about it was when we found out that he had sold the newspapers on his plan." Thus did the efforts of the committee, of the consultant, of advisers in and outside the community become identified as the efforts of one man.

Necessary to the plan that was developed was the willingness of the Medical Center to buy the lands and buildings of Crestview and Doctors' Memorial for use in the center, possibly for a medical hospital or for dormitories. With the four million that might be realized from such a sale plus the six million from a drive and two million from Hill-Burton funds, there would be enough to do the job. The consultant spoke with officials in the Medical School and found some interest. Then the chairman discussed the matter with the head of the Medical Center. They were given assurance that the center would approve but that final approval depended upon acceptance in the community, since the Medical School did not want to force something that would create a hostile local environment.

The plan called for the sale of Doctors' and Crestview's lands and buildings and the legal merging of three teams—Crestview, Central, and Doctors'. Central's building would continue to be used, but for long-term rather than acute care. Each of these teams would lose its identity, its very existence as a team under this plan. The fourth team in the game, St. John's, would be left unscathed; in fact, as in the First Committee's report, it was to have a new residence and school of nursing added. Recommendations also covered other hospitals, but the central considerations were those affecting the four teams whose play we are recounting.

By way of preparing the community generally and the supporters of each team, the Second Committee's general plan was announced without details to press and radio officials. State, county, and city officials had been kept generally acquainted with developments along the way. Following these discreet public announcements, the committee met with each hospital board and administrator at the offices of the company headed by "Mr. Industrialist," the committee chairman. At these meetings the boards were encouraged to approve the plan. A great deal of pressure was put on them to approve it. This took the form of "working on" industrialists and others who, in the case of Crestview, had wives on the board or, in the case of the other hospitals, themselves served on the boards. Finally, all boards approved the plan "in principle," and these decisions were transmitted to the chairman in writing. The chairman thought his task was nearly over. He reports asking each hospital to appoint a committee to work with the Second Citizens' Committee in developing the specific details and effectuating the plan.

But at this point, active resistance was met. The battle for survival was joined. If there is a cardinal principle of this game, it is that survival is the first, even if minimal, goal of each team. With it, everything is possible; without it, nothing is. This is not peculiar to the hospital game. Seldom, in any sphere of endeavor, does an organization fail to struggle against a threat to its existence. Mergers take place in commerce and industry just as they do in baseball; but the teams and the players usually have little to say concerning these decisions about ownership and sale because stockholders or higher levels of a formal organization are the ones who have control. But even here there is resistance, as shown by the furor caused by the move of the New York Giants to the West Coast.

Now, faced with a common threat, the teams united in a common effort. At a meeting at which the chairman of the Second Committee presented his report to the committees each hospital had appointed, a former state senator ("one of the best lobbyists we've ever had from this area," according to a community leader) rose on behalf of the Doctors' Memorial board to question whether the hospital had approved the plan. Then he turned the discussion over to a representative of Central's board who talked and talked until the chairman of the Second Citizens' Committee, who had written documents establishing as much, rose in impatience to state that there was no question that the boards had approved. But the former senator was on his feet to say that even if such approval had been given by a majority of the board of Doctors', a legal vote with a two-thirds majority was required for merger or sale. Then he threw the bomb; he was sure that seven of the eighteen board members would oppose a merger. The meeting adjourned.

The Second Citizens' Committee met immediately following the general meeting. As the chairman put it: "It was clear that we had run into a serious block. Crestview and Central were all right, but as soon as they saw Doctors' waivering, they began to waiver too." There was a discussion as to strategy, with the result that "certain people were assigned to certain people." As an example of this procedure, a prominent Catholic layman was assigned to "work on" an influential Catholic citizen who was among the "old," loyal members of Doctors' board. This board member was the brother-in-law of the man assigned to "work on him," and a member of the power structure (though a slightly deviant member, as we shall indicate). Another prominent Catholic citizen was also encouraged to talk to this reluctant member of Doctors' board. Apparently, "working on" someone as the committee practiced it meant, sociologically speaking, putting the person acting as loyal board member in conflict with as many of the central roles in his role-complex as possible. Under such pressure, this particular board member reportedly told the chairman that he didn't know himself why he was against the plan. This was hardly calculated to please this iron-willed man so bent on a rational economic solution to the hospital problems of Urban Center. The hapless board member reportedly changed his mind in favor of the committee and then changed it back. The board of Doctors' held a vote, and, true to the senator's prediction, the merger failed by one vote—eleven for, seven against.

But more than one vote was lacking. The determination of these seven board members to sustain Doctors' Hospital was symbolic of something broader. In the hospital-support game, as it now is played in our local communities, the teams have considerable strength, for they are legally incorporated units independent of stockholders, holding companies, or other super-hierarchies. This is not to say that they are completely independent; far from it. This very case and other work suggest the degree to which the voluntary hospital is dependent upon and subject to the control of elements in its environment.[9] However, each hospital team in Urban Center had certain elements that enabled it to resist this outside control over its own destiny.

Each hospital had a name and an identity. These, as Simmel has pointed out, are some of the minimal but essential elements for group maintenance.[10] Associated with these identities were many players on each team (including former patients, employees, students of nursing, and so on) who found themselves interested in a given hospital. In turn, members helped to give the team its characteristics. These enabled it to make certain moves. We shall examine these actions, characteristics, and special ties to the environment in some detail, for in meeting a threat to its very existence a team calls forth its strongest qualities and players.

Crestview had its administrator who had served for nearly two decades. As a graduate of one of the most influential nursing schools in the country, she worked well with the well-placed

members of her women's board. It is not a usual thing for
women to have control over such a powerful and prestigious
institution.[11] Jealously guarding their unusual position, the
women of Crestview presented strong opposition to the pressure
from their husbands, who were generally members of the Board
of Councilors. It is reported that some serious family arguments
developed when the Second Committee assigned "certain people
to certain people" and husbands began "working on" wives.
However, the medical staff of Crestview was perhaps less concerned than the staffs of Central and Doctors', for their relations
to the Medical School were somewhat closer and they could
expect to be taken in by the Medical School and receive appointments without difficulty in any new hospital resulting from a
merger. Eventually, Crestview went along.

Curiously enough, once this Second Citizens' plan was no
longer possible because of the essential opposition of other hospitals, Crestview's willingness to give up all support as a separate entity in the name of the larger unit—the community—may
have preserved a degree of support for this team that it might
not have received in the long run if it had bitterly opposed the
plan at this juncture.

One other hospital was in the happy position of going along.
For St. John's, there seemed to be nothing to lose either way.
In fact, the Second Committee's report called for "a new residence and school of nursing" for this team. This is not to say
that there was nothing at stake for St. John's. It recognized
the value of having tie-ins with the Medical School, even though
it wanted to assure its own control over its medical staff. But
with the plan to merge three hospitals and the sale of two
hospitals to the Medical School, there would be some chance
that the Medical School would break its relationships with St.
John's, thereby subtracting the prestige and legitimation of the
organization and making it more difficult to get interns, residents,
and adequate staff generally. Thus, St. John's was not disinterested, but there was no essential threat to its support as in
the other cases.

Like Crestview and Doctors', Central's identity and existence
were at stake. The report recommended that it continue as a

building, serving long-term patients in conjunction with the new hospital that would be built. But a hospital team is far more than a building. Without its own name or team members, and with a change in its function, it could not be said to have survived. This obvious implication of the plan was strongly resisted. The administrator, although aging and shortly to retire at the time of the committee's report, had served as administrator of this hospital for many years and had, according to informants, "a tremendous emotional investment in that hospital." The board had among its members a few very influential people who supported the plan of the Second Committee and brought this hospital to an expression of approval "in principle." But as one knowledgeable person put it, "Apparently the little people got together and outnumbered the big people." One of these "little people" (in this context, "little" means without great power in the community at large) was a widow, a member of an old family, whose husband had left $100,000 to Central Hospital. She knew in her heart that her husband had given that money to Central and not to any community hospital plan forced upon the community by newcomers. Thus, Central called the plan in question at the general meeting described above.

Perhaps Doctors' had the greatest team spirit of all. Here we can distinguish between internal support and external support, if we wish, and note that the two do not necessarily go together. The administrator had given long service to the hospital. From the day of its founding, she was with the hospital, working as a clerk for the "rebel" doctor who was principally responsible for starting it. Under his tutelage and with immense ability of her own, this woman became an administrator in her own right, and established a reputation that carries on today long after the death of her dear friend and former chief. Never having married, and having devoted her adult life to Doctors' Memorial, there was little chance that she would willingly abandon the team or see its identity transformed. Furthermore, the board had a core of men whom one can best define as indigenous. The industrialists who were added as the present phase of the game got under way, beginning in 1950, were

relatively unidentified with the hospital. When the plan of the
Second Committee was defeated by one vote, all eleven of
these new members resigned, leaving the original board of
seven members. Those who "stuck to their guns" under such
pressure were indeed the old-timers on the board. Three of them
were physicians whose work was entirely in Doctors'. Two of
these had their offices in the hospital and were close associates
of the founders. Another member of the board had been a
business partner of the founder. Along with other members of
his law firm, he had helped the founder set up "my baby," as
he referred to the hospital in an interview. He had served on
the board for many years. Another had devoted many years
to the hospital and was repaid in part by having his crippled
son well cared for in the hospital for a number of years. Although
he had paid considerable sums to the hospital for the care of
the boy, in part this was repaid because his firm carried the
insurance accounts of the hospital. Still another member was
the only Democrat (in fact, he was a delegate to a recent party
convention) in this Republican stronghold who received enough
nominations to place in the "most nominated" leadership group
of Urban Center.[12] Although he works with and plans with
other private financial and industrial leaders in Urban Center,
he has an identification with the "man on the street" and he
sees Doctors' Hospital as one that tries to serve the "man on
the street." The last of these old-time board members was a
druggist who, it is said by some (but this is not established),
was a main supplier of the hospital's drug needs.

Other players were also highly identified with this team. The
medical staff with a higher proportion of general practitioners
felt comfortable in Doctors', which was more relaxed than those
teams more closely associated with the Medical School. As the
head of the staff put it, "This hospital isn't like the cut-and-dried
places that some of the others are." The auxiliary was devoted
to Doctors'. The nursing school, its graduates, and the activities
of its alumni and friends provided most of the considerable
amount of newspaper space the hospital got. This rewarded
these players individually and aided the hospital in its public
relations efforts. With its family approach and heavy personal

investments on the parts of key players, this team could not afford to abandon the game in favor of merger.

Aside from the high involvement of their players, these teams had other features that allowed them to oppose the strong threat presented by the Second Committee's plan. The point has been made that one way a hospital or any other organization has of controlling its dependence upon elements in its environment is through "creating" a favorable public image.[13] But as the study of this game suggests, there may be no such thing as a generally favorable hospital image that each team tries to represent. Or, if there is, then it still appears to be the individual variation on the theme that assures a team of its own fans and supporters and is among its most valuable resources in playing the support game.

The large cities typically have many hospitals, and in time a division of work may occur among them. For example, one hospital may take the majority of medical indigents, thus easing the financial strain on the others. A hospital may acquire a specialist who becomes famous for a particular type of surgery and thus come to emphasize the surgical arts. Another hospital may gain a reputation for being patronized by the very rich, or a particular religious group. Physicians, patients, and townspeople generally become acquainted with the reputation of local hospitals and choose among them accordingly.[14]

It is this division of labor and development of special images and connections to the community that we would highlight here as explaining the strength of each team in meeting the threat posed by the merger plan of the Second Citizens' Committee.

As part of this case study of the hospital-support game in Urban Center, a survey was made of 280 persons in the metropolitan area.[15] In addition a number of key informants, including board members and members of the several citizens' committees, were interviewed. From the responses of these groups it is possible to draw a kind of composite picture of each team and point out how it is "plugged in" to its own supporters in the environment.

St. John's is "the Catholic Hospital." Community leaders were asked their ideas of how St. John's came through the ten-year hospital struggle so well. A number of reasons were offered: its proximity to major industrial plants, where immediate attention to accidents might be needed; its status as the oldest hospital in town, which would give it firmer roots than the others; its general religious character, which would protect it from attacks that could be interpreted as prejudice; the "free" service of the nuns, which enlists the sympathy of persons who feel that hospitals are too expensive. (Some took this service as indicative of extra devotion to the care of the patient.) While each of these factors may have played a role in St. John's support, a number of them are associated with its being "the Catholic hospital." As each of our informants noted, the significance of this depended upon the large proportion of the population who thought of St. John's first or chose it first because they are Catholic.[16] Indeed, our survey data show this. As compared with the other three teams, Catholics composed a larger proportion of the groups that named St. John's first, preferred it to others for both major and minor treatment problems, and had been in it as patients.[17]

When these data are coupled with the firm Catholic, and therefore nonmergeable, identity this team held among hospital planners on the various citizens' committees, it would appear that it was firmly rooted in at least this one part of the community. It also had special connections to "middle"-class,[18] middle-income people, to Irish and Latins; and a higher proportion of its patients were women than was true for the two low-support teams.

Crestview had its strength in its relationship to the "middle" and "upper" classes. This was reflected in the strong board and the "upper" class auxiliary that served it. As one respondent described it, "Crestview gets the people who take themselves seriously socially." Compared with the other teams, the "upper" classes were better represented among the groups naming this team first, among those preferring it to others for major and minor treatment problems, and among those who had been in it as patients. Like St. John's, a larger proportion of Crestview's patients were women than was true for the low-support teams.

Central was characterized as a comfortable "neighborhood hospital." As one leader put it: "Central is in a certain part of town, but they have wonderful service there. Smart people who aren't too sick would take it over the others." Being somewhat smaller, it had a more limited service area and was identified by many as belonging to a particular ecological segment of the city. Those living in this segment were not rich nor were they extremely poor, though they tended in the latter direction. Among those naming it first, a higher proportion were "lower" class than was true for the other hospitals. Those preferring Central were not particularly identifiable in class terms, but those who reported having been there as patients were over-representative of the "lower middle" and "lower" classes.

Doctors' was as clearly identified as any of the teams. "It is," as several expressed it, "the hospital for the man on the street." It was also seen as "the hospital with a heart," one that cared for the person as much as for the ailment. Perhaps this went along with the fact that it had the highest percentage of general practitioners on its staff and had a relaxed, unofficious air about it. The "lower-middle" and "lower" classes gave special character to those naming this team first, those expressing a preference for it, and those who had been patients there. These groups had a considerably higher proportion of Protestants than was true for any other team. Among those who had been patients at Doctors', a higher proportion were in the sixty-and-over age group.

The reciprocal of special fans, of course, was the special composition of each team. Consonant with it being "the Catholic hospital," that is, the hospital most known, used, and preferred by Catholics, St. John's, to state the obvious, was owned and controlled by a Catholic sisterhood. Sisters were active in administration and nursing, and religious objects were to be seen in the hospital. Medical-staff policies and emphases regarding tube tying, abortions, and saving of a newborn's life in preference to the mother's of course reflected the religious doctrines held by the legal controllers of the team. Though medical-department heads were not all Catholic, most of them were. In spite of such special emphases, their teaching relationships were maintained with the Medical School, making "high-powered" care available. It had an air of efficiency and excellence mixed with a "lower-middle"-class emphasis on painted furniture and portable-pay T.V.

Crestview, on the other hand, capped its building with bell and dome and offered a white-pillared entrance opening onto a circular drive that provided access for taxis and an occasional chauffeured car. Although in the same tight location as Doctors', its parking lot had space for more cars. Its staff was the duplicate of the Medical School Hospital's staff. Almost all were board-certified specialists. The emphasis was on high-powered facilities, equipment, and care. As the administrator put it, "The emphasis here, of course, is on serious cases. When somebody comes in with something, we give them everything we've got. We get to the TLC [tender loving care] later. But we try to work that in."

Central appeared to offer flexibility and special attention. There was particular emphasis on nursing and on special arrangements to suit the patient who demanded them. In part, this may have been an inheritance from the homeopathic days when the team had to struggle for patients in a hostile "regular" medical world. Until a recent "tightening up," as one staff member put it (ordered to regain the hospital's accreditation), there were a number of general practitioners on the staff who subsequently left. Ties to the Medical School were minimal, but existed in that several of the staff also held clinical professorships. However, for anything serious, patients had to be referred to Crestview or the Medical School Hospital. Thus it would appear that neighborhood ties were held, up to certain limits placed upon the hospital by its equipment and the severity of a patient's illness.

Doctors' Hospital emphasized "things of the heart." The upwardly mobile, "lower-middle"-class girls who took their work in its nurses' training school developed intense loyalty to the hospital that continued into the alumni stage. These girls served the team in the capacity of student nurses; thus nursing care was abundant and attention to the patient's desires was foremost. The building and equipment were far from the best.

Although money was spent on paint and fixing, only so much could be done with an old, converted, crowded apartment building. Some of the medical staff had appointments in the Medical School, the wards of Doctors' providing them much-needed clinical material. The tie to the Medical School was a real one, but it was modified by a history of rebellion against the school. The fact that a considerable number of the medical staff at Doctors' were general practitioners who might not meet the Medical School's requirements for appointments and who might do work the school would not allow if it were in complete control made for a more distant relationship between this team and the Medical School than was true for Crestview and St. John's.

Thus it would appear that where the emphasis could not be placed on specialized, high-powered care, it was placed on TLC and personal attention. It seems reasonable to hypothesize, on the basis of what our data show with regard to the differentiation of Central and Doctors' according to social class, that the "lower-middle"- and "lower"-class person may be more attracted to this type of care than he is to the highly specialized variety offered by Crestview and to a degree by St. John's. Of course, the role of doctors in the channeling of patients and the availability in terms of cost, convenience, and so on, of different types of physicians to different segments of the population would be important to consider. Undoubtedly physicians are important players in this game and form a part of the system. It is for this reason that we have pointed to the concentration of general practitioners in the two low-support hospitals.[19]

We are now in a position to understand how these special ties and characteristics aided these hospitals in their particular moves in the over-all strategy of resistance.

Doctors' moves are the clearest. As already noted, the seven indigenous board members formed a united front, and the plan was defeated on that basis alone. But following the meeting at which Central filibustered and Doctors' declared the plan illegal, there was still much work to be done. There was a general mobilization of the devotion and feeling that team members had for the hospital. While the Citizens' Committee was sending "certain people to work on certain people," Doctors' was spreading the word that "autocratic tycoons were ramming *their* plan down the community's throat and destroying its hospital system." Another part of the message was that "Mr. Industrialist," the forceful head of the Second Citizens' Committee, was trying to build a hospital of cold efficiency where everybody would be a number and tender loving care would be absent. In spite of intense struggle, there was one theme common to Doctors', the other teams, and the elite public represented by the Second Citizens' Committee—the "community good."

By the time the Citizens' Committee had encouraged various organized parts of the public to announce their support for its plan, Doctors', and by this time Central, and to some extent Crestview, were effective in their campaign. The point about an autocratic approach to planning was effective, for it matched many persons' impressions of the chairman of the Second Committee. As another community leader put it, "Just between us, he had a good idea and got the best consultation, but he operated as a chairman of his company; he asked for opinions, but they weren't supposed to make any difference." Credence was lent to this line of argument by the fact that Doctors' particularly, but to some extent Central too, were identified with and tied to "the man on the street." What tremendous wells of sympathy can be aroused by any organization so identified that decides to fight the top elements of the community! The point about cold efficiency was also effective with the special supporters of Doctors' and Central who might expect personal care and attention as the major emphases of a good hospital, since these were given so central a place in the two hospitals they preferred.

Even though they might be "tied in" to some of the sociologically less dominant elements, it would appear that the strongest bulwarks of these teams were their attachments to some special parts of the social environment. Each team would normally play to as broad an audience as possible and would certainly maintain in public that it was serving "the whole community." But in time of threat, as a last resort, the team can depend upon its own special fans even though they do not have the loudest voices or the fullest pockets. What effect these special ties and this strategy of resistance had on support in the long run can be judged better as we proceed with our account of the game.

THE THIRD PERIOD

With the failure of this plan, the community was divided. This was nothing new for Urban Center. Its system of voluntary leadership and control, though it may have many things to its credit, has also provided a long list of frustrations and failures in community planning. Indecisive battles had been fought over schools, water facilities, and a mental-health board. Twenty years ago a woman willed a million dollars to the community for a new art museum. With battles involving the boards of the old museum and the university museum, Urban Center is still without a new art center. But following the demise of the Second Citizens' Hospital Planning Committee, community spirit was at a particularly low ebb. A news report stated in March, 1957:

The city was left to wallow in a tragic aftermath of recrimination, suspicion and bitterness engendered by the long struggle. . . . For a long time after the demise of the Citizens' Hospital Committee last May, no representative group would come forward to lead in planning. Any community leaders who had not yet taken an active part were wary of setting themselves up as targets for the kind of vitriolic attack suffered by their predecessors. . . . Thus hospital planning went underground.

While each team had defended itself against the pressures of the elite public to go out of business as a separate entity, it was another matter for any one team to get positive support for its dreams of expansion. In a very real sense, the community was back where it started in 1950 when all teams put in their bids for support. Now, however, the facilities had deteriorated further and were more crowded, and the Medical School had lost its patience with delaying to build a new Medical School Hospital until the city got its plans worked out so that the city would not lose its Hill-Burton priority.

While the pieces were strewn, the teams were not idle. Knowing full well that another game period was under way, they prepared. Each readied building plans of its own. In addition, Doctors' pushed ahead in its drive to label the plans of the Second Committee as authoritarian, arbitrary, and separated from the desires of the common people. In doing so, it was able to enlist the sympathy of some of the secondary power figures in town, people who were not happy on other grounds about the way the "manufacturers' association" did things. Immediately after the resignation of the eleven new "downtown" industrialists, Doctors' drew to its board the financial secretary of the steelworkers' local who was also the president of the Industrial Union Council of the AFL-CIO in the Urban Center area.

The last period of this phase of the game began in earnest in February of 1957. At this point, one of the editors of a local paper was to be admitted to the Medical School Hospital for minor surgery. Signals got mixed, and he was placed in one of the more inadequate rooms in the building, "a small, odd-shaped cubbyhole with slanting ceiling somewhere on the top floor." He reportedly didn't even undress. He simply left the hospital and flew to Washington where his son-in-law, a physician, was able to see that he got proper treatment. Shortly after his return, a week-long series of articles on the deplorable conditions in the hospitals appeared, including a picture of over twenty pregnant women waiting in a narrow, crowded, dingy corridor for their prenatal care. This series also included a presentation of the plans of each hospital which, as we have noted, they had been readying for just such an occasion.

These plans were not strikingly different from those submitted in 1950. In essence, each team "offered" to meet the community's need for new beds by additions or replacements of its own facilities. Crestview's plan called for a $4.7 million expansion of its facilities—a three-story addition and a new ten-story wing. Doctors' offered two plans: one to rebuild its own facilities on their present site, including the land they had been slowly buying up; the second, to build a new medical center with one of the units to be a new Doctors' Hospital. This latter plan, it was estimated by one informant, though no figure was given in the article, would have cost a minimum of $10 million. Other estimates ran higher.

The series ended with a statement by the mayor that the hospital situation was the greatest social and economic problem faced by the city and that within three weeks he would offer a decisive plan "to break the log jam." Thus municipal government entered the picture when "citizen cooperation," as we may euphemistically call it, failed to produce a plan that could be carried out. But the mayor tossed the ball back to the voluntary leaders of the community, for the plan that he said he would offer proved to be the appointment of the Third Citizens' Hospital Committee.

This committee operated quite differently from the second one. It too brought in an outside consultant widely recognized as an authority in hospital affairs, but it also invited many different groups and individuals to appear before it. The chairman was a home-town boy who had risen from a modest background to become a junior partner in the most powerful law firm in town, again the firm of "Mr. Urban Center."

Various people, including two physicians, one of them the chairman's brother, claim authorship of the plan the committee announced in November, 1957, only six months after its formation. It would appear that the plan did originate close to the county medical society. For in the series of newspaper articles appearing in March of 1957, before the committee's official formation, considerable space was given to a plan presented to the Community Chest by the county medical society that, in effect, was the same as that adopted by the Third Committee. It called for an entirely new three-hundred-bed community hospital without requiring any of the existing hospitals to merge. It further recommended that $1,250,000 be given to St. John's for the construction of a new nurses' home. This proposal, it will be recalled, had been made by each of the previous committees. Various comments were heard in many of the interviews carried out in this research to the effect that this addition to St. John's was the "power structure's pay-off to the Catholic hierarchy for their support of any over-all plan and fund drive they might come up with." As one of the backers of the plan put it: "However that may be, it worked out fine for us. We gave them [the Catholics] $1,250,000, and they contributed $3 million in the drive."

A drive was held under the direction of a professional fund-raising firm. Large amounts were contributed by corporations. To make clear what pressure was exerted to make the drive succeed, what the wife of a former vice-president of one of the firms said can be reported: "We were handed a slip saying what we were expected to contribute and that the company would match the total amount given by employees. My husband objected privately, but it was a demand, not a suggestion." The drive succeeded, bringing in $7.5 million where $6 million had been the goal.[20]

The three hospitals that had earlier resisted merger felt themselves by-passed, as they were, in spite of the Third Committee's recommendation that existing hospitals be kept in operation. As a part of effecting its plan, the committee received the endorsement of various organized parts of the general public. This time, the committee's campaign *vis-à-vis* the general public was well organized. The hospitals, however, did not take this lying down.

Crestview took immediate steps to obtain funds, and began adding a new wing, costing $850,000, that would include a special deep-ray therapy unit. Doctors' enlisted the support of various dissident groups. One of the board members of Doctors', a heavy contributor to his church, reportedly spoke to his minister. That church, an influential member of the Council of Churches, kept the Council from endorsing the Third Committee's plan. An official of a radio station and an editor of one of the papers who had earlier been on Doctors' board came out against the new hospital plan. The A. F. of L. local approved the plan, but the C.I.O. came out against it. In addition, the latter local union had booklets printed and carried out a publicity campaign recommending that a new Doctors' Hospital be constructed. But the community leaders were playing for keeps this time. The union man on Doctors' board was shortly promoted to management, and the union reconsidered its position.

The game is not over yet. But the phase we are dealing with drew to a close as the various teams resigned themselves to admitting two more teams into the league, a new Community Hospital and a new Medical School Hospital. They readied themselves to meet the stiff competition they would face. Crestview will not be seriously affected. Its ties to the Medical School may become so integral that it may have to give up some of its earlier characteristics and begin offering more in the way of teaching material rather than emphasizing service to "upper-middle"- and "upper"-class elements of Urban Center. St. John's may lose its affiliation with the Medical School or find it attenuated, especially if both Crestview and the new Community Hospital develop primary medical-school relationships. But these developments, if they occur, will not seriously threaten the existence of these teams.

For Doctors' and Central, however, the new teams will be serious competitors indeed. In fact, several persons close to the struggle over the years expressed the opinion that, in effect, *the plan of the Second Committee, bitterly as it was fought, was nevertheless carried out in the end by the Third Committee.* As they point out, Doctors' facilities are old and so are Central's. Indeed the latter, being to some extent a neighborhood hospital, will be directly affected, for the new Community Hospital, a veritable builder's dream, will open in the same general area of the city. Central appears to have resigned itself to becoming a long-term care institution, if it continues at all. But Doctors' is still fighting valiantly. It held a fund drive among its own staff and friends of the hospital at the time of the community drive for the new hospital and raised the surprising sum of $300,000. This is being spent, along with other money, on renovations and improvements. But the outlook is dim, for when the new hospital opens, Doctors' can expect to find building-code inspectors from the State Welfare Department on its doorsteps. As one community leader put it, "I've got enough in my files to close Doctors' today." Thus there will be a Medical School complex composed of Crestview and the Medical School Hospital, a Catholic hospital—St. John's—and the new Community Hospital. When "Mr. Industrialist" drew a map of his plan for this investigator, that was what it looked like.

Discussion and Conclusions

While it has limitations,[21] the game analogy has allowed us
to examine the characteristics, environmental connections, and
actions relevant to the goal of gaining support *as if* this were
what the hospital business "were all about." It focused our attention on important factors that appear to affect the outcome
of the game. The teams themselves were regarded as the central
units in competition with one another for the potential support
available in the environment. The character of the community
and its stage of development were seen as affecting the way the
game was played: in the stage of transition, "newcomers" to the
power structure might not carry out major community projects
as well as a combination of old and new might; the class divi-
sions of the community allow some organizations to find strength
to resist the elite's plans in taking support from "lower"-class
segments of the population; changing cultural expectations regarding medical care place the team not connected with the
Medical School at a disadvantage over the long run; and so on.
Though these teams involve many players of many different
types, it was clear that certain ones were more heavily involved
with gaining support than were others. It also became clear that
emotional characteristics of the players, such as degree of identity with and attachment to a team, appeared to be of considerable importance, even though such things could not easily be
included in any abstract calculus of this game.[22] The apparatus
was clearly important—the condition of buildings and equipment, availability of land and facilities, and location in the
ecology of the community were all of some importance. The
nonmaterial apparatus was also of importance, "the things these
teams stood for," and the consequent images they presented.

The supporters on all levels were important. Clearly the elite,
especially the industrial, financial, and legal leaders, were central
in the final channeling of support in one direction rather than
in another. But support is more than a matter of funds; the elite
public as represented in the various citizens' committees found

that it had to go through organizations to try to reach the general public for support of the various plans. The teams continually appealed to their own special supporters in the elite and general publics and to the public in general through news stories in the press and on the radio. The rules of the game are important for the outcome. Certain things like direct advertising in the papers could not be done. Self-determination on the part of each team, which is legally recognized in the laws of incorporation, could not be violated by the elite public no matter how strong the pressure. Like the rules of the game, the time periods also help to structure the game. Those the observer sees are somewhat arbitrary. But, as with most of social life, there is an apparent ebb and flood of activity. While the rules determine what can be done with whom, the periods of the game determine when it will be done.

As far as strategy is concerned, one important point is that the teams seek to represent the core values of the surrounding community, particularly those of the elite public. Cooperation among and coordination of facilities are becoming more and more central as heavy supporters regard the growing complexities and costs in the health field. For this reason, numerous committees and councils are set up,[23] but at a certain point the teams part ways and revert to what is perhaps the most fundamental strategy of all—the differentiation of the team from others *vis-à-vis* the environment.[24]

This differentiation takes place in a host of ways. Some ties to any part of the environment are better than none. In times of extreme threat, the team can call on its special supporters even if they are not among the strongest—"any port in a storm." However, to obtain positive support it is better to be connected with the stronger elements of the community. Ties to certain elites have already been mentioned. Other connections also appear to be important. The two poorly supported hospitals depended more on the "lower" classes in general for recognition, use, and favorable attitudes. It would seem that the internal characteristics of each organization mesh with these connections. The two teams that offered "high-powered" medicine, yet were not entirely under the control of the Medical School (where teaching and research might tend to take precedence over treatment and care), were preferred and had more links to the power structure and to the "middle" and "upper" classes.

The factor of religion suggests a way in which our framework should be broadened. Although it comes perilously close to being tautological, and although the terms may resist precise measurement, the following hypothesis is suggested by this case study: that organization will be better supported than another if the elements in the environment with which it is mainly identified and with which it has the most connections are more dominant than those with which the other organization is identified and connected. The term "dominant" cannot be defined in simple terms. What is meant is the ability of a segment of the population to control the flow of resources in the community. In these terms, Protestants may be more dominant than Catholics even though the latter predominate in numbers. But at some point, as was certainly true in Urban Center, Catholics may become dominant, especially as they rise in the class structure and gain organization and awareness of themselves as able to control resources. The difficulty with this hypothesis is that one would have to have a test of "ability to control the flow of resources" that is independent of control over the flow of resources to any pair of organizations one would compare. Nevertheless, this interpretation appears to lend understanding both to the favorable support position of St. John's (which was tied into a dominant religious element and through it to the power structure) and to that of Crestview (which was tied into the "higher" classes and the power structure).

The strategy of differentiation has important implications for hospital planning in a situation such as Urban Center. Clearly, even if it is not tied firmly to the most dominant elements of the community, each team appears to have its own fans on whom it can count in a tight spot. This makes each organization extremely intransigent and resistant to coordinating and planning efforts that may threaten its existence—even though it is not the most well-supported organization. Realizing this, and with the experience of years of struggle behind them, the leaders of Urban Center have established a hospital planning council as

an important part of the Community Chest. Similar developments have taken place in other metropolitan centers. In some
cities, Pittsburgh, Chicago, and St. Louis, for example, a formal
organization, supported by the major sources of funds in the
community, has been set up with a technical staff to do research
on community hospital needs and recommend support or non-
support for various projects. However, such organizations have
definite limits. First of all, if motivated mainly by an interest
in saving money, such as "Mr. Industrialist" expressed in our
case, the community's health and hospital needs may be no
better served than under the present rules of the game. Second,
these organizations generally limit themselves to hospital planning. They leave aside questions of the integration of nursing
homes and mental and other special hospitals with the general
hospital; the development of home-care, rehabilitation, and outpatient programs; the training and supply of health personnel;
and other problems of the health-care system. Third, such planning organizations at present represent mainly the private financial and industrial segment of the community. This is perhaps
the major element that must be behind such efforts, but official
health-agency personnel, other professionals, and other power
segments of the community must be represented if such organizations are to be effective. Fourth, even if constituted in
the best possible manner, such hospital planning organizations
are not able officially and formally to change the rules of the
hospital-support game. They do not have the degree of control
that a legally constituted hierarchy has over subordinate segments. Thus, each team is still legally able to fall back on its
own fans.

Under the present rules of the hospital-support game, it is
difficult to see how the much-trumpeted notion of the hospital
as a community health center can be actualized. While an important part of the game's strategy is to announce that the hospital is serving "the whole community," and while no doubt
each hospital does do so to a considerable degree, an equally
important part is to gain attachments to particular segments of
the community and to compete with other teams in this respect.
Thus, questions of domain, of the number of extramural pro-

grams, of which hospital will house the health department, of which will have ties to the Medical School, and so on, are difficult to decide as the game is now played.

NOTES

1. Gordon R. Cumming, "Revitalizing Hospital Planning," *American Journal of Public Health,* 51 (August, 1961), pp. 1158–1162; Milton I. Roemer and Robert C. Morris, "Hospital Regionalization in Perspective," *Public Health Reports* (October, 1959), pp. 916-922; Ray E. Brown, "Let the Public Control Utilization through Planning," *Hospitals,* 33 (December, 1959), pp. 34-39, 108-110, reprinted in *Areawide Planning for Hospitals and Related Health Facilities,* Report of the Joint Committee of the American Hospital Association and the United States Public Health Services (U.S. Government Printing Office, 1961); "Community Planning, a Report on the Schivitalla Symposium, St. Louis, Mo., 1961," *Hospital Progress,* 42 (August, 1961), pp. 89-98.

2. Milton I. Roemer and E. A. Wilson, *Organized Health Service in a County of the United States* (Washington, D.C.: U.S. Public Health Service Publication No. 197, 1952); S. M. Gunn and P. Platt, *Voluntary Health Agencies: An Interpretative Study* (New York: Ronald Press, 1945); Richard Carter, *The Gentle Legions* (New York: Doubleday, 1961); Bradley Buell, "Administrative Problems of the Community as a Whole," in *Third Conference on Administrative Medicine* (New York: Josiah Macy, Jr. Foundation, 1952), pp. 149-157.

3. Norton Long, "The Local Community as an Ecology of Games," *American Journal of Sociology,* 64 (November, 1958), pp. 251-261.

4. This process of the old order giving way to the new is fairly general in our urban communities. See Maurice Stein, *Eclipse of Community* (Princeton, N.J.: Princeton University Press, 1960).

5. This interpretation of developments is made from our own studies of boards and the history of hospitals and the community generally and from the work of colleagues in Urban Center. Their cooperation is hereby gratefully acknowledged. For a similar analysis of developments in an urban center, see Aileen D. Ross, "Philanthropic Activity and the Business Career," *Social Forces,* 32 (March, 1954), pp. 274-280.

6. As Merton notes, the medical school also plays this role of guarding ideals against the unruly world of practice for medical practitioners themselves. Robert K. Merton *et al., The Student-Physician* (Cambridge: Harvard University Press, 1957).

7. Both the chairman of this committee and the head of the law firm who approached him claim to have had a major hand in choosing the committee members even though the committee was not successful. Perhaps choosing people for such work is a major way of showing power.

8. However, one of the old-time members of Doctors' board who served as the outgoing president of the Chest at the time of the committee's formation was formally made a part of the nominating committee that presumably selected the members of the Second Citizens' Hospital Committee (according to the public report that issued from the Second Committee's

work). Yet this person reported that "Mr. Industrialist" was entirely responsible for the selection of committee members.

9. Max Shain and Milton I. Roemer, "Hospitals and the Public Interest," *Public Health Reports*, 26 (May, 1961), pp. 401-410. For a discussion of the concept of organizational autonomy, see S. N. Eisenstadt, "Bureaucracy and Bureaucratization, a Trend Report and Bibliography," *Current Sociology*, 7:2 (1958), entire issue, pp. 99-164, especially p. 114.

10. *The Sociology of Georg Simmel*, Kurt H. Wolff, trans. and ed. (New York: The Free Press of Glencoe, 1950).

11. N. Babchuk *et al.*, "Men and Women in Community Agencies," *American Sociological Review*, 25 (June, 1960), pp. 399-403. A member of one of the citizens' committees put it this way: "That's grown to be too big a business and too complex an operation for these ladies to run. More than that, it's not a place for sentimentality. These people have lost themselves in that organization. Crestview board women have been around for years. It was the thing to do to be on that board."

12. The most nominated leaders were determined by asking a large number of knowledgeable people to name the most influential people in Urban Center. Nominations were then tallied and an arbitrary cutoff point used to determine "ins" and "outs." This is the man referred to earlier in an example of the Second Committee's "working on" certain individuals.

13. Charles Perrow, "Organizational Prestige: Some Functions and Dysfunctions," *American Journal of Sociology*, 66 (January, 1961), p. 335.

14. Temple Burling, Edith M. Lentz, and Robert N. Wilson, *The Give and Take in Hospitals* (New York: G. P. Putnam's Sons, 1956), p. 15. In summing up their consideration of hospital-community relations, these authors note: "Hospitals, like people, take on a character and a personality. Some attributes arise from the regional or local setting and its traditions and customs. . . . Once it [the community] forms an impression of the character of the hospital, that interpretation clings and is very hard to change. Thus historical events influence the present by providing a framework within which it is comprehended" (pp. 24-25).

15. Generally complete interviews were obtained from 79 per cent of this sample of persons, and short "emergency" interviews were completed with another 14 per cent. Thus on some items better than 90 per cent response was obtained. Numerous training sessions were held, including demonstration in the use of carefully drawn maps and instructions for the selection of households and individuals within households as well as instruction as to variation of call-back times. In spite of such instructions and agreed-upon payment schedules for return calls, there apparently was a tendency for the interviewer to interview the person who came to the door; this was usually the housewife. There was also a slight tendency for higher socioeconomic households to be selected, though our results on this characteristic are not discrepant enough to exclude the possibility that they are due to random sampling error. Since it involves comparisons internal to our sample, we can answer the question "For whom does a given hospital hold a favorable image?"

However, the question "Which hospitals are regarded more favorably by the population of Urban Center in general?" can be answered only tentatively. Recognizing this limitation, it can be noted that the two high-support teams, St. John's and Crestview, each drew approximately twice as many first mentions as did the low-support teams, Central and Doctors', when the sample was asked, without prior cues, "What hospitals are there in Urban Center?" There was little difference among these teams in being mentioned at all. Likewise, there was little difference among them in the proportion of the sample that had been hospitalized in each, though Central lagged slightly behind—perhaps because of its smaller capacity. When it came to preferences, however, there were interesting differences. Whereas, no general difference existed between high- and low-support hospitals when treatment for a minor problem was considered, for a major illness a larger proportion of the sample would prefer to go to the high-support hospitals. Thus St. John's and Crestview may have a more prominent place in the community in general, and it may be that there is somewhat greater favor shown for them "when the chips are down," as in the serious illness. But this probability cannot be too firmly embraced because of possible biases in our sample that we have noted.

16. According to different estimates, the population is between 45 and 65 per cent Catholic. Of the 93 per cent of our general community sample for which we had information on religious preference, 41 per cent were Catholic. This was the metropolitan area as a whole, however. For Urban Center proper, our sample showed 47 per cent Catholics and 34 per cent in the rest of the metropolitan area. Thus the impressionistic estimates we obtained on this question may be based more on the city proper, though it also is possible that our sample is slightly underrepresentative of Catholics.

17. These statements are based on inspection, but the percentage differences are substantial. For lack of space, the figures are not given here but are available on request to the author.

18. The index for this is described in A. B. Hollingshead, the Index of Social Position, Yale University, processed. In what follows the "upper" classes we refer to are I's and II's; the "middle," III's; "lower-middle," IV's; the "lower" V's.

19. For a full treatment of this question of patient preferences, see Eliot Freidson, *Patients' Views of Medical Practice* (New York: Russell Sage Foundation, 1961). While the numbers involved are small, it is interesting to note that those in our sample with no religious preference and those of the Jewish faith confined their hospital care to the two well-supported hospitals—St. John's and Crestview, more of them going to Crestview than to St. John's. Again, this suggests a connection between one's pattern of life and consultation of certain types of physicians who in turn place one in a given kind of hospital. There are instances, however, in which persons change their physician in order to receive treatment in a given hospital in which the doctor has no privileges. Thus the connection between hospital and patient may be fairly direct in some cases.

20. This success was, it might be noted, in spite of the lack of generosity of physicians. As one lay leader put it: "They'd tell us, 'I'm pretty well set at X [one hospital or another]. I don't need a new hospital.'" This informant continued: "We found doctors earning $40–50 thousand a year who gave $26 or $50. They are god damned poor community citizens when it comes to giving either time or money." But many physicians did not see the proposed new hospital as anything but a threat. Having a secure place on one or more of the existing teams, why should they greet another

competing team enthusiastically? And with all the talk of high standards in the new hospital, what would be the chances of the average practitioner gaining a berth on that team? Because they couldn't be sure, enthusiasm and contributions were not high among most physicians. This did not stop the industrial and financial interests who by this time were fed up with "the hospital mess."

21. We have a responsibility to mention these. For one thing, the game places considerable emphasis on the goal of support, and may leave the impression that this is "what hospitals are all about." This is obviously not the case, and suggests more emphasis on the total system. See Amitai Etzioni, "Two Approaches to Organizational Analysis," *Administrative Science Quarterly* 5 (September, 1960), pp. 257-278. This emphasis on goals is related to a second problem—the emphasis on conscious, rational decisions. Even though we recognized this at the outset, the tendency has been to interpret moves in this manner even though many of them may have "just happened." Third, the competitive aspect of the game breaks down when the teams join to meet a common problem. Coalition raises the question of a team's boundaries. The assignment of players to teams is also problematic. Were the eleven industrialists coopted onto Doctors' board on that team or were they always playing for the elite public? Another problem may be more one of method than of framework. It is difficult to establish the rules of the game in studying only one case, as one cannot see thereby what is never done.

22. But there is a point about individual actions that needs emphasis. The actions of any one individual, although they are important when operating in concert with others and in a certain context, are dependent for their significance upon the general community system that channels support to one team rather than to another. Whether such actions be those of a medical-staff member, an administrator, a board member, a community leader, or those of a "man on the street," their effect in and of themselves appears minimal. Thus, our attention is drawn to the community system, the place of each team in the system, and the means by which resources are channeled within the community. As we have seen, even the resources deriving from outside the community, such as those available from Hill-Burton and those available to the Medical School, were dependent upon the local community structure for the "what," "where," "when," and "how" of their use.

23. A somewhat jaundiced, though perhaps insightful, view suggests that these councils and committees function to "cool the mark out." In his studies of "fleecing," Erving Goffman discovered that when "con" men "take" a customer (the mark), they generally leave someone behind to appease the person and prevent him, as much as possible, from calling the police. In the hospital-support game, the public, and perhaps the elite public particularly, is beginning to feel like "the mark." Committees and councils of health agencies do the "cooling out."

24. See Ray H. Elling and Sandor Halebsky, "Organizational Differentiation and Support, A Theoretical Framework," *Administrative Science Quarterly*, 6 (September, 1961), pp. 185-209.

4

Goals and Power Structures

A HISTORICAL CASE STUDY

CHARLES PERROW

In this paper I shall examine the relationship between organizational goals and the power structure of a voluntary general hospital. My discussion has several purposes:

1. To provide an institutional history of one hospital that is believed to be illustrative in many respects of developments in American voluntary general hospitals.

2. To demonstrate how the goals of the hospital have changed over the years in response to changes in technology and community needs, which brought about changes in the power structure of the organization.

3. To assess the consequences of the current goals and power structure for the character of the organization.

The theory that will guide my analysis of the history of the hospital has been presented at greater length elsewhere.[1] Briefly,

I should like to acknowledge my indebtedness to Philip Selznick for the viewpoint that will be apparent in this paper, and to Sheldon Messinger for valuable criticism of an earlier version, which appeared as Part I of "Authority, Goals, and Prestige in a General Hospital," unpublished Ph.D. dissertation, University of California, Berkeley, 1960.

Date_____

WHILE Y

M_____

of_____

Phone_____

TELEPHONED		PLEASE CALL	
CALLED TO SEE YOU		WILL CALL AGAIN	
WANTS TO SEE YOU		URGENT	

Message_____

_____

_____

_____

_____

Operator

it hypothesizes that, over the long run, an organization will be controlled by those individuals or groups who perform the most difficult and critical tasks. The characteristics of this dominant group (social background, career, ideology or point of view, personal interests, and so on) will determine major operating policies and thus organizational goals.

Difficult tasks are those that cannot be routinized and/or assigned to persons of low skill levels. A task is critical not just because the organization would cease functioning if it were not performed—many tasks are of this sort—but also because it represents the distinctive problem the organization faces because of its stage of development, condition of the market, internal operations, and so forth. Several task areas are listed below that are likely to be both difficult and critical for organizations at different times: [2]

1. Securing inputs in the form of capital or operating subventions.

2. Securing acceptance in the form of basic legitimation of activity.

3. Providing production skills where these are nonroutine and highly specialized.

4. Coordinating the activities of organizational members.

5. Coordinating relations with other organizations, clients, or consumers.

All these tasks may be important in any one organization, but not all are likely to be equally important at any point in time. The importance of a particular task area will depend upon the technology employed, the market for the goods or services, and the stage of growth of the organization. An emphasis upon any one (or upon a combination of two or more) will tend to give controlling power to the group that fulfills the task.[3] The distinctive characteristics of that group with controlling power will shape operating policies and major decisions such that organizational goals will be altered. For organizations with certain characteristics it is possible for two or more groups to share power and thus to share the determination of goals. When this occurs, it has a distinctive consequence for the character of the organization, as will be discussed later.

Historically, the dominant task areas in voluntary general hospitals are asserted to change over time in a sequence that is believed to be typical, and to reflect changes in technology and the needs of the community. Put briefly, an era of trustee control, emphasizing capital investments and community acceptance of hospitals, is followed by a period of control by doctors based on the increasing complexity and importance of their skills. At present there is a trend toward domination by the administration because of the mounting complexity of hospital activities and the increasing contact with health agencies proliferating outside the hospital. Obviously, not all hospitals will go through this sequence or go through it in this order. The sequence is an "ideal type" based on the assumption that in most cases the predicted relationship between the independent and dependent variables will not be upset by intervening variables. Thus, technology and community needs will generally dictate changes in the power structure, but particular historical circumstances may delay changes or produce "premature" ones. Similarly, the power structure will generally dictate the operative goals of the organization, but intervening variables may upset this relationship. The concept of "operative goals" has been dealt with elsewhere; [4] briefly, it refers to the actual goals pursued by the organizations as revealed in operating policies and routine and critical decisions, rather than simply "official" goals as set forth in authoritative public pronouncements.

We shall now examine the history of "Valley Hospital" in "Middleplains" in these terms. Valley Hospital is the pseudonym for a general hospital organized under Jewish auspices. At the time of the study (1957–1958) Valley Hospital had over 300 beds and was generally considered to be the best voluntary hospital in the city and region. It is located in a large metropolitan area in the western half of the United States.

Trustee Domination (1885–1929)[5]

The first stage of the development of the hospital, from its incorporation in 1885 until 1929, reflected the importance of capital and legitimization. Medical science at the turn of the century was still primitive, and the doctor neither required nor controlled many facilities. With a simple technology and little interinstitutional interdependence, the coordinating functon was easily performed by trustee or a former nurse, bookkeeper, and so on. However, securing capital was crucial for a new organization, and legitimization was especially important since capital had to be donated rather than invested. In later periods the legitimacy of the organization was to become self-evident to the contributing public, and while trustees were needed to ensure that community interests were protected from fraud or malfeasance, their role was not so critical as other roles. Initially, however, legitimacy was not so self-evident.

Valley Hospital established itself as primarily a charity hospital. Its stated purpose was to afford "surgical and medical aid, comfort and protection in sickness to deserving Israelites and others." While this was a common basis for legitimacy in the East, where most hospitals established in the nineteenth century were for the poor, it was less common in the western parts of the country. Western communities began to build hospitals when patients with means began to utilize them. Since they relied heavily upon paying patients, they provided few free beds. Local governments set up hospitals for the poor. Valley Hospital, however, was influenced by the ideology of eastern hospitals, and especially the Jewish ones that were set up on a half-pay, half-free basis. Its first permanent building contained 27 free beds and 23 pay beds. The income from the latter would help meet the cost of the former. When a new building was constructed in 1914, of the 134 beds initially installed, 83 were for free patients and 57 for paying patients. By contrast, all other voluntary hospitals in the city, including the university hospital, provided a total of only 34 free beds. Not only was Valley Hospital unique in its concern with the poor; it provided nearly as much

free care for non-Jews as the rest of the hospitals combined.
Between 1914 and 1929 non-Jews accounted for from one-
quarter to one-third of the free days of care.

How could such an effort be legitimated? The goal of providing care for "needy Israelites and others" was related to the
position of Jews in the community. Relative to Jews in most
urban communities, the Jews in Middleplains had enjoyed an
enviable status. They had been among the earliest and most
respected settlers. They prospered with the city and were con-
spicuous for their sense of community welfare. Prominent Jews
founded the first two welfare organizations, contributed to
cultural institutions and civic organizations, and served as
public officials.

With this high degree of integration, the founders of Valley
Hospital felt it was not only their duty to "care for their own"
—a matter of some importance where dietary and other religious
proscriptions and observations were involved—but also to make
a contribution to the community in general. Indigent Jews should
not be a burden on the community, and the facilities should be
open to all. The pay beds were explicitly designed to provide
income that would support the "real work" of the hospital, as
care of the needy was frequently designated.

But the donors were asked to make a sectarian contribution
in a city where they generally supported nonsectarian activities,
such as the university hospital. Significantly, the fund-raising
drive for the large 1914 building foundered badly until a very
large gift was received from a donor living in Europe—someone
who was not involved in the highly integrated Middleplains
community. Another problem proved to be the very presence of
free beds. According to repeated passages in the annual reports
from 1914 to 1929, private patients refused to be cared for in a
hospital that had an outpatient department and free beds. To
combat this feeling the president of the board of trustees stressed
each year in the annual report that the charity and private wings
were physically separated. Despite subventions from Jewish
charities and later from the Community Chest, the hospital had
chronic financial problems throughout the period.

There is no doubt that the affairs of the hospital were dominated by the trustees during this period. Annual reports and other documents make it clear that the serious problems were financial support and community acceptance; problems of medical care or administration are not mentioned during this period. One president held office for twenty years, from 1906 until 1927. He and other trustees intervened in most phases of the operation, making daily tours and firing people on the spot, ordering work to be done here or there, and often having the expenses charged to themselves directly. They borrowed money under their own names to meet pressing bills. It was "their" organization. The president probably had a great deal to say about medical policies also; his brother was chief of staff from 1915 to 1929. According to present informants, he dominated the medical staff as absolutely as the president dominated the organization as a whole. At the time such authority was typical of hospitals, as indeed of many other organizations.

Doctors, other than the chief of staff, apparently had little status in the organization. The most powerful committee appears to have been the outpatient department committee of the board of trustees, concerned exclusively with free care. In annual reports, appreciation is expressed to virtually all groups in the hospital except the medical staff until 1916. After that a routine paragraph is inserted in the president's report referring to the doctors' "fine cooperation" with the trustees and the superintendent.

There is no reason to believe that standards of care were anything more than adequate for the times, despite occasional claims that the hospital was becoming one of the finest medical institutions in the country. Indeed, it may have fallen behind other hospitals in the area in several respects near the end of this period, for a revolution in medical care was under way but had not touched the hospital. For the trustees, one may conjecture, the hospital was less a medical institution than a symbol of their contribution of time, money, and effort to community welfare. This changed radically after 1928; in keeping with changes in technology and community utilization, control passed to the medical staff, and the hospital altered its goals substantially.

Medical Domination (1929–1942)

Four basic changes occurred at the beginning of the next period. The medical staff replaced the trustees as the controlling group. The emphasis upon free care declined greatly, and service was oriented toward paying patients. Technical facilities were expanded, and the quality of care was improved. Finally, the hospital sought prestige in terms that the medical profession recognized: through research.

These changes are directly related to the technical advancement of medical science. The first thirty years of the century saw the rise of many new specialties and complex techniques. Medical schools were reorganized, and efforts were made to control standards of care in hospitals. With technical advances making hospitals a place in which to be cured rather than just cared for, people who could pay for their care came to use them more.[6] This in turn changed the interests and status of the doctor. He had little vested interest in charity patients, and was less inclined to see the "real work" of the hospital as care of indigents. He did have a vested interest in paying patients, and thus in the hospital that provided beds where he might treat them. Furthermore, the increasing importance of his complex skills augmented his status in the hospital, and his control of medical and surgical therapies provided him with a basis for the control of decision making.

In 1927 the president of the board of trustees retired after twenty years in that position; his brother retired as chief of staff two years later. Referring to a new president of the board who took office in 1929, a physician-chronicler, writing in the 1936 Annual Report, recalls the change:

In 1929 a new and energetic leader assumed command of Valley Hospital's Ship of State. . . . In his desire to make a bigger and better hospital he worked untiringly and well. He realized that Valley Hospital should mean something more than *merely a habitat for the indigent sick*. Encouraged by an ambitious medical staff under the able leadership of Dr. ———, a move was started to create a real medical center. [Emphasis supplied.]

The change in goals was apparent. The new president increased the hospital's deficit in the first year by $130,000, by renovating and modernizing the facilities, in particular the facilities for private patients. In addition, he gave the new chief of staff a free hand in creating an entirely new field of activity at the hospital—research. Laboratories were built, with building and operating costs coming out of the hospital's operating budget, further increasing the deficit. In his brief, blunt section of the 1930 Annual Report the new president turned to the community: "Bequests and donations have averaged $18,900 per year for the past five years. This amount is insufficient to maintain the hospital as it is organized at present."

He then announced that a million dollars would have to be raised. The physician-chronicler in 1936 admiringly referred to this move as "a preposterous and almost impertinent idea." For one thing, the depression was upon them, and for another thing, leaders of the integrated, comfortable Jewish community of Middleplains were known for their opposition to large fund-raising campaigns for sectarian causes. However, the appeal was now for services to private patients and for the magic word "research." The community as a whole responded to the appeal, and three-quarters of a million dollars was raised.

The allocation of the funds reflected the changing emphasis. Thirty per cent of the original goal was to go into a loan fund so that the "white-collar sick" could pay the hospital and physician for their care; this reflected both a concern with the changing clientele and a concern with income from private patients. Thirty per cent was to go for research, and 40 per cent for debt retirement. Because the million-dollar goal was not reached, the proportion going to the loan fund had to be cut to 11 per cent, but research still received 29 per cent of the money raised.

The composition of the board of trustees was also changed; three directors resigned, and the size of the board was increased from fifteen to twenty-four. Thus, half of the new board would consist of new members. They were younger in age and presumably sympathetic to the new developments. The women's auxiliary—traditionally concerned with small fund-raising projects and needy patients—was also reorganized, and younger women were brought in.

The changes in the board and the auxiliary did not reflect an increase in their power; in fact there was a dilution of that power. They were to meet less frequently and merely approve the actions of the medical staff. Once the new president had completed the reorganization of the hospital, he himself resigned, and full control passed to the chief of staff and the heads of the various medical departments. In contrast to previous trustees, the president's interest in the hospital was not proprietary, husbanding and hovering over a thing of his own creation. Autocratic and forceful, he stepped in long enough to ensure that, in his own words, "Valley Hospital may become a true medical center of which we may all be proud, and take a place comparable to Jewish hospitals in other cities."

The instrument of this regeneration, the new chief of staff, was a prominent surgeon who had long been associated with the hospital and with one of the university hospitals in the city. Reportedly he was a great teacher and a great researcher, but had been denied sufficient official recognition at the university hospital because he was a Jew. He had little scope for his talents at Valley Hospital until he became chief of staff. Once in that position he dominated the hospital for well over a decade. In contrast to previous reports, the 1930 Annual Report bustles with enthusiasm. An "intimate history" of the hospital, written by a physician, closes with the significant words:

The future looks bright. It is in the hands of Valley Hospital's able *younger* men, *lay and medical*. The advance of medical science means new laboratories, new equipment and the *higher ideal* that it is just as important to create a great medical center where scientific work may be done by earnest young men as it is to have an efficient place for treating the sick poor. [Emphasis supplied.]

Not only are "earnest young men" to receive new laboratories, equipment, and research facilities; they are also to have a say in medical staff government. A section of the report on organization of the staff mentions that they will be represented on the key advisory committee.

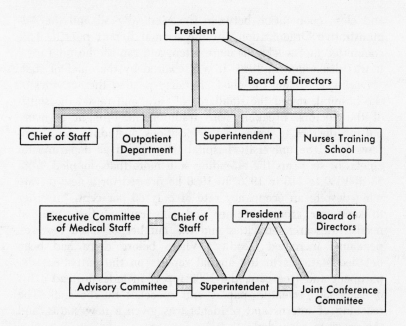

Figure 4-1
Probable organization of Valley Hospital for the 1920's (top).
Organization of Valley Hospital, 1930 (from Annual Report).

Lest anyone not be clear about the changes, an elaborate organization chart is presented (Figure 4-1). In contrast to the probable chart of the first period, presented here for comparison, the executive committee of the medical staff, the chief of staff, the president and board of trustees are all on the same level of authority. Conspicuously absent is a line connecting the chief of staff and the president. Furthermore, the mechanism for co-ordinating actions of the trustees and medical staff officials—the joint conference committee—is on a lower level, along with the administrator. This suggests the autonomy the medical staff sought. The effective decision-making group for the hospital proved to be the "advisory committee," consisting of the most powerful departmental chiefs and some younger doctors. The superintendent met with it once a week to ensure "excellent and close cooperation between the Medical Staff and the Administrative Organization," as the Annual Report puts it. This committee met weekly or more often, and ran the hospital until it was disbanded in 1943. It was chaired by the chief of staff.

During his reign, the chief of staff expanded the activities of the hospital, raised the standards of care, and raised the status of the doctors. Breaking with tradition, he brought in many outside doctors to serve in key positions, including some non-Jews from the university hospital who served as departmental chiefs. In six years the attending staff more than doubled, from 53 in 1930 to 116 in 1936. In 1936 he pressed for a new private wing despite an occupancy rate of only 66 per cent, "in order to keep our group together and take care of their medical needs." Research activities and the number of hired research personnel increased steadily. Where before there had been detailed statistics in the annual reports on the outpatient department and free care, the 1936 report includes instead a list of some 300 scientific papers and speeches by the staff. The teaching of interns and residents was given a new status, and the program expanded.

The "higher ideal" of a great medical center focused upon scientific work took its toll upon the presumably lesser ideal of "treating the sick poor." A part-payment scheme and close financial screening were instituted in the outpatient department. Despite the depression, the minutes of the board of trustees reflect concern with "fostering bad habits of dependency" and the "detection of chisellers" through scrutiny of bank accounts. Nevertheless, the hospital acquitted itself well during the depression. Outpatient department visits trebled. Despite woefully inadequate support from non-Jewish agencies, 37 per cent of free or part-pay patients ("clinic patients") were non-Jews. Yet the proportion of free or part-pay *in*patients continued to decline steadily, and private patients increasingly spilled over into the segregated wing during these years. After the depression the war years brought more prosperity to the community, and thus the need was less desperate. Yet the hospital did not serve the potential patients in the immediate neighborhood—a Negro slum that by now had surrounded the hospital. Free care declined so sharply that during the early 1940's the limited medical education program was threatened by inadequate "teaching material"—that is, clinic patients. Care given in the outpatient department came under prolonged and scathing criticism in the early 1940's by a respected member of the medical board, but to no avail. The department deteriorated medically and administratively in the late 1930's and throughout the next period.

There were other consequences of medical domination, at least according to informants who were on the scene. The autocratic rule of the chief of staff allowed him to have his personal complement of nurses and priority on the best rooms; he could also dictate which operations he wished to perform, regardless of whose patient it was.[7] Other departmental chiefs had similar, though lesser, perquisites. Favoritism was reportedly practiced in promotions within the medical staff and in access to desirable patient rooms. While standards of care had been raised in many respects, as compared with the pre-1930 situation, there was still no effective system of policing abuses or establishing that surgeons were qualified to perform specific therapies. As we have noted, medical responsibility was particularly derelict in the area of outpatient treatment for indigents, and the teaching that went on in this department was strongly criticized.

There was little to prevent such abuses. The doctor is an individual entrepreneur, selling his services for a profit. His income is affected by the facilities he commands in the hospital, his freedom from scrutiny, and by the price he must pay for facilities in the form of reciprocal duties such as teaching or committee work. Reliance upon professional ethics, even buttressed by the atmosphere created by teaching and research activities, is not sufficient in itself to guarantee a disinterested, ethical, non-economic point of view. Nor will it prevent abuses stemming from the enormous concentration of power in the hands of the chief of staff and department heads who also control the hospital. A constitutional system limiting these powers, establishing reasonable criteria for promotion within the staff, and allowing younger men a voice in medical staff policies was needed. Also needed was more effective representation of the interests of the patients and the interests of the organization as a whole. The patient is in a poor position to represent himself. At the minimum, hospital resources should be allocated on the basis of medical needs. Regarding the organization itself, the vested interests of doctors in administrative routines established under their control could, and perhaps did, forestall innovations that could improve patient care. Routines set by doctors are often designed to meet their convenience and reinforce their status. Unless efficient use is made of all personnel and the hospital quickly adapts to changing needs and technologies—administrative as well as medical—it will not long command community respect and support.

The Administrative Challenge (1942–1952)

The next period in the hospital's history saw a determined effort by a new administrator to meet some of these requirements, and the subsequent period saw them more firmly established. In the period from 1942 to 1952 a new administrator, basing his power upon the increased importance of internal administration, rationalized the procedures, improved business practices, placed the medical staff on a constitutional basis that defined their official powers, and even raised medical standards. These are not inevitable goals growing out of increasing administrative power, but they are possible ones.[8]

Until 1942 the superintendent had been a relatively passive figure in the organization: a low-status lieutenant of first the trustees and then the doctors. He kept records, supervised plant operation and maintenance, and carried out the directives of his superordinates with regard to the nursing service, outpatient department, equipment purchases, room rates, and so forth. He, or she, was recruited from the nursing service, administrative departments such as accounting, or from business or voluntary organizations in the community.

However, administrative problems were increasing. The

weekly minutes of the "advisory" committee in 1940 and 1941 show that many complex internal matters of an administrative nature had to be handled by the departmental chiefs. In addition, relations with other hospitals, welfare agencies, voluntary and governmental standard-setting agencies, and the community in general became more complex. When the incumbent superintendent died in 1942, it was decided to bring in someone who had been trained specifically for hospital administration.

In addition, it was decided that he should be a doctor. It is likely that this was intended to ensure that medical interests would remain paramount even though the administrator would have more power. A medically trained administrator would understand the needs of the doctors, and maintain the emphasis upon research and private patients. Such men were available. Some physicians had completed their internships during the depression years and gone immediately into the administrative field; some of these had received training in the newly established schools of hospital administration. The new administrator had such training and had subsequently served as assistant administrator in a large and highly respected Jewish hospital in the East.

The administrator had no quarrel with the emphasis upon private patients, teaching, and research, for these goals reflected changing community demands and professional requirements. He did, however, take issue with the operating policies established by the doctors, and sought to curtail their power through several means. He immediately interposed himself between the medical staff and the trustees. Whereas before the trustees had followed the wishes of the medical staff, the administrator, by channeling all communications through his office, was able to block recommendations from the medical staff, and initiate recommendations from the trustees. The latter gave him respect and authority both because of his administrative experience and his medical degree. He reduced the frequency of advisory committee meetings and finally had them abolished; the committee was succeeded by a medical staff committee without a representative of the trustees as an official member. In addition, the joint conference committee (consisting of representatives of the medical board and the board of trustees) rarely met. Thus contact between the two boards was effectively curtailed. One of the most frequent criticisms by doctors of this administrator in 1957 was that he spoke to the trustees as a representative of the doctors, and to the doctors as a representative of the trustees.

Trustees were even unable to get in touch with second-level administrative personnel directly. For example, women on the board had been accustomed to taking a direct hand in the affairs of the outpatient department, but the administrator ordered all communications to go through his office. Communication became so centralized that a management engineering firm studying the hospital in 1951 found twenty-five people reporting directly to the administrator.[9]

Authority, as well as communication, was centralized in the administrator's office. Working with a very loyal administrative staff—which grew ever larger, to the consternation of the doctors —he intervened in areas where doctors or board members were wont to have the first and final say. The screening policies of the outpatient department became more stringent, and he intervened in nursing policies, which doctors were accustomed to setting. Close control of many administrative functions, such as equipment purchases, medical-records procedures, nursing assignments, applications for admission to the attending staff, and procedures for admitting and billing patients, gave him considerable power over the doctors. In each of these cases their interests, directly or through their private patients, were vitally affected.

Doctors as well as the nonmedical staff in 1957 recalled how the administrator increasingly referred to the hospital as "my hospital," and spoke of "my beds" and "my lab." Revealing evidence of this was found in a draft of a speech which the administrator gave before the medical staff. In it, the reference to "my efforts" to maintain standards is penciled out and the more diplomatic phrase "our mutual efforts" is written in; similarly, the "frequent" cooperation from the medical staff is changed to the "constant" cooperation. Shortly after he arrived, the administrator had his title changed from superintendent to "director." However, the doctors persisted in referring to him as the superintendent, or at best, the administrator. As late as 1951 some memoranda of the medical staff have the word "director" crossed out and "administrator" submitted.

These items were symptoms of both a mounting tension between the medical staff and the M.D. they had hired as administrator, and his steady effort to gather power from them. The most serious issue, where the administrator stepped far beyond his official role but was somewhat within bounds of his status as a physician, was the attempt to improve standards of care. About two months after his arrival, he told a surgeon that the surgeon could not perform an operation because he was unqualified. This struck at the heart of medical staff autonomy, and the surgeon resigned. The advisory committee discussed this grave matter at length: after all, the administrator was not even a surgeon. The minutes reveal that the administrator pointed out that in the hospital he had come from the staff was assigned surgical privileges on the basis of their training and skill; not every surgeon could perform any operation. Two years later he succeeded in instituting this plan for the surgical staff. Valley was the first hospital in the city to do so.

Besides attempting to raise standards in this and many less dramatic ways, the administrator reorganized the medical staff within a year of his arrival. Actually, he gave it its first effective organization. The first constitution and bylaws were drawn up, clearly spelling out the relationship of the medical staff and its officials to the rest of the hospital, and specifying the internal structure of the staff and procedures for promotion. An executive committee was established that met monthly with the administrator attending. Responsibilities were outlined for other committees. An unsuccessful move was made at this time, though not necessarily at the instigation of the administrator, to place constitutional limits upon the powers of the chief of staff by limiting his term to three or four years, rather than retirement age.

The administrator's relations were as good with the board of trustees as they were bad with the medical staff. The trustees, never very active when the hospital was controlled by the chief of staff, relied heavily upon the administrator, and supported his recommendations for change. They had little reason to be dissatisfied. "Sound business practices" were introduced; rates rose regularly; during the war years the hospital operated at close to capacity, and the clinic load was kept small. A sizable deficit was paid off and even a surplus accumulated.

The medical staff had not acquiesced in the shift of power that was taking place; tensions were mounting during the war years, and are reflected in various committee minutes. But many of the staff were in the service, and those at the hospital were extremely busy. After the war ended, another distraction postponed the seemingly inevitable showdown—a fund-raising drive and the building of a new private wing. Occupancy was high; private patients filled most of the wards designed for clinic patients; laboratory services were inadequate. Though the trustees had appointed a committee to look into the possibilities of a new wing, nothing had transpired for some time. Finally, in 1945, several officials of the medical staff donated approximately 5,000 dollars apiece for a new building. The trustees had little choice but to start a fund-raising drive. The medical staff as a whole contributed heavily, both on their own and through friends and patients, and thereby laid a substantial claim to continuing or expanding their influence in the hospital. Though the total drive did not meet its goal, over 4 million dollars was raised. A large new wing, with extensive laboratory facilities, brought bed space to around 300 beds. It was opened in 1951 and was the most advanced in design and function in the region.

The completion of the building coincided with a crisis in the hospital that culminated in both a reorganization of the medical staff and the resignation of the administrator. After the war many younger doctors returned to the hospital with considerable experience and advanced training. Training in specialties had been formalized in American medicine, and physicians and surgeons were less dependent upon departmental chiefs for training and promotion. Thus the basis for some of the older autocracy and paternalism had been lost. Returning veterans were impatient of the autocracy that still existed in the medical staff, and sought more representation of their points of view and recognition for their accomplishments. The chief of staff who had led the hospital in the 1930's had retired; his successor was clearly in the autocratic tradition, but had lost many of his prerogatives to the administrator. Furthermore, the reorganization of the medical staff that the administrator had brought about in 1944 provided constitutional means for bringing about changes. Some changes were discussed by the medical board, but a group of younger men were impatient with the slow progress. They formed an ad hoc committee, dubbed the "vigilante committee," and demanded authority to conduct a survey. This prodded the board to further action. Tensions ran so high that at one point a prominent surgeon on the board resigned in protest over the dictatorial powers of the chief of staff.[10]

Out of this turmoil some drastic changes were made. The most important were as follows. The age limit of departmental chiefs was reduced from sixty-five to sixty. Furthermore, their tenure was limited to a maximum of fifteen years. The tenure of the chief of staff was reduced from retirement at age sixty-five to *three years*—a drastic reduction in power for the office that once had uncontested rule of the hospital, and had continued to rule the medical staff during the last ten years. Furthermore, procedures were established enabling the staff to force the medical board to review the qualifications of a departmental chief or chief of staff if indicated. Finally, medical board representation was given to the members of staff who were not chiefs of departments; three were to be elected by the staff as a whole for a one-year term. The new policies automatically retired the chief of staff and four of the sixteen departmental chiefs. One other major change was directed at the administrator. Henceforth, the chief of staff was to be a voting member of the board of trustees. Thus, the administrator was no longer to be the sole spokesman for the medical staff on the board of trustees.

The "vigilante committee" found these changes were already made by the time they presented their report on "the state of the hospital." They approved of them heartily, though they did not think all of them went far enough. Their report notes that the questionnaire to the staff indicated they were nearly unanimous in agreeing that the tenure of the chief of staff should be drastically limited. They found nearly three-quarters of the staff dissatisfied with teaching material in the outpatient department, 70 per cent dissatisfied with a specific department for which the chief of staff bore considerable responsibility, and 54 per cent dissatisfied with the administrator. From 30 to 40 per cent of the respondents were also dissatisfied with the cashier, nursing superintendent, nurses in general, and clinical services— all areas over which the administrator now exercised considerable control.

The administrator came under direct fire in their discussion of "the place of the administrator in the over-all organization of the hospital." They charged that he had poor personal relations with all but close subordinates and that he lacked sound business principles. Most important, and striking at the heart of the administrative challenge, they found a "progressive assumption of responsibilities and authorities properly belonging to the attending medical staff." In submitting their qualifications for an ideal administrator, they indicated they had had enough of doctors as administrators, and they testified to a basic shift in hospital goals: "Above all he must never lose sight of the fundamental fact that Valley Hospital is a facility to enable the doctors to care for their patients. His primary background and training should be in the field of business and administration." A trustee generally sympathetic to the committee and its findings wrote a memorandum on their report that took issue with their statement that the hospital is a facility to enable doctors to care for their patients. He wrote: "*The fundamental fact* is that Valley Hospital is a facility for the care of patients who are unable to pay for its services in whole or in part, and to afford training and facilities for hospitalization for a group of doctors who might otherwise not find ready access to other institutions."

This philosophy applied prior to 1930, but the new "private wing," the decline in clinic cases, and the drift of former attending men to other hospitals signified change. Jewish physicians could practice or train anywhere in the city now; the goal of the hospital was no longer service to the needy; and the hospital was, in important respects, primarily a "facility" for the physician.

As the report of the vigilante committee was being filed, there occurred, as one document put it, the "spontaneous resignation" of the administrator. Thus the main contestants of the ten-year struggle left the field: the chief of staff and the administrator. Coincidentally, the six-year term of the president of the board of trustees was just ending. This left the hospital without a dominant group or individual. Thus that "fundamental prize" in organizational life, the evolving character of the organization,[11] was open to seizure.

The power of the administrator had increased remarkably, relative to that of the doctors, in this period. However, the importance of the doctor's skills to the organization had not declined in absolute terms, and the doctors retained much of their organizational advantage. That is, they still had an efficient, relatively disciplined internal organization with a committee system that allowed access to all facets of hospital organization. Short of a drastic routinization of their skills and a collapse of their internal government, they could still demand a say in major policy formation.[12] On the other hand, the importance of administrative skills was not likely to decline, but to continue to increase. Only the trustees were out of the contest, for the time being.

A new administrator might pursue an aggressive and debilitating war with the medical staff until he either broke its power (an unlikely event) or was forced to resign. An ineffectual administrator might allow the medical staff to regain its full power, and he would serve as a "housekeeper"—in the argot of hospital administrators. Or a skilled administrator, appreciative of the power and importance of the medical staff, could avoid another open contest while judiciously expanding his own influence. This latter is what happened. For the administrator to expand his power, however, he found it necessary to activate the trustees and utilize their support in critical issues. But he also found that, once activated, the trustees also began to set policy. Thus, within a few years, all three major groups were active in hospital affairs, and no one of them could dominate. Before examining this period in detail, we shall discuss the phenomenon of "multiple leadership" in more general terms.

Multiple Leadership (1952–1958)

While social scientists have been reluctant to consider the possibility of an organization without some *de facto* single source of power, it is possible for two or more groups to share power and leadership, to divide up the organization into segments where each has control. This division of labor regarding the determination of goals and the power to achieve them is what we shall call multiple leadership. It is different from fractionated power where several groups have small amounts of power in an unstable and temporary situation. With multiple leadership there are a small number—perhaps two or three— of recognized centers of power. It is different from a contest of power, for the groups do not seek—at least over the short run —to vanquish each other, but recognize each other's sphere of interests. Nor is it the same as decentralized authority, where specialized units have autonomy. In such a case units are free to operate as they choose only up to a point, when it becomes quite clear that there is a centralized authority. In multiple leadership there is no single ultimate authority in fact, even though there is in the official constitution.

Multiple leadership, as a stable system of goal determination and policy setting, is most likely to be found in organizations where there are multiple goals and where these goals lack precise criteria of achievement and allow considerable tolerances with regard to achievement. Organizations with a single goal or a clear hierarchy of goals provide little basis for multiple leadership. Multiple leadership arises because important group interests diverge, and each group has the power to protect its interests. Interests that command loyalty sufficient to threaten competing interests are not likely to be trivial but will be linked to or have consequences for organizational goals. Organizations that have precise performance standards and allow little tolerance in achievement cannot easily allow the accommodation of diverse group interests that is found with multiple leadership.

These considerations have two consequences: the accommodation of group interests in such a situation can easily lead to organizational drift, ambiguity of purpose, and opportunism. Furthermore, the important lubricant of such a system is some kind of facilitating leadership, someone who keeps explosive issues from erupting too often and maintains easy, comfortable relations among the groups. For the threat to multiple leadership is open confrontation of competing interests that could lead to a debilitating power struggle and vanquishment of one or more groups.

A hospital is a likely site for multiple leadership because its goals are generally multiple—trustees, doctors, and the administration may all have diverse and conflicting goals. Furthermore, performance criteria are not rigorous. Accreditation means only that minimal requirements are met; beyond that there is much room for dispute, and few accepted judges.[13] For multiple leadership by doctors, administration, and trustees to develop at Valley Hospital it was necessary that the administrator consolidate and extend his power, that the power of the doctors be reduced, and that of the trustees be increased. The personal qualities of the new administrator immediately gained for him the respect of the doctors and the trustees. He was highly intelligent, articulate, and well informed on hospital, medical, and administrative matters. He spoke and wrote well and published in hospital journals. These qualities and his interest in the social aspects of medicine also made him respected and sought after by community groups and his professional society. His charm, wit, and facility in interpersonal relations perhaps meant even more within the hospital, for he contrasted sharply with the previous administrator. He was the natural target for complaints upon almost any hospital matter, but the barbs appeared impotent, for he could parry and disarm with facility. One physician compared him with the previous administrator, neatly summing up both assets and deficits of the administrator in the doctor's eyes:

When you went in to see Dr. ———— you knew he was going to say no to whatever you asked, and say it in a way to make your blood boil. He might, occasionally, do what you asked, but he always said no. With this one, he always says yes. Often he doesn't do what he agreed to do, but you feel a lot better about it somehow.

The administrator made himself accessible to the medical staff in many ways. His office door, in contrast to that of his predecessor, was always open, and this impressed the doctors more than any other single thing—they could always have a few minutes of his time. Furthermore, he made a practice of socializing with them informally in the wards, in the corridors, coffee shop, lab and X-ray departments, and the doctors' lounge. He also attended almost every meeting of a medical staff committee during the first year—a prodigious feat, as the writer knows from experience, for there are a great many of them. Here he heard their complaints and problems, presented the administrative point of view, and attempted at least to pacify the medical staff where he could not fully satisfy them. He also began a monthly newsletter that became so successful that it later expanded into a regular bulletin with reports from the administrator, chief of staff, and the president of the board of trustees. The equal priority of these reports effectively symbolized the emergent multiple leadership.

The doctor on the attending staff has some very specific interests in the hospital. He must conserve his time so that he may see as many patients as possible. Thus he demands convenient nursing schedules, easy access to the hospital and to patients within it, convenient record dictating arrangements, prompt and accessible technical services, and no interference from visitors or hospital personnel. He also demands excellent service for his patients, special favors for many, and a congenial patient environment. Finally, he requires that his status be upheld in dealings with nurses, administrative personnel, and

other paramedical personnel, residents, interns, and other doctors. The administrator tended to these matters assiduously. A
great deal of administrative staff time went into serving the
doctors, and the effects were rapidly evident. One year after
his arrival the administrator (now always called the "director"
by the doctors) was praised by the medical board. The minutes
noted that "for the first time Valley Hospital has increased its
percentage of occupancy while other hospitals in the city have
shown a decrease. The director was praised by the medical
board for the evidence of improved relationships he has brought
about between the administrative staff and personnel of the
hospital toward the medical staff." A questionnaire to the doctors
in the next year indicated that 95 per cent felt that patient care
had improved, and 35 per cent volunteered such comments as
"very much" or "considerably."

It was not only necessary that the administrator demonstrate
his interest in the doctors' welfare, and promote good "human
relations"; he had also to work with them, either attempting to
achieve their ends or his own. He adroitly utilized the precedent
of medical staff participation in hospital affairs. Parking problems, a chronic complaint of the staff, were given to the "Good
and Welfare Committee" of the medical staff for recommendations with the administrator's blessing. Thus doctors on the
committee became responsible for policing violations by other
doctors. When the formulary of the OPD was being abused,
and the pharmacy complained to the administrator about waste
and inconvenience, the medical staff committee on drugs and
patient care got the problem and policed the doctors. The
operating-room superintendent (a nurse) could do little about
surgeons who were late for scheduled operations, but when
the problem was properly presented to the medical staff surgical committee they set up penalties and enforced them.

Of course, the medical staff also interfered in matters the
administration felt were beyond their province. Medical staff
committees would countermand orders from the administration
to nurses. Registered nurses took their complaints about the
encroachment of practical nurses to a medical staff committee,
who demanded action, before even approaching the administra-

tion. Failure to include the medical staff of the obstetrics department in so trivial an administrative decision as a change in the technique of photographing newborn babies created a prolonged and noisy crisis in the hospital. Cooptation on some matters had blurred the boundaries of legitimate power, which are constantly under dispute anyway. This ambiguity, coupled with the jealously guarded prerogatives of the doctors, presented problems demanding extraordinary skill on the administrator's part if he was to increase his power and not alienate the doctors.

Administrative power rested not only on internal administration. Increasingly the hospital had become involved in a complex network of organizations involved with health, from a women's club seeking a speaker to the giant prepaid insurance firms. These contacts had consequences for the internal affairs of the hospital, and the administrator was in a position to shape these consequences and even to seek out new relationships with organizations in the environment. For example, by establishing a contract with an agency providing care for crippled children or victims of particular diseases, the hospital might need to establish additional facilities, which then could be justified before the board of trustees. Such a program could require more control over medical procedures such as standards, medical records, or the extent of psychiatric or social service consultations. This would increase his control over the doctors. In time a wide range of institutions and voluntary organizations had formal relations with the hospital—special health agencies such as the associations for tuberculosis, cerebral palsy, polio; institutions such as the university hospitals, nurses-training schools, the city hospital association; governmental units, commissions and study groups, and so forth. As the official link between the environment and the organization, the administrator could shape the impact of such contacts on the hospital. He could establish relationships that became firm commitments in time, binding the hospital to a course of action with implications the doctors and trustees might not even be aware of.

REDUCTION IN MEDICAL STAFF POWER

The administrator found favor in the doctor's eyes because he attended to many of their needs. This provided him with support for various programs, and tended to reduce opposition to other programs. However, it was also necessary for the power of the medical staff to be reduced. They conveniently contributed to this reduction themselves by extending the constitutional revolution that commenced in 1951. While continuing to respect and like the new administrator, they were aware that his power was increasing. Yet no strong leadership emerged as a serious challenge to the administrator on basic matters involving more than the doctors' convenience or status.

The constitutional revolution that brought in the new administrator continued unabated during the first two years of office. Younger members of the medical staff succeeded in having an amendment to the bylaws adopted that required that two of the three elected members of the medical board should sit on the nominating committee for new chiefs of departments or the chief of staff. As the original amendment that was proposed put it, "under the present method, the President of the Medical Board [the chief of staff], who is also a member of the Board of Trustees, could either perpetuate himself in office for three years or could name his successor, or could be influenced by the Board of Trustees to that end." This apprehension was not without substance. Correspondence indicates that the previous chief of staff, under pressure from the trustees, had "agreed upon" his successor. The new chief of staff did not continue in the autocratic tradition; indeed, for a time, a supporter of the previous chief attempted to create a competing center of power through his role as chairman of the executive committee—a position heretofore held by the chief of staff. The rebellious medical board refused to accept the actions of the executive committee without prolonged debate, and even then sometimes reversed them. In fact, recommendations of the chief of staff, as president of the medical board, were also defeated at times. This was unheard of in the past, and further signified a break-down of authority. Trivial matters that were decided without question under the previous system became hotly contested issues, splintering the board. Other more basic issues that might not have been raised now were debated.

One of these involved departmental representation. The medical board was made up primarily of the chiefs of sixteen departments, each one having a vote. Yet eight of these departments had an average size of only six doctors, while the chief of medicine represented sixty-two doctors, and the chief of surgery, thirty. The chief of dermatology, for example, admitted that there was no logical reason why his department with seven members should have a vote equal to the chief of medicine or surgery, especially since it admitted no patients. The seventeen members of the "professional departments" (anesthesiology, pathology, and radiology) were represented by three chiefs who had rather direct financial interests in the hospital since their income was geared to the amount of work their departments did. Some doctors resented this degree of representation and power.

Periodically there were struggles to reduce the size of the board, increase it by adding more elected members, drop specific departments, or include new ones. The division of interests and opinions within the medical staff on this matter left it exposed to intervention by the administrator and the trustees. On one occasion, the administrator and trustees looked with favor upon the absorption of a small department by a larger one, which had the effect of removing a potent critic of their policies from the medical board. On another occasion they succeeded in having a new, complex technique removed from a large department and placed in a separate department. Some doctors opposed the establishment of this technique since it would compete with their own techniques and require enormous facilities. Its departmental status enabled it to survive and grow. By rallying the opponents and proponents of small departments on each of these issues, the administration could capitalize on the division within the medical staff.

On another occasion the administrator and the trustees felt

that a fifteen-year tenure for a departmental chief was too long. A poor chief might do a great deal of harm in that time. Three years earlier an elected member of the board had tried to require that, at the least, the performance of a departmental chief be reviewed very five years. His amendment was defeated, yet the matter had been broached and some support had been found. In the meantime a member of the board of trustees had quietly become an "observer" on the nominating committee. In this capacity he informally proposed such a review. The medical board balked, and there was considerable tension. But finally the board of trustees made it clear that the medical board had no choice; they should recommend such a review. Without the division in the medical board, such a move would have been unthinkable.

ACTIVATION OF THE TRUSTEES

As long as the medical staff dominated the hospital, the trustees remained inactive. When the contest of power between the doctors and the administrator erupted in 1951, they were forced into involvement. Yet there is no evidence that they wished to play any substantial role once that crisis was passed. Indeed, for some time afterward, most board committees were inactive and board meetings poorly attended. The trustees continued to help bring in donations and bequests, and symbolized the fiscal responsibility of the nonprofit institution. Gradually, however, the board members became involved in the affairs of the hospital. The new board president showed a lively interest in hospital problems and a keen appreciation of the complex processes at work. He had considerable knowledge of health matters and social medicine, and was in a position to devote most of his time to voluntary organization in the community. The administrator and president worked closely together and were in almost daily contact. The administrator retained the initiative, but the president saw to it that the board gave their approval when the two men agreed upon some step. In this manner the administrator was able to find support for the policies that otherwise might have been blocked by the doctors, such as their review of the performance of departmental chiefs every five years.

The enthusiasm of the administrator for his job, the interest of the board president, and the discussions of policy matters enlivened board meetings and stimulated interest. The issues were carefully prepared and presented by the administrator and president, leaving them in control, but once again the board was participating in hospital affairs. The board had reason for placing its confidence in the administrator. Relations with the physicians had improved remarkably; the hospital was gaining considerable prestige through programs designed to meet patient needs; from a deficit of $62,500 before depreciation in 1952 the hospital showed its first surplus in years in the very next year. Some costs were cut and new methods brought economies, but the cost of new services for patients and doctors probably offset these. The real cause of prosperity was the rise in occupancy. The hospital became an attractive place for doctors to bring patients, and patients were likely to request that they go to Valley Hospital rather than one with a slightly lower rate. Occupancy over the next few years rose from one of the lowest in the city to the highest of all voluntary, non-university hospitals.

In 1957 the term of the president ended, and a new one was elected. The new president did not have as much time to give to the hospital, and did not have a close personal interest. Thus, he reorganized the board and activated the many committees. They would, henceforth, make policy decisions that would be reviewed by the executive committee of the board (which had not met for years prior to this). The board, as a whole, would now meet only quarterly since it had little to do. As a consequence, the careful regulation of board activities and interests broke down. The board had not been completely dominated by the administrator. Members had balked at some of his proposals, chiefly those involving financial outlays, but they had exercised this power only occasionally, and the president, as the representative of a conservative approach to long-range planning, had defined these occasions. But now the board was "turned loose," so to speak, in all areas of hospital activity. Medical staff committees covered all vital areas of hospital activity, from nursing practices to long-range planning, paralleling the administrative organization. Now the activated committees of the board of trustees constituted still another "parallel organization." The administrator found policies scrutinized that had never before been discussed by the board. Committees sought out the views of doctors and personnel, and queried the administrator at length. Time-honored fiscal practices were criticized by nationally respected business leaders, lawyers, and judges on the board ("You're doing it with mirrors," the chairman of the finance committee once said in exasperation with fiscal policies). Planned equipment purchases, remodeling, and new services received careful scrutiny (and increasingly unfavorable action) in the light of a baffling financial statement and overdue bills. The board found that while the hospital had presumably been in financial straits for some time, extensive additions to the plant and considerable remodeling and updating of facilities had taken place over the years. Actually, it would appear that the administrator had been extremely resourceful and had served the interests of the organization well. But he was confronted now on the one hand with standards of accounting developed in business and industry, and on the other with a viewpoint that did not share his ambitious plans.

In some respects, it should be noted, the involvement of the trustees served the administrator's ends. Board members of long years of service made their first tour of the dilapidated outpatient department and had to face the prospect of either discontinuing the service or revamping it and admitting full-pay patients. They realized the need for stable, long-term means of financing capital improvements, and took steps in this direction. They also came to view sympathetically the need for a long-term care unit, increased medical social services, and an expanded preventive-medicine program. Since the administrator favored these plans, and the doctors were at best lukewarm, trustee support was welcome.

Goals, Decision-Making, and Multiple Leadership

By 1958 multiple leadership fully included the trustees as well as the administrator and the doctors. Where each group has veto power, how do decisions come to be made and the direction of the organization shaped? First, of course, all three groups might agree upon the desirability of an action and be fully aware of its long-range implications. There were many areas of common agreement and they suggested obvious lines of action. Action could also be taken if supported by two of the groups and not meeting the *unified* opposition of the third. Thus, because of a division in the medical staff, a group of doctors could not prevent the establishment of a new program, but they could delay it and jeopardize its future. Because trustees were not unified in their opposition to a major fund-raising drive (they held different images of the role of the hospital in the community), it was apparent that a drive would soon take place because of medical and administrative pressures. This form of decision-making is obviously not a preferred one. Large resources might have to be expended to protect a decision of this nature if even a minority of one group opposed it.

Neither of these forms of decision-making is especially distinctive, but three others appeared to be favored under a system of multiple leadership. Each involved the sacrifice of an assessment of long-term consequences in favor of short-term harmony and parochial gains. The first was predicated upon the fortuitous convergence of unrelated and diverse short-term interests. Thus, a new floor could be added to the 1951 building because it expanded the scope and size of the hospital—an interest of the administrator; would provide more facilities for treating private patients—a concern of the doctors; and the objections of conservative trustees were met because it could be financed out of the "profits" of private care on the floor, and a low-interest loan could be secured. However, this decision meant a deflection of effort and resources from areas of presumably greater need, such as the outpatient department, or house staff quarters, or new specialized services. These were matters where interests did not converge. The new floor would also overtax existing laboratory and other supporting facilities, thus committing the hospital to another round of expansion. Another form of action was relatively simple, but frequent. One group could make a minor decision completely within its province, but the ramifications of that decision would come to involve other groups. By then, however, commitments and investments precluded any turning back. By having medical, administrative, and community spheres of action segregated to prevent conflict, the consequences for the organization as a whole, and thus the interests of all three groups, went unreviewed.

The third form of action was related to the above, but required successive approval of controversial steps, each of which either appeared to be minor, or became so entangled with the investments and commitments of earlier steps as to make a veto very difficult. It appears that this form of action enabled a modest research proposal by one man to culminate rapidly in a facility that was remarkable for a three-hundred-bed hospital —a highly specialized surgical suite that was practically unique in the country, consumed much valuable space, and required a huge investment and a large operating budget. At each step of the way, either trustees or the medical board voiced misgivings, but the ramifications of earlier steps made a veto impossible. Once established, however, the unit was attacked by some members of the medical board and board of trustees. They realized the long-run implications of the program in terms of investment, operating costs, demands for publicity by local donors, critical reaction to such publicity by other key groups, uncertain research productivity, and the insistent pressure for therapy of unproved and unpredictable value as opposed to careful research. "Does a hospital of this size, using community funds, have any *right* to build such an elaborate facility?" one trustee asked, in summing up the problem. By then the question was rhetorical.

These three forms of action or policy setting—the fortuitous convergence of interests, segregated decision-making, and the piecemeal accumulation of small victories—are distinctive in that they avoid the open confrontation of conflict of interests. Open conflict would threaten established prerogatives and powers. Where there is disagreement upon goals, but power to pursue separate goals, a group may stand to lose more from open conflict than it stands to gain. Multiple leadership rests upon relatively segregated spheres of interest with accommodation in the overlapping areas; it puts a premium on harmony. The kind of decision-making favored under such a system has two consequences. First, there is no guarantee that precarious values will be protected. While they will be given lip service by all groups, they stand, by definition, outside the interests of the ruling groups. One of the responsibilities, even luxuries, of leadership is to support difficult, unpopular, and irritating programs that nevertheless embody values accepted by the organization. Without a monopoly of power, such a task is difficult for a ruling group. Thus, at Valley Hospital, the needs of the outpatient department—an important factor in achieving the official goal of providing a high level of medical care—found few supporters. Ironically, the initial funds for the surgical suite mentioned above were diverted from a much needed remodeling of the dilapidated outpatient building. The department suffered from budgetary deprivations, administrative indifference, and medical neglect.[14]

Another consequence of the accommodation of group interests under multiple leadership was the avoidance of long-range planning. Planning could expose conflicting interests. A long-range assessment of a proposed line of action might doom it to a peremptory veto from one group. This exposed the organization to vagrant and opportunistic pressures that could dictate the direction of growth or the restriction of effort.[15] Only the "something for everyone" plan could succeed, and this had to avoid the assessment of long-range consequences. Outwardly the hospital might prosper, but perhaps for reasons that had little to do with its avowed goals, and even at the expense of those goals.[16] By avoiding the questions of what is its distinctive competence and its responsibility, the organization is no longer a means for achieving goals that are rationally established and publicly offered for community inspection and support.

NOTES

1. Charles Perrow, "The Analysis of Goals in Complex Organizations," *American Sociological Review*, 26 (December, 1961), pp. 854-866.

2. These are not meant to be exhaustive or empirically mutually exclusive. They will, however, serve our purposes here and probably would serve for many other types of organizations.

3. For various reasons this is only a tendency; e.g., a group may be prevented from gaining power in some situations, or may not use the power that is potentially theirs.

4. Perrow, *op. cit.*

5. The data for the period 1887 to 1936 comes primarily from annual reports of the hospital. A brief history of the hospital under preparation by a physician was also valuable, as were extensive interviews with doctors and trustees regarding the early periods. Beyond 1936 more complete records of official minutes are available, and for the 1940's and 1950's there were also voluminous correspondence, memoranda, and a variety of other documents, as well as interviews and observations that were made in 1957 and 1958. The author had access to all material and to all meetings of the administrative and medical staffs and the board of trustees. Some dates and minor particulars have been altered throughout to help ensure anonymity. My indebtedness to the personnel, and especially the administrator, of the hospital studied is enormous.

6. In 1914 free patients accounted for well over half of the inpatient days of care at Valley Hospital; even by 1919 this was true of only 43 per cent. By 1930, despite the depression, the figure was 37 per cent, and by the end of the period (1942), it was 30 per cent.

7. The story has it that each morning upon arrival he received two things: a list of quotations on stock he was interested in and a list of all surgery scheduled for that day. Actually, since he was an excellent surgeon, the patients of other surgeons may have benefited from his proprietary behavior.

8. For some alternative ones, see the author's "The Analysis of Goals in Complex Organizations," *op. cit.*

9. For an excellent analysis of the relationship between policy and communication in a different setting, see Richard McCleery, *Policy Change in Prison Management* (Governmental Research Bureau: Michigan State University, East Lansing, 1957).

10. Demands for changes in representation, policies, and administrative power have occurred in many hospitals, and indeed are frequent in voluntary organizations in general. Michael Reese Hospital in Chicago had crises in 1921 and again in the middle 1950's, occurring under physician-administrators and concerned with similar problems. See Lucy Freeman,

Hospital in Action (Chicago: Rand McNally, 1956), pp. 170-223. Wessen
mentions one in Hartford Hospital in the early 1930's (Albert F.
Wessen, "The Social Structure of a Modern Hospital," unpublished Ph.D. dis-
sertation, Yale University, 1951, p. 157). Lentz describes one in Detroit's
Crittendon Hospital in the late 1920's (Edith M. Lentz, "The American
Voluntary Hospital as an Example of Industrial Change," unpublished
Ph.D. dissertation, Cornell University 1956, p. 48).

11. Philip Selznick, *TVA and the Grass Roots* (Berkeley: University of
California Press, 1953), p. 181.

12. Doctors need not dominate even where their skills are critical.
Trustees or the administration may be so well organized and vigilant as
to keep them in a subordinate state; the hospital may command such scarce
and powerful resources—e.g., a prestigeful affiliation with a medical school,
or scarce bed space in an area that is chronically "underbedded"—as to
ensure their dependent state; or, finally, the medical staff itself may find it
impossible to organize effectively to challenge the power of the controlling group.

13. Many service organizations have these characteristics, and one
would expect examples of multiple leadership to be found there. But
these characteristics might also be found in large, public-relations-conscious
businesses or industrial organizations where a variety of goals can be
elevated to such importance that power must be shared by the representatives of each.

14. This is apparently a common fate of such departments. Cf. Jerry
Solon *et al.*, "Staff Perceptions of Patients' Use of a Hospital Outpatient
Department," *Journal of Medical Education*, 33:1 (January, 1958), p. 18.
At the close of the field study at Valley Hospital, steps were finally taken
to improve medical care in the department because of various pressures.

15. On this general problem, see Philip Selznick, *Leadership in
Administration* (Evanston, Ill.: Row, Peterson, 1957).

16. Valley Hospital did prosper and served the community as well as
or better than any of its competitors, in the author's judgment. But we
are judging it here by its own ideals and pronouncements, and attempting
to detect the consequences of its form of leadership. The official goals of
patient care, teaching, research, and preventive medicine all suffered by
reason of the conflicting interests of the three groups. For documentation,
see Perrow, "Authority, Goals, and Prestige in a General Hospital," unpublished Ph.D. dissertation, University of California, Berkeley, 1960.

5

The Hospital and
Its Negotiated Order

ANSELM STRAUSS

LEONARD SCHATZMAN

DANUTA EHRLICH

RUE BUCHER

MELVIN SABSHIN

Introduction

In the pages to follow, a model for studying hospitals will be sketched, along with some suggested virtues of the model. It grew out of the authors' research, which was done on the premises of two psychiatric hospitals. The reader must judge for himself whether a model possibly suited to studying psychiatric hospitals might equally well guide the study of other kinds of hospitals. We believe that it can, and shall indicate why

The writing of this chapter is part of a larger project studying psychiatric hospitals, which is being carried on at the Institute of Psychosomatic and Psychiatric Research and Training of Michael Reese Hospital under the State of Illinois Mental Health Fund, Program 1737.

at the close of our presentation; indeed, we shall argue its usefulness for investigating other organizations besides hospitals.

Our model bears upon that most central of sociological problems, namely, how a measure of order is maintained in the face of inevitable changes (derivable from sources both external and internal to the organization). Students of formal organization tend to underplay the processes of internal change as well as overestimate the more stable features of organizations —including its rules and its hierarchical statuses. We ourselves take our cue from George H. Mead, who some years ago, when arguing for orderly and directed social change, remarked that the task turns about relationships between change and order:

How can you bring those changes about in an orderly fashion and yet preserve order? To bring about change is seemingly to destroy the given order, and yet society does and must change. That is the problem, to incorporate the method of change into the order of society itself.[1]

Without Mead's melioristic concerns, one can yet assume that order is something at which members of any society, any organization, must work. For the shared agreements, the binding contracts—which constitute the grounds for an expectable, nonsurprising, taken-for-granted, even ruled orderliness—are not binding and shared for all time. Contracts, understandings, agreements, rules—all have appended to them a temporal clause. That clause may or may not be explicitly discussed by the contracting parties, and the terminal date of the agreement may or may not be made specific; but none can be binding forever— even if the parties believe it so, unforeseen consequences of acting on the agreements would force eventual confrontation. Review is called for, whether the outcome of review be rejection or renewal or revision, or what not. In short, the bases of concerted action (social order) must be reconstituted continually; or, as remarked above, "worked at."

Such considerations have led us to emphasize the importance of negotiation—the processes of give-and-take, of diplomacy, of bargaining—which characterizes organizational life. In the pages to follow, we shall note first the relationship of rules to negotiation, then discuss the grounds for negotiation. Then, since both the clients and much of the personnel of hospitals are laymen, we wish also to underscore the participation of those laymen in the hospital's negotiative processes. Thereafter we shall note certain patterned and temporal features of negotiation; then we shall draw together some implications for viewing social order. A general summary of the argument and its implications will round out the paper.

A Psychiatric Hospital

Before discussing negotiation in hospitals, it will help to indicate two things: first, what was engaging our attention when research was initiated; and, second, the general characteristics of the hospital that was studied.[2] At the outset of our investigation, three foci were especially pertinent. The first was an explicit concern with the professional careers of the personnel: Who was there? Where did they come from? Where did they think they were going in work and career? What were they doing at this particular hospital? What was happening to them at this place? A second concern was with psychiatric ideology: Were different ideologies represented on the floors of this hospital? What were these ideologies? Did people clearly recognize their existence as well as did their more articulate advocates? And anyway, what difference did these philosophies make in the lives and work of various personnel? A third focus consisted of the realization that a hospital is par excellence an institution captained and maintained principally by professionals. This fact implied that the nonprofessionals who worked there, as well as those nonprofessionals there as patients, must manage to make their respective ways within this professionalized establishment. How, then, do they do this—and vice versa, how do the professionals incorporate the nonprofessionals into their own schemes of work and aspiration? These directions of interest, and the questions raised in consequence, quickly led us to perceive hospitals in terms to be depicted below.

A Professionalized Locale

A hospital can be visualized as a professionalized locale—a geographical site where persons drawn from different professions come together to carry out their respective purposes. At our specific hospital, the professionals consisted of numerous practicing psychiatrists and psychiatric residents, nurses and nursing students, psychologists, occupational therapists, and one lone social worker. Each professional echelon has received noticeably different kinds of training and, speaking conventionally, each occupies some differential hierarchical position at the hospital while playing a different part in its total division of labor.

But that last sentence requires elaboration and amendment. The persons within each professional group may be, and probably are, at different stages in their respective careers. Furthermore, the career lines of some may be quite different from those of their colleagues: thus some of our psychiatrists were just entering upon psychoanalytic training, but some had entered the medical specialty by way of neurology, and had dual neurological-psychiatric practices. Implicit in the preceding statement is that those who belong to the same profession also may differ quite measurably in the training they have received, as well as in the theoretical (or ideological) positions they take toward important issues like etiology and treatment. Finally, the hospital itself may possess differential significance for colleagues: for instance, some psychiatrists were engaged in hospital practice only until such time as their office practices had been sufficiently well established; while other, usually older, psychiatrists were committed wholeheartedly to working with hospitalized patients.

Looking next at the division of labor shared by the professionals: never do all persons of each echelon work closely with all others from other echelons. At our hospital it was notable that considerable variability characterized who worked closely with whom—and how—depending upon such matters as ideological and hierarchical position. Thus the services of the social worker were used not at all by some psychiatrists, while each man who utilized her services did so somewhat differently. Similarly some men utilized "psychologicals" more than did others. Similarly, some psychiatrists were successful in housing their patients almost exclusively upon certain wards, which meant that, wittingly or not, they worked only with certain nurses. As in other institutions, the various echelons possessed differential status and power, but again there were marked internal differences concerning status and power, as well as knowledgeability about "getting things done." Nor must it be overlooked that not only did the different professions hold measurably different views—derived both from professional and status positions—about the proper division of labor; but different views also obtained within echelon. (The views were most discrepant among the psychiatrists.) All in all, the division of labor is a complex concept, and at hospitals must be seen in relation to the professionalized milieu.

Ruled and Unruled Behavior

The rules that govern the actions of various professionals, as they perform their tasks, are far from extensive, or clearly stated or clearly binding. This fact leads to necessary and continual negotiation. It will be worth deferring discussion of negotiation per se until we have explored some relationships between rules and negotiation, at least as found in our hospital; for the topic of rules is a complicated one.

In Michael Reese, as unquestionably in most sizable establishments, hardly anyone knows all the extant rules, much less exactly what situations they apply to, for whom, and with what sanctions. If this would not otherwise be so in our hospital, it would be true anyway because of the considerable turnover of nursing staff. Also noticeable—to us as observers—was that some rules once promulgated would fall into disuse, or would periodically receive administrative reiteration after the staff had either ignored those rules or forgotten them. As one head nurse said, "I wish they would write them all down sometimes"—but said so smilingly. The plain fact is that staff kept forgetting not only the rules received from above but also some rules that they themselves had agreed upon "for this ward." Hence we would observe that periodically the same informal ward rules would be agreed upon, enforced for a short time, and then be forgotten until another ward crisis would elicit their innovation all over again.

As in other establishments, personnel called upon certain rules to obtain what they themselves wished. Thus the nurses frequently acted as virtual guardians of the hospital against some demands of certain attending physicians, calling upon the resources of "the rules of the hospital" in countering the physicians' demands. As in other hospital settings, the physicians were only too aware of this game, and accused the nurses from time to time of more interest in their own welfare than in that of the patients'. (The only difference, we suspect, between the accusatory language of psychiatrists and that of internists or surgeons is that the psychiatrists have a trained capacity to utilize specialized terms like "rigid" and "overcompulsive.") In so dredging up the rules at convenient moments, the staff of course is acting identically with personnel in other kinds of institutions.

As elsewhere, too, all categories of personnel are adept at breaking the rules when it suits convenience or when warrantable exigencies arise. Stretching the rules is only a further variant of this tactic, which itself is less attributable to human nature than to an honest desire to get things accomplished as they ought, properly, to get done.[3] Of course, respective parties must strike bargains for these actions to occur.

In addition, at the very top of the administrative structure, a tolerant stance is taken both toward extensiveness of rules and laxity of rules. The point can be illustrated by a conversation with the administrative head, who recounted with amusement how some members of his original house staff wished to have all rules set down in a house rule book, but he had staved off this codification. As will be noted more fully later, the administrative attitude is affected also by a profound belief that care of patients calls for a minimum of hard and fast rules and a maximum of innovation and improvisation. In addition, in this hospital, as certainly in most others, the multiplicity of medical purpose and theory, as well as of personal investment, are openly recognized: too rigid a set of rules would only cause turmoil and affect the hospital's over-all efficiency.

Finally, it is notable that the hospital must confront the realities of the attending staff's negotiations with patients and their families—negotiations carried out beyond the physical confines of the hospital itself. Too many or too rigid rules would restrict the medical entrepreneurs' negotiation. To some degree any hospital with attending men has to give this kind of leeway (indeed, the precise degree is a source of tension in these kinds of hospitals).

Hence, the area of action covered directly by clearly enunciated rules is really very small. As observers, we began to become aware of this when, within a few days, we discovered that only a few very general rules obtained for the placement of new patients within the hospital. Those rules, which are clearly enunciated and generally followed, can, for our purposes, be regarded as long-standing shared understandings among the personnel. Except for a few legal rules, which stem from state and professional prescription, and for some rulings pertaining to all of Michael Reese Hospital, almost all these house rules are much less like commands, and much more like general understandings: not even their punishments are spelled out; and mostly they can be stretched, negotiated, argued, as well as ignored or applied at convenient moments. Hospital rules seem to us frequently less explicit than tacit, probably as much breached and stretched as honored, and administrative effort is made to keep their number small. In addition, rules here as elsewhere fail to be universal prescriptions: they always require judgment concerning their applicability to the specific case. Does it apply here? To whom? In what degree? For how long? With what sanctions? The personnel cannot give universal answers; they can only point to past analogous instances when confronted with situations or give "for instance" answers, when queried about a rule's future application.

The Grounds for Negotiation

Negotiation and the division of labor are rendered all the more complex because personnel in our hospital—we assume that the generalization, with some modification, holds elsewhere—share only a single, vaguely ambiguous goal. The goal is to return patients to the outside world in better shape. This goal is the symbolic cement that, metaphorically speaking, holds the organization together: the symbol to which all personnel can comfortably, and frequently point—with the assurance that at *least* about this matter everyone can agree! Although this symbol, as will be seen later, masks a considerable measure of disagreement and discrepant purpose, it represents a generalized mandate under which the hospital can be run—the public flag under which all may work in concert. Let us term it the institution's constitutional grounds or basic compact. These grounds, this compact, are never openly challenged; nor are any other goals given explicit verbal precedence. (This is so when a hospital, such as ours, also is a training institution.) In addition, these constitutional grounds can be used by any and all personnel as a justificatory rationale for actions that are under attack. In short, although personnel may disagree to the point of apoplexy about how to implement patients' getting better, they do share the common institutional value.

The problem, of course, is that when the personnel confront a specific patient and attempt to make him recover, then the disagreements flare up—the generalized mandate helps not at all to handle the specific issues—and a complicated process of negotiation, of bargaining, of give-and-take necessarily begins. The disagreements that necessitate negotiation do not occur by chance, but are patterned. Here are several illustrations of the grounds that lead to negotiation. Thus, the personnel may disagree over what is the proper placement within the hospital for some patient: believing that, at any given time, he is more likely to improve when placed upon one ward rather than upon another. This issue is the source of considerable tension between physicians and ward personnel. Again, what is meant by "getting better" is itself open to differential judgment when applied to the progress—or retrogression—of a particular patient. This judgment is influenced not only by professional experience and acquaintance with the patient but is also influenced by the very concept of getting better as held by the different echelons. Thus the aides—who are laymen—have quite different notions about these matters than do the physicians, and on the whole those notions are not quite equivalent to those held by nurses. But both the nurses and the aides see patients getting better according to signs visible from the patient's daily behavior, while the psychiatrist tends to relate these signs, if apprehended at all, to deeper layers of personality; with the consequence that frequently the staff thinks one way about the patient's "movement" while the physician thinks quite otherwise, and must argue his case, set them right, or even keep his peace.

To turn now to another set of conditions for negotiation: the very mode of treatment selected by the physician is profoundly related to his own psychiatric ideology. For instance, it makes a difference whether the physician is neurologically trained, thus somatically oriented, or whether he is psychotherapeutically trained and oriented. The former type of physician will prescribe more drugs, engage in far more electric shock therapy, and spend much less time with each patient. On occasion the diagnosis and treatment of a given patient runs against the judgment of the nurses and aides, who may not go along with the physician's directives, who may or may not disagree openly. They may subvert his therapeutic program by one of their own. They may choose to argue the matter. They may go over his head to an administrative officer. Indeed, they have many choices of action—each requiring negotiative behavior. In truth, while physicians are able to command considerable obedience to their directives at this particular hospital, frequently they must work hard at obtaining cooperation in their programing. The task is rendered all the more difficult because they, as professionals, see matters in certain lights, while the aides, as laymen, may judge matters quite differently—on moral rather than on strictly psychiatric grounds, for instance.

If negotiation is called for because a generalized mandate requires implementation, it is also called for because of the multiplicity of purpose found in the hospital. It is incontestable that each professional group has a different set of reasons for working at this hospital (to begin with, most nurses are women, most physicians are men); and of course colleagues inevitably differ among themselves on certain of their purposes for working there. In addition, each professional develops there his own specific and temporally limited ends that he wishes to attain. All this diversity of purpose affects the institution's division of labor, including not only what tasks each person is expected to accomplish but also how he maneuvers to get them accomplished. Since very little of this can possibly be prefigured by the administrative rule-makers, the attainment of one's purposes requires inevitably the cooperation of fellow workers. This point, once made, scarcely needs illustration.

However, yet another ground of negotiation needs emphasizing: namely, that in this hospital, as doubtless elsewhere, the patient as an "individual case" is taken as a virtual article of faith. By this we mean that the element of medical uncertainty is so great, and each patient is taken as—in some sense—so unique, that action round and about him must be tailor-made, must be suited to his precise therapeutic requirements. This kind of assumption abets what would occur anyhow: that only a minimum of rules can be laid down for running a hospital, since a huge area of contingency necessarily lies outside those rules. The rules can provide guidance and command for only a small amount of the total concerted action that must go on around the patient. It follows, as already noted, that where action is not ruled it must be agreed upon.

One important further condition for negotiation should be mentioned. Changes are forced upon the hospital and its staff not only by forces external to the hospital but also by unforeseen consequences of internal policies and negotiations carried on within the hospital. In short, negotiations breed further negotiations.

Lay Personnel and Negotiated Order

Before turning to certain important features of negotiation, we shall first discuss the impact of laymen—both personnel and patients—upon the hospital's negotiated order. A special feature of most hospitals is that, although administered and controlled by professionals, they also include among their personnel considerable numbers of nonprofessionals. This they must, for only in the most affluent establishments could floors be staffed wholly with professionals. The nonprofessionals set special problems for the establishment and maintenance of orderly medical process.

To suggest how subtle and profound may be the lay influence, we give the following illustration as it bears upon negotiated order. The illustration pertains to the central value of our hospital: returning patients to the outside world in better shape than when they entered. Like everyone else, the aides subscribe to this institutional goal. A host of communications, directed at them, inform them that they too are important in "helping patients get better." Yet none of the professionals ascribe an unduly important role to the aides: in the main, aides are considered quite secondary to the therapeutic process. The aides do not agree. They do not contest the point, because in fact the point does not arise explicitly: yet our own inquiry left no doubt that most aides conceive themselves as the principal agent for bringing about improvement in most patients. The grounds of their belief, in capsule form, are as follows:

Working extensively with or near the patients, they are more likely than other personnel to see patients acting in a variety of situations and ways. The aides reason, with some truth, that they themselves are more likely to be the recipients of patients' conversations and even confidences, because of frequent and intimate contact. They reason, with common sense, that no one else can know most of the patients as well as do the aides. ("I always know more than the nurses and the doctors. We are with the patients almost eight hours, whereas the nurses and doctors don't come in. The nurse reads the charts and passes the medicine.") With due respect to the best nurses—and some are greatly admired—nurses are too busy with their administrative work; and lazy ones just never leave the office! As for the physicians: not only do they make evident mistakes with their patients, and spend scarcely any time with them, but they must even call upon the nurses and aides for information about their patients.

Actually, aides have no difficulty in comprehending that they themselves cannot give shock treatment—only the physicians know how to do that—but we found that our aides could not, with few exceptions, make a clear distinction between what the doctor does when he helps the patient "by talking" and what they themselves do when they talk with him. Even the aides who have worked most closely with head nurses do not really comprehend that a substantial difference exists between talking and psychotherapy. Hence aides believe that everyone may contribute toward patients' improvement, by acting right toward them and talking properly with them. The most that aides will admit is: "Sometimes the patients will really talk more about their problems with the doctor than they will with us. Sometimes it's vice versa." But on the whole those who talk most with patients are the aides.

It does not take much imagination to anticipate what this view of the division of labor implies for the aides' handling of patients. However frequently the aides may attend staff meetings, however frequently they listen to psychiatrists talk about the problems of patients and how to handle patients, they end by perceiving patients in nonpsychiatric (nontechnical) terms and use their own kinds of tactics with patients. Aides guide themselves by many common-sense maxims, and are articulate about these when questioned about how they work with patients. The professional staff generally regards good aides as being very "intuitive" with patients; but aides are probably no more intuitive than anyone else; it is that their reasoning is less professionalized. Lest this seem to be a characterization of psychiatric aides alone, we hasten to add that aides on medical services seem to us to think and operate in similar ways.

Turning briefly now to how these nonprofessionals affect the processes of negotiation, one may begin by stating that, like anyone else, they wish to control the conditions of their work as much as possible. Of course, they must negotiate to make that possible: they must stake claims and counterdemands; they must engage in games of give-and-take. Among the prizes are: where one will work, the colleagues with whom one will share tasks, the superiors under whom one will work, and the kinds of patients with whom one will deal. Illustrating from one area only, that of controlling superiors: aides have various means of such control. These include withholding information and displaying varying degrees of cooperativeness in charting or in attending meetings. Aides also are implicated, as are the nurses, in negotiations with the physicians—except that the head nurse tends to carry on the necessary face-to-face bargaining. Since aides have their own notions about how specific patients should be handled and helped, they may negotiate also with the nurses in order to implement those notions. Nurses and physicians, in their turn, need to transact negotiations with the aides: while the physicians usually work through the head nurse, on occasion they may deal directly with an aide. In any event, professionals and nonprofessionals are implicated together in a great web of negotiation. It does not take much imagination to see that this world, and its negotiated order, would be different without nonprofessionals.[4] More important: unless one focuses upon the negotiated character of order, he is most unlikely to note the above kinds of consequential actions and relations.

The Patients and Negotiated Order

The patients are also engaged in bargaining, in negotiative processes. (As some public-administration theorists have put it, clients are also part of the organizational structure.) Again, a significant aspect of hospital organization is missing unless the clients' negotiation is included. They negotiate, of course, as laymen, unless they themselves are nurses or physicians.[5] Most visibly they can be seen bargaining, with the nurses and with their psychiatrists, for more extensive privileges (such as more freedom to roam the grounds); but they may also seek to affect the course and kind of treatment—including placement on given wards, amounts of drugs, and even choice of psychiatrist, along with the length of stay in the hospital itself. Intermittently, but fairly continually, they are concerned with their ward's orderliness, and make demands upon the personnel—as well as upon other patients—to keep the volume of noise down, to keep potential violence at a minimum, to rid the ward of a troublemaking patient. Sometimes the patients are as much guardians of ward order as are the nurses, who are notorious for this concern in our hospital. (Conversely, the nursing personnel must also seek to reach understandings and agreements with specific patients; but sometimes these are even collective, as when patients pitch in to help with a needy patient, or as when an adolescent clique has to be dealt with "as a bunch.")

An unexpected dividend awaits anyone who focuses upon the patients' negotiations. An enriched understanding of their individual sick careers—to the hospital, inside it, and out of it —occurs. In the absence of a focus upon negotiation, ordinarily these careers tend to appear overly regularized (as in Parsons)[6] or destructive (as in Goffman).[7] When patients are closely observed "operating around" the hospital, they will be seen negotiating not only for privileges but also for precious information relevant to their own understandings of their illness. We need only add that necessarily their negotiations will differ at various stages of their sick careers.

What William Caudill [8] and Erving Goffman have written of as patient culture is roughly equivalent to the demands and expectations of the patients; but their accounts require much supplementation by a conception of patients entering, like everyone else, into the over-all negotiative process. How demands and claims will be made and met, by whom, and in what manner—as well as who will make given demands and claims upon them, how, and in what manner—are of utmost importance for understanding the hospital's structure. When patients are long-term or chronic, then their impact upon structure is more obvious to everyone concerned; but even in establishments with speedy turnover, patients are relevant to the social order.

Patterned and Temporal Features of Negotiation

To do justice to the complexity of negotiative processes would require far more space than can be allowed here. For present purposes, it should be sufficient to note only a few aspects. In our hospital, as elsewhere, the various physicians institute programs of treatment and care for their patients. Programming involves a mobilization and organization of action around the patient (and usually involves the patient's cooperation, even in the psychiatric milieu). Some physicians in our hospital had reached long-standing understandings with certain head nurses, so that only a small amount of communication was necessary to effectuate their treatment programs. Thus a somatically oriented psychiatrist typically would attempt to get his patients to those two wards where most electric-shock treatment was carried out; and the nurse administrators there understood quite well what was expected in handling "their type of patients." It was as if the physician were to say "do the usual things" (they sometimes did)—little additional instruction being needed. We ourselves coined the term "house special" (as opposed to "à la carte") treatment, to indicate that a patient could be assigned to these wards and handled by the ward staff without the physician either giving special instructions or asking for special favors. However, an original period of coaching the nurses and of reaching understandings was necessary. Consequently when personnel leave, for vacations or permanently, then arrangements must be instituted anew. Even with house-special treatment, some discussion will be required, since not every step of the patient's treatment can be imagined ahead of time. The nurses are adept (as in nonpsychiatric hospitals) at eliciting informa-

tion from the physician about his patient; they are also adept
both in forcing and fostering agreements about action vis-à-vis
his patient. We have watched many a scene where the nurse
negotiates for such understandings, as well as many staff meetings that the nurses and aides consciously convert into agencies
for bringing recalcitrant physicians to terms. When physicians
choose, they can be equally concerned with reaching firm agreements and understandings.

It is important that one realize that these agreements do not
occur by chance, nor are they established between random
parties. They are, in the literal sense of the word, patterned.
Thus, the somatically oriented physicians have long-standing
arrangements with a secretary who is attached to the two
wards upon which their patients tend to be housed; this secretary does a variety of jobs necessitated by these physicians'
rather medical orientation. The more psychotherapeutically
minded physicians scarcely utilize her services. Similarly, the
head nurses and the administrative residents attached to each
ward reach certain kinds of understandings and agreements,
which neither tends to establish with any other type of personnel. These latter agreements are less in evidence when the
resident is new; then the nurse in some helplessness turns to
the next highest administrative officer, making yet other contracts. Again, when an attending physician is especially recalcitrant, both resident and nurse's aide seek to draw higher
administrators into the act, negotiating for support and increased
power. This kind of negotiation occurs with great predictability:
for instance, certain physicians because of their particular philosophies of treatment use the hospital in certain ways; consequently, their programs are frequently troublesome for the
house staff, who must then seek to spin a network of negotiation around the troublesome situation. When the ward is in
high furor, then negotiative activity of course is at its most
visible!

In sum: there is a patterned variability of negotiation in the
hospital pertaining to who contracts with whom, about what, as
well as when these agreements are made. Influencing this variability are hierarchical position and ideological commitments,

as well as periodicities in the structure of ward relationships (for instance, because of a rotational system that moves personnel periodically on and off given wards).

It is especially worth emphasizing that negotiation—whether characterized as "agreement," "understanding," "contract," "compact," "pact," or by some other term—has a temporal aspect, whether that aspect is stated specifically or not by the contracting parties. As one listens to agreements being made in the hospital, or watches understandings being established, he becomes aware that a specific termination period, or date line, is often written into the agreement. Thus a physician after being accosted by the head nurse—who may in turn also be responding to her own personnel—may agree to move his patient to another ward after this specific ward has agreed "to try for two more days." What he is doing is issuing to its personnel a promissory note that if things don't work out satisfactorily, he will move his patient. Sometimes the staff breaks the contract, if the patient is especially obstreperous or if tempers are running especially high, and transfers the patient to another ward behind the back of the physician. However, if the patient does sufficiently better, the ward's demands may subside. Or interestingly, it often happens that later both sides will negotiate further, seeking some compromise: the staff, for instance, wishing to restrict the patient's privileges or to give him stronger drug prescriptions, and the physician giving in on these issues to gain some ends of his own. On less tender and less specific grounds, the physician and the head nurse may reach nodding agreement that a new patient should be handled in certain ways "until we see how he responds." Thus there exists a continuum running from specific to quite nonspecific termination dates. But even those explicit and long-term permissions that physicians give to nurses in all hospitals—such as to administer certain drugs at night without bothering to call upon the physicians—are subject to review and withdrawal along with later qualified assent.

It should be added that the very terms "agreements" and "understandings" and "arrangements"—all used by hospital personnel—point up that some negotiations may be made with

full explicitness, while others may be established by parties
who have scarcely talked. The more implicit or tacit kinds of
contracts tend to be called "understandings." The difference can
be high-lighted by the following contrasting situations: when
a resident suggests to a nurse that an established house rule
temporarily be ignored, for the good of a given patient, it may
be left implicit in their arrangement that he must bear the
punishment if administration discovers their common infraction.
But the nurse may make this clause more explicit by demanding
that he bear the possible public guilt, otherwise she will not
agree to the matter. It follows that some agreements can be
both explicit and specific as to termination, while others are
explicit but nonspecific as to termination, and so on. What might
be referred to as "tacit understandings" are likely to be those
that are neither very specific nor very explicitly discussed.
When a physician is not trusted, the staff is likely to push him
for explicit directives with specific termination clauses.

Negotiation, Appraisal, and Organizational Change

We come now to the full import of the above discussion, for
it raises knotty problems about the relationships that exist between the current negotiated order and genuine organizational
change. Since agreements are patterned and temporal, today's
sum total of agreements can be visualized as different from
tomorrow's—and surely as quite different from next week's.
The hospital can be visualized as a place where numerous agreements are continually being terminated or forgotten, but also
as continually being established, renewed, reviewed, revoked,
revised. Hence at any moment those that are in effect are considerably different from those that were or will be.

Now a skeptic, thinking in terms of relatively permanent or
slowly changing structure, might remark that from week to
week the hospital remains the same—that only the working
arrangements change. This contention only raises the further

question of what relationship exists between today's working agreements and the more stable structure (of rules, statuses, and so on).

With an eye on practicality, one might maintain that no one knows what the hospital "is" on any given day unless he has a comprehensive grasp of what combination of rules and policies, along with agreements, understandings, pacts, contracts, and other working arrangements, currently obtains. In any pragmatic sense, this is the hospital at the moment: this is its social order. Any changes that impinge upon this order—whether something ordinary like a new staff member, a disrupting event, a betrayed contract; or whether unusual, like the introduction of a new technology or a new theory—will call for renegotiation or reappraisal, with consequent changes in the organizational order. Mark the last phrase—a new order, not the reestablishment of an old, a reinstituting of a previous equilibrium. This is what we remarked upon earlier as the necessity for continually reconstituting the bases of concerted action, or social order.

That reconstituting of social order, we would hazard, can be fruitfully conceived in terms of a complex *relationship between the daily negotiative process and a periodic appraisal process.* The former not only allows the daily work to get done; it also reacts back upon the more formalized—and permanent—rules and policies. Further elaboration of this point will follow, but first the following illustration taken from our field notes should be helpful. For some time the hospital had been admitting an increased number of nonpaying adolescent patients, principally because they made good supervisory subjects for the residents. As a consequence, the hospital began to get the reputation of becoming more interested in adolescents than previously; also, some attending physicians were encouraged to bring adolescents for treatment to the hospital. Their presence on the wards raised many new problems, and led to feverish negotiative activity among the various actors implicated in the daily drama. Finally, after some months of high saturation with an adolescent population, a middle-level administrative committee formally recognized what was happening to the institution. The committee recognized it primarily because the adolescents, in the mass, were much harder to handle than an equal number of adults. Yet the situation had its compensatory aspects, since adolescents remained longer and could be given more interesting types of therapy. After some debate, the committee decided that no more adolescent patients would be admitted after an additional stated number had been reached. The decision constituted a formal proclamation, with the proviso that if the situation continued, the policy should be reviewed at high administrative levels in light of "where the institution was going." The decision was never enforced, for shortly thereafter the adolescent census dropped and never rose again to such dangerous heights. The decision has long since been forgotten, and if the census were again to rise dangerously, doubtless a new discussion would take place rather than an evocation of the old rule.

But this is precisely how more long-standing policy and many rules become established in what conventionally is called "hospital structure." In turn, of course, the policies and rules serve to set the limits and some of the directions of negotiation. (This latter proposition is implicit in much of our foregoing discussion on rules and negotiation as well as the patterning of negotiation.) We suggest that future studies of complex relationships existing between the more stable elements of organizational order and the more fleeting working arrangements may profit by examining the former as if they were sometimes a background against which the latter were being evolved in the foreground—and sometimes as if the reverse obtained. What is needed is both a concentrated focus upon, and the development of a terminology adequate to handle, this kind of metaphor. But whether this metaphor or another, the question of how negotiation and appraisal play into each other, and into the rules or policies, remains central.

Summary and Implications

As remarked at the outset of this paper, the reader must judge for himself whether a model possibly suited to studying psychiatric hospitals might equally guide study and understanding of other types of hospitals. The model presented has pictured the hospital as a locale where personnel, mostly but not exclusively professionals, are enmeshed in a complex negotiative process in order both to accomplish their individual purposes and to work—in an established division of labor—toward clearly as well as vaguely phrased institutional objectives. We have sought to show how differential professional training, ideology, career, and hierarchical position all affect the negotiation; but we have also attempted to show how nonprofessionals may affect the total process. We have outlined important relationships between daily working arrangements and the more permanent structure.

We would argue that this mode of viewing hospitals can be very useful. One reason is that it directs attention to the interplay of professionals and nonprofessionals—*as* professionals and nonprofessionals rather than just in terms of hierarchical position. It forces attention also upon the transactions of professionals, among echelons and within echelons. Properly carried out, the approach will not permit, as in many studies, a focus upon the hospital without cognizance of how the outside world impinges upon what is going on within the hospital: a single hospital, after all, is only a point through which multiple careers stream—including the patients' careers. As suggested in the opening page, the approach also pins one's gaze upon processes of change, and of stability also, providing one assumes that "no change" must be worked at within the organization. Among other considerations, it allows focus upon important internal occurrences under the impact of external pressures as well as of internal changes within the establishment. Whatever the purely specific characteristics of psychiatric hospitals as compared with nonpsychiatric ones, it is evident that most of the latter share certain features that make them amenable to our approach. Hospitals are evolving as institutions—and rapidly. They are locales where many different kinds of professionals work—and more are joining the ranks. The very heterogeneity of personnel and of professional purpose, along with the impact of a changing medical technology, bespeaks the kind of world sketched above.[9]

But what of other organizations, especially if sizable or complex—is this kind of interactional model also relevant to them? The answer, we suggest, is strongly in the affirmative. Current preoccupation with formal organization tends to underplay—or leave implicit—the interactional features underscored in the foregoing pages.[10] Yet one would expect interactional features to jump into visibility once looked for systematically. We urge that whenever an organization possesses one or more of the following characteristics, such a search be instituted: if the organization (1) utilizes personnel trained in several different occupations, or (2) if each contains an occupational group including individuals trained in different traditions, then (3) they are likely to possess somewhat different occupational philosophies, emphasizing somewhat different values; then also (4) if at least some personnel are professionals, the latter are likely to be pursuing careers that render them mobile—that is, carrying them into and out of the organization. The reader should readily appreciate why those particular characteristics have been singled out. They are, of course, attributes of universities, corporations, and government agencies, as well as of hospitals. If an organization is marked by one or more of those characteristics, then the concept of "negotiated order" should be an appropriate way to view it.[11]

NOTES

1. "The Problem of Society—How We Become Selves," *Movements of Thought in the Nineteenth Century* (Chicago: University of Chicago Press, 1936), pp. 360-361.

2. Two psychiatric hospitals were studied, but only one will be discussed here, namely, the psychiatric wing of Michael Reese Hospital in Chicago. (The other hospital was a state mental hospital that, like most, was maintained and run, though not administered at the very top, by nonprofes-

sionals. Indeed, it is just this that causes many psychiatrists to despair of such establishments.) The psychiatric wing of Michael Reese is in a separate building, administered with considerable autonomy. It consists of five wards, altogether containing about ninety beds. The psychiatric hospital is organized for quick turnover of private patients: their average length of stay is only one month. There is a high ratio of personnel to patients, with many nurses and aides, as well as one resident administrator assigned to each ward. Over 100 men are on the attending staff, of whom about thirty use the hospital with some frequency. The hospital is well regarded both by the general and psychiatric community. It has the reputation of being a psychoanalytically-oriented establishment—many of its attending staff are analysts or analysts-in-training—but on any given day actually a considerable number, if not the majority, of patients will be those of psychiatrists not especially sympathetic to the analytic viewpoint.

3. Melville Dalton's book, *Men Who Manage* (New York: Wiley and Sons, 1959), is crammed with such instances. See especially pp. 104-107.

4. In passing, it is worth suggesting that many physicians do not regard nurses as true professionals either and that this affects their transactions with nurses. Their denial of professional status affects what they will ask a nurse to do, how they will utilize her services. Stated another way: if she believes herself to be a professional, and he either denies or is dubious about her claim, then, in common parlance, "there will be problems." It happens to be one of the most common problems in American hospitals, as many nurses, at least, know.

5. In all hospital settings, when the latter appear the situation becomes, as the staff says, "complicated"—complicated because they make additional, or at least additionally different, demands upon the personnel.

6. Talcott Parsons and R. Fox, "Illness, Therapy, and the Modern Urban American Family," *Journal of Social Issues*, 7 (1952), pp. 31-44.

7. Erving Goffman, "The Moral Career of the Mental Patient," *Psychiatry*, 22 (1959), pp. 123-142.

8. William Caudill *et al.*, "Social Structure and Interaction Processes on a Psychiatric Ward," *American Journal of Orthopsychiatry*, 22 (1952), pp. 314-334; Erving Goffman, "On the Characteristics of Total Institutions," *Proceedings of the Symposium on Preventive and Social Psychiatry* (Washington, D.C.: Walter Reed Army Institute of Research, 1957).

9. Without drawing the same conclusions, W. S. Sayre, a professor of public administration, has suggested similar features of modern hospitals: "In the health and medical professions together in a hospital these stresses between *organization* and *profession* are made the more complex by a multiplicity of professions, a multiplicity of values and perspectives not easily reconciled into a harmonious organization. . . . The hospital would seem to be an organizational setting where many semi-autonomous cooperators meet for the purpose of using common services and facilities and to provide services to each other, but in a loosely integrated organizational system." See his "Principles of Administration," *Hospitals* (January 16 and February 1, 1956).

10. Dalton, *op. cit.*, has made the same criticism of this literature.

11. Julius Roth's yet unpublished research on tuberculosis hospitals similarly emphasizes negotiation, although he is less concerned with social order.

6

Patterns of Bureaucracy among Hospital Staff Physicians

MARY E. W. GOSS

This paper approaches the study of physicians on hospital staffs within the framework of the sociology of bureaucracy and the professions. That framework contains a rich variety of problems for research and analysis, not the least of which stem from an apparent incompatibility between bureaucratic and professional norms. Accordingly, after a brief review of norms that conflict in principle, attention is here focused on how, in practice, reconciliation may take place through structural mechanisms that minimize strain. The resulting organization of professionals is characterized in terms that utilize and extend Gouldner's

---

Much of the present essay was first presented as part of a report by the author entitled "Physicians in Bureaucracy: A Case Study of Professional Pressures on Organizational Roles," unpublished Ph.D. dissertation, Columbia University, 1959. For valuable aid in analyzing the problems under review I am indebted to Robert K. Merton, George G. Reader, Hans L. Zetterberg, and Charles R. Wright. David Caplovitz generously made available unpublished survey data from his own investigation of physicians ("Student-Faculty Relations in Medical School: A Study of Professional Socialization," unpublished Ph.D. dissertation, Columbia University, 1961).

classification of bureaucratic patterns, and problems for further research are considered.

Throughout, the propositions advanced represent provisional hypotheses of limited scope in that they refer specifically to the formal organization of authority and the division of labor among physicians, and are based primarily though not exclusively on empirical examination of the situation of physicians on the staff of a single large teaching hospital in the United States.[1] Other patterns might well prevail in different types of hospitals and in different countries. Nevertheless, the propositions direct attention to a somewhat murky aspect of the organization and functioning of hospitals, and simultaneously invite investigation in the various settings where professionals work.

Bureaucracy and the Professional

The type of organization that Max Weber [2] described as bureaucracy has long appeared to be at odds with the work requirements, norms, and values of professionals. Weber's conception of bureaucracy is well known; in brief, it is a rational, efficient organization of statuses, characterized by hierarchical authority, division of labor on the basis of specialized competence, systematic rules, and impersonality.[3]

The professional, however, is a recognized master of a particular body of knowledge and practice as a result of prolonged and specialized intellectual training, and he is committed to using his knowledge and skills in accordance with standards set by the profession to which he belongs.[4] Far from condoning the hierarchical authority roles characteristic of bureaucracy, the work norms of professionals emphasize self-government for the profession as a whole and autonomy for each practitioner within the limits laid down by the profession. Further, hard-and-fast bureaucratic rules that apply to all alike do not allow for dealing with the exceptional case, and it is precisely the exceptional case that professionals, more than many other occupational groups, are likely to encounter in the course of their work. While the professional is enjoined to treat all alike according to need, and in this sense to be impersonal and to abide by general rules, his impersonality must always be conditioned by his judgment as to the needs of the particular case under consideration; the "rules" he must take into account are those of the profession rather than of any particular bureaucracy. Only in the realm of specialization and the division of labor does there seem to be agreement between bureaucratic standards and professional norms; as specialists themselves, professionals are committed to the division of labor according to specialized competence. However, as has been indicated, they are also committed to self-government, and therefore they may set aside the requirement of trained, specialized competence in the case of administrative activity.

Taking note of such contradictions as well as of the growing number of professionals who work in apparently bureaucratic contexts, students of the professions have repeatedly stressed the need for empirical research to determine the kinds of adjustments or alternative tensions that occur when the two are confronted.[5]

In considering the kinds of adjustments or tensions that may ensue, what has been learned in other contexts has been less often stressed. Recent research in the sociology of complex organization [6] indicates that actual patterns of bureaucratic structure and operation are less rigid and more variable than the ideal type Weber outlined and that his conception of bureaucracy needs to be extended accordingly. Similarly, research in the sociology of the professions [7] suggests that there are wider ranges of permissible behavior open to professional persons than might be assumed from their ethical codes or public statements. Together, the two sets of observations imply that there may be somewhat more room for mutual adjustment of professional norms and bureaucratic standards than has generally been supposed.

Studies that specifically investigate this possibility are not plentiful.[8] No doubt partly because of the nature of the particular cases examined, available analyses and studies have tended to focus either on the professional *or* on the organizational structure as the major site for adjustments or tensions. Thus, for example, Merton,[9] Field,[10] Wilensky,[11] and Ben-David [12] have paid primary attention to the impact of bureaucratic requirements on professional norms, values, and behavior. Parsons,[13] Wilson,[14] and others,[15] however, have reversed this focus and attended more to the problem of how the professional's demands may affect the over-all network of roles that constitutes bureaucratic organization. Neither approach logically excludes the other, of course, and it is not unreasonable to assume that both are ultimately required for adequate understanding of the issue under consideration.

Professional Medical Staff as an Object of Study

With specific reference to the professional group this paper concerns—physicians—several recent sociological investigations of American hospitals [16] explicitly or implicitly suggest that in such a setting physicians affect the organizational structure more than they are affected by it. These investigations indicate that, while physicians are not generally employed by the hospital, they are functionally necessary for the hospital's continued operation; though they are ordinarily "production" workers rather than administrators, by virtue of their profession they enjoy higher prestige than those in other occupations who may officially operate the hospital; and even though physicians hold staff positions that are nominally outside the line organization of authority in the hospital, their qualifications as medical experts enable them to exert influence and authority with regard to the behavior of all levels of hospital personnel. They are, in other words, in a strategic position to enforce their professional demands, and it would seem that the burden of adjustment—or its alternative, unresolved tension—consequently falls heavily on their co-workers in the hospital: nurses, technicians, administrators, trustees, and other personnel. As Harvey Smith [17] has remarked, the formally bureaucratic structure of hospitals actually involves "built-in conflicts," with physicians and their professional norms more often than not emerging the victors.[18]

Such findings turn attention to the structure of the hospital's professional medical staff itself as a fruitful area for inquiry, and to organizational arrangements in which physicians are formally responsible for supervision and coordination of the work of other physicians. There are few empirical sociological studies of this kind of situation,[19] yet there is reason to believe they would provide valuable information for students of the professions and of complex organization alike. For in such instances the factor of professional medical training, together with the prestige and authority it entails relative to other occupations, is automatically held constant, with the result that differences in this regard cannot be utilized to explain or account for the nature of the structure (as they have been in the case of the hospital as a whole). The mutual impact of professional norms and organizational requirements can therefore be examined in fairly "pure" form; adjustments or tensions that are inherent in the supervision and coordination of professional work can be singled out from those that are merely artifacts of lay persons' attempts to control the activities of experts.

Precisely because a professional medical staff is occupationally homogeneous, it might be expected that their organizational role relationships would exhibit more adjustments than tensions [20] and that professional norms would dictate organizational roles. But it would be a mistake to assume that no adjustments need occur or that the norms that govern physicians' intraprofessional relationships in private practice will find their exact counterpart in an organizational setting. As Wilson has indicated with respect to the organization of teachers in American universities, the sheer facts of size and the need for coordination of many complex activities make complete individualism and autonomy on the part of each professional impossible.[21] And regarding physicians who work in bureaucratic settings, both Field [22] and Ben-David [23] present evidence that suggests that under certain circumstances organizational pressures play an important part in molding the roles of these professionals. Studying a group of physicians employed by the Sick Fund of the General Federation of Labor in Israel, Ben-David found that "the transfer of responsibility from the individual doctor to the institution was apparently perceived by the doctors as a loss of status," [24] which in turn led to apathy with respect to the professional role or, alternatively though less frequently, to an inappropriately great emphasis on either the "service" or "science" components of the professional role in an effort to achieve higher status.[25] In Soviet Russia, as Field notes, the medical profession is currently trained by and under the direct control of the government. In deciding who is sick and who is well, who needs medical treatment and who does not, Soviet physicians must take into account the stated needs of the government for manpower. To the extent that these physicians make such decisions according to governmental dictum rather than their own professional judgment, they are plainly relinquishing their professional role obligation to render unbiased service to patients.

Nevertheless, it is the thesis of this paper that at least in large teaching hospitals in the United States, the professional norms and values of physicians set distinct limits on how organizational needs for policy-making, coordination, and supervision will be met, and thus markedly affect definition of the organizational roles of the physicians involved. Organizational pressures exist, of course, but their impact is regularly tempered by built-in professional counterpressures, to the extent that the latter appear highly significant in accounting for the nature of physicians' organizational roles. Though evidence for this thesis is largely qualitative, it bears review in the absence of more rigorous and extensive data.

Potential Strains and Mechanisms for Their Resolution

Study of physicians in a large teaching hospital [26] indicates that, where there might have been conflict between bureaucratic standards and the professional values of physicians, there were instead institutionalized structural mechanisms that served to reconcile potentially discordant elements in ways that were approved by physicians as well as functional for their work. The mechanisms also served to give the organization a distinctive character, a character of a type that Weber did not explicitly describe but that perhaps most closely approximates what Logan Wilson has called "semi-bureaucracy." (As will be suggested, this type appears to combine what Gouldner has identified as the "representative" pattern of bureaucracy as well as what will be identified here as "advisory bureaucracy.")

AUTHORITY

As is commonly believed and as was found to be the case in the teaching hospital investigated, physicians place high value on assuming personal responsibility and exercising individual authority in making professional decisions. Accordingly, their role expectations emphasize independence in the realm of professional work. The hierarchical authority structure characteristic of bureaucratic organization as delineated by Weber clearly conflicts with such role expectations, since there, in the interest of the organization as a whole, decisions are commonly subject to direction, review, and possible revision by those who hold superordinate positions in the hierarchy.

To find that physicians held positions in the hospital that were officially hierarchically organized [27] seemed, therefore, to constitute evidence for the existence of bureaucracy, and consequently for the anticipation that there would be continuing conflict or strain as a result of curtailed individual authority. Yet conflict was not apparent, and closer examination of role relationships between those who were formally superordinate and formally subordinate provided a provisional explanation.

Individual authority in making professional decisions was not curtailed, by virtue of the fact that the hierarchy of positions entailed two different types of control relationships that varied according to whether the area of work was professional or administrative in nature. Only in the realm of administration did the supervisory hierarchy refer to a set of formal *authority* relationships, that is, to the right to make decisions with which subordinates have an obligation to comply. In the realm of pro-

fessional work, the hierarchy referred to formal role relationships that are most properly termed *advisory,* that is, the right
to give advice that subordinates are obliged to take under critical review, but not necessarily to follow in making their decisions. It may be emphasized that this was not merely a matter
of differences in the phrasing of requests in the two areas, but,
at least among those who had attained the rank of assistant
resident or higher, of differences in expectations regarding compliance as well.

Formal sanctions for physicians' behavior in the hospital existed primarily in the form of possible promotion or dismissal
from the staff. Anticipated informal praise or criticism from associates and superiors, however, appeared to constitute a much
more potent force in molding the physicians' conduct. Noncom-
pliance with a suggestion offered by a supervising physician
about a professional matter generally meant, therefore, that the
responsible physician had weighed the suggestion and had concluded that, nevertheless, his own course of action would not
be open to criticism when all the relevant facts were taken into
account.

Thus with respect to the organization of authority among physicians, a major mechanism for reconciling bureaucratic standards with professional values would seem to be a dual control
system within a single hierarchy of positions. Structured authority relationships in the area of administration make coordination of effort possible and relatively predictable; structured
advisory relationships in the realm of professional work allow
systematic supervision and yet leave intact each physician's individual authority. (Formal advisory relationships do not, of
course, permit the same degree of predictability as formal
authority relationships; the former introduce an element of uncertainty that is largely absent in an effective authority relationship. However, as a later section will suggest, such relative
uncertainty and unpredictability may not be so dysfunctional for
the achievement of organizational aims as has sometimes been
thought.) A single hierarchy that encompasses both kinds of
control relationships not only tends to ensure maintenance of

professional norms and values; it also serves to reduce the likelihood of formulating conflicting policies in the two areas of work.

However, it would also seem that these control relationships cannot be effectively maintained except under certain conditions that, subject to more extensive investigation, may therefore be viewed as subsidiary mechanisms for reconciling bureaucratic standards with professional values in the realm of control.

Among these conditions, available data suggest that where *professional* supervision—that is, the formal advisory relationship —is concerned, the qualifications of those who are assigned to supervise must be taken into account, as must the supervisor's opportunity to obtain information on which to base advice. Even though the supervisor offers only advice rather than orders, in the nature of the supervisory situation (and in contrast with the consultation situation where advice is given only upon request) the supervisor's advice is often unsolicited. Regardless of the qualifications of the supervisor, physicians are likely to interpret unsolicited advice as an adverse reflection on their professional competence. Nevertheless, because they are trained to value competence and at the same time to believe that no physician is so proficient as to be right all the time or equally informed about every area of medicine, they are likely to experience supervisory advice as helpful and to review it carefully *if* they respect the supervisor as their professional peer or superior.

In the medical subculture, this means that the supervisor must first of all be a physician. But in addition to this basic qualification, commanding the respect necessary for unsolicited advice to be critically reviewed (though not necessarily followed) requires that the supervising physician be known to be at least as competent, if not more competent, in the science and art of medicine than those whom he supervises. Judging the competence of physicians is not a cut-and-dried, easily codified procedure, even when it is done by fellow physicians trained in the same medical specialty. Yet as informal interviews and survey data suggest,[28] there are certain attributes that most physicians consider important and that they regularly seem to take into account in judging the professional competence of a colleague: diagnostic skill, knowledge of medical facts as well as of therapy, and, to a lesser extent, interpersonal skills in dealing with patients.

Commanding respect as a supervisor of professional work would also seem to depend somewhat on the formal rank of the supervisor in the organization; when this is as high or higher than the ranks held by the physicians who are supervised, respect is more likely. Although there is no definite empirical evidence as to the relative significance of formal rank versus professional competence as bases for respect, it appears that in the eyes of physicians in the United States, rank may well be less important than demonstrated professional competence.[29] Finally, and quite apart from these two kinds of qualifications, the supervisor must have appropriate information that is specific to the case at hand; if he has not had the opportunity to examine personally the patient whom his advice concerns, he is in danger of losing respect unless the advice is confined to relatively routine aspects of patient care.

Because the same physicians who served as supervisors of professional work also served as administrative officers in the hospital that was studied, it was impossible to examine independently what supervisory qualifications might be necessary in order for effective control relationships to exist in the realm of administration as contrasted with professional work. However, there was some indication that formal rank is considerably more important in the administrative context than in the context of professional activity, provided the rank is held by a physician.

Although physicians consider administration to be a nonprofessional activity that requires no particular training or skill, they nevertheless recognize that seemingly administrative decisions may sometimes have close bearing on their professional work; accordingly, there is pressure toward filling administrative positions with men who can be counted on to know, understand, and abide by professional norms and values in formulating and carrying out organizational policy.[30] It may be that all such men *need* not be physicians; if they are physicians, however, it would

seem that they stand a greater chance of maintaining effective
authority relationships with the professionals under their charge,
since they tend to know "automatically" what administrators
who are nonphysicians must sometimes learn laboriously: the
probable limits of their authority in administrative matters. It
is not, in other words, so much the extent of the physician-
administrator's professional competence that secures compliance
with his administrative decisions as it is his intimate and first-
hand knowledge of the medical subculture, which usually enables him to know in advance what decisions he may make with
assurance that they will be accepted. Apparently, the more
closely the content of an administrative decision approaches the
realm of professional work and the less routine the decision is,
the greater is the demand that the decision be made by a
physician-administrator rather than by a nonphysician of the
same rank.

DIVISION OF LABOR

The demand for physicians as administrators conflicts, however, with the bureaucratic norm of dividing organizational work
on the basis of specialized competence; although the physician
is trained to be a specialist in medical knowledge and practice,
only rarely is he a trained specialist in administration. More significantly, the demand also conflicts with a professional norm, in
that to engage in administrative work represents a departure
from the professional ideal of patient-care, teaching, and research as the major types of work appropriate for a doctor.
Consequently, physicians tend to view administration as a less
prestigeful kind of work and are not, by and large, highly motivated to be administrators. Nevertheless, it would seem that
some proportion must be administrators if effective authority
relationships are to be maintained and if the value physicians
place on professional self-government is to be upheld.

They need not, however, be full-time administrators, and in
this observation lies the key to the organizational mechanism
that at least partly resolves the problem: institutionalization of
administration as a part-time occupational role for a minority

of the physicians who work on the staff, a minority who hold salaried, full-time positions. Through this arrangement, the majority of the physicians in the organization are left free to pursue more strictly professional work objectives, and the minority who do engage in administration are not thereby forced to abandon the professional work for which they were specifically trained. The latter group may, of course, face the problem of balancing their professional and administrative role obligations in terms of time.[31] But because there exist among physicians informal norms concerning the proportions of time that are appropriate to devote to each type of obligation, the existence of tensions in this respect tends to be minimized though not entirely eliminated. Further, the fact that they are salaried, full-time staff members enhances the probability that they will be motivated to live up to their administrative role obligations, although clearly other motivating forces must also be explored and taken into account.

This analysis of structural mechanisms for reconciling bureaucratic standards with professional values and norms is far from complete, based as it is on examination of selected aspects of only two areas of potential strain—authority and the division of labor—in one particular organization. Yet these areas are vital in characterizing and differentiating various types of formal organization, and thus the analysis draws attention to the problem of how to classify, in meaningful sociological terms, the kind of staff organization that has been described: a kind in which physicians apparently are not only able but willing to work without experiencing noticeable strain. The analysis also raises the problem of why this kind of staff organization does not always occur among physicians, and, more generally, among professionals in other fields who work in an organized context. These problems are considered below.

Patterns of Bureaucracy

Plainly, the staff organization described is neither a "pure" case of bureaucracy *nor* of a "company of equals." As has been suggested, professional pressures prevent the former, while organizational pressures prevent the latter. Rather, closely interwoven in the organization are both bureaucratic and egalitarian elements: hierarchical authority roles in the administrative sphere exist along with individual authority roles in the professional sphere; formal rank receives emphasis as the basis for effective control relationships in one context while professional competence is emphasized in another context; specialization and division of labor occur generally but not particularly in connection with administrative work.

Since the organization under review was academic as well as medical, it is not surprising that the net result of this interweaving appears to approximate the semibureaucratic pattern that Logan Wilson found to be more or less characteristic of faculties in American universities.[32] In outlining this type of structure, he attended mainly—though not exclusively—to the locus of control, and thus placed semibureaucracy somewhere between the "company of equals" pattern and the hierarchical authority pattern described by Weber as characteristic of bureaucracy. Recognized but given less systematic attention by Wilson were possible variations in the type of control exercised within a semibureaucratic framework, as well as the question of how such types might vary in predictable ways according to the area of work considered.[33] Yet in characterizing an organization of professionals, the present analysis suggests that these dimensions also need to be considered explicitly.

In this connection, Gouldner's analysis of patterns of bureaucracy [34] provides a useful extension of Weber's work, and though he apparently did not specifically intend it as such, of Wilson's as well. On the basis of his examination of work relationships among the personnel in an industrial plant that mined

and processed gypsum, Gouldner differentiated three patterns
of bureaucracy: "mock," "representative," and "punishment-
centered." All three types involve division of labor, a hierarchy
of positions, and rules; what distinguishes one type from another
are not these gross bureaucratic features but the relative presence
or absence of particular sets of conditions within this broad
framework. As Gouldner indicates, in mock bureaucracy rules
are neither enforced by those in superordinate positions nor
obeyed by those in subordinate positions; joint violation and
evasion of rules is buttressed by the informal sentiments of
participants; and as a consequence there is usually little conflict
between the two groups. In punishment-centered bureaucracy,
however, rules are either enforced by those in superordinate
positions or those in subordinate positions, and evaded by the
other; enforcement occurs through punishment and is supported
by the informal sentiments of either the superordinate or subordinate group; consequently relatively great tension and conflict are entailed. Finally, in representative bureaucracy rules
are both enforced by those in superordinate positions and obeyed
by those in subordinate positions; there is joint support for the
rules, buttressed by informal sentiments, mutual participation,
initiation, and education of those in both groups; and as a
result a few tensions but little overt conflict occur.[35]

In discussing the relative prevalence of the representative pattern as compared with the punishment-centered pattern, Gouldner suggests that "it may be wise to adopt the working hypothesis
that representative bureaucracy in industrial settings operates
in a 'social space' whose contours, opportunities, and barriers
are defined and shaped by punishment-centered bureaucracy."[36]
It may, however, be equally wise to apply this hypothesis in
reverse to academic and other professional work settings. For
of the three types, it is representative bureaucracy that, more
than the other two, appears to specify further what Wilson meant
by a semibureaucratic pattern and, at the same time, to portray
in part the sort of organization that has been outlined here.[37]
In addition, however, to anticipating that representative bureaucracy will be more prevalent among professionals than will the

punishment-centered type, the co-existence and relatively high prevalence among professionals of a fourth type of pattern—*advisory bureaucracy*—is proposed.

This type does not involve, as do the three outlined by Gouldner, organizational "rules" that are "enforced" or "unenforced" by those in charge, or that are "obeyed" or "evaded" by those in subordinate positions. Rather than rules, specific technical knowledge and guiding principles for the application of this knowledge represent the content-focus of advisory bureaucracy. Further, in advisory bureaucracy the counterpart of enforcement of rules is the formal obligation of those in superordinate positions to give advice based on technical knowledge, while the counterpart of obedience is the obligation of those in subordinate positions to take such advice under critical review when making relevant decisions. If, after critical review, the recipient of advice chooses not to follow the advice, he nevertheless remains an organizational member in good standing; so long as he can justify his contrary decisions in terms of appropriate technical knowledge and principles he is neither punished nor viewed as in need of further education.

The advisory pattern is bureaucratic, however, in that it entails a formal hierarchy of positions as well as impersonality; other things being equal, precedence in the hierarchy rather than friendship confers the right to give unsolicited advice. The advisory pattern is specifically similar to *representative* bureaucracy in that it is apparently responsible for some tensions but little conflict between those in charge and those in subordinate positions. Factors associated with the avoidance of conflict would also seem to be similar to those that Gouldner suggests [38] are involved in representative bureaucracy. That is, the body of technical knowledge and principles for application are shared by both groups and legitimated by their values; the advisory relationship does not violate either group's values; deviance from accepted technical principles is viewed as correctable through education instead of punishment, since it is seen as a result of ignorance or accident rather than willful error; and finally, such deviance impairs the status of both superordinates and subordinates, while conformity to the principles either maintains or improves the status of both.[39]

In short, the advisory pattern has much in common with the representative pattern as far as certain hypothesized social and cultural antecedents, correlates, and consequences are concerned. Indeed, there is reason to believe that in organizations of professionals, the two patterns may necessarily supplement each other. Gouldner, however, was not faced with an organization composed primarily of professionals, but rather with an organization in which trained experts were few and unusual. In outlining bureaucratic patterns, therefore, he understandably did not dwell on the possibility of a formal hierarchy of influence that might parallel and be functionally associated with a formal hierarchy of authority.

To suggest that there is a type of bureaucratic pattern that involves neither hierarchical authority nor specific rules may appear to be a contradiction in terms, in that, following Weber, these features have often been considered defining characteristics of bureaucratic organization. However, the bureaucracy that Weber describes is an ideal type, which, as Blau has cogently pointed out,

includes not only definitions of concepts but also generalizations about the relationships between them, specifically the hypothesis that the diverse bureaucratic characteristics increase administrative efficiency. Whether strict hierarchical authority, for example, in fact furthers efficiency is a question of empirical fact and not one of definition.[40]

On the basis of such reasoning, the advisory pattern here outlined qualifies for at least provisional inclusion as one of the complex sets of factors that may, under certain circumstances, promote efficiency in achieving organizational aims.[41]

Certainly, it has not been empirically demonstrated that the pattern is *in*efficient, especially in organizations such as universities, hospitals, and research units, where the presence of professionals is required in order to fulfill adequately the organization's objectives. More generally, the *organizational* functions and dysfunctions of the advisory pattern remain largely unexplored, and it is only in the light of empirical investigation of these matters that sound conclusions could be drawn concerning the pattern's efficiency or inefficiency.

Thus whether the pattern is called a type of bureaucracy, an aspect of semibureaucracy, or something else entirely would seem to be less important, in the long run, than its identification as a probable characteristic of professional staff organization whose prevalence, antecedents, correlates, and consequences require further empirical research and analysis. In this respect, comparative studies of organized professional staffs are clearly necessary, and inquiry concerning functional and dysfunctional consequences of the pattern for the professionals themselves, for their nonprofessional work associates, for their clients, and for the over-all organization in which they work is particularly desirable.

The Problem of Explanation

Comparative studies are also necessary in order to clarify the conditions that determine whether one or another type of organizational pattern will prevail among physicians as well as among other professionals. How does it happen, for example, that both advisory and representative bureaucracy were institutionalized among the physicians on the hospital staff that has been described here, while among physicians in Soviet Russia these patterns were evidently considerably less prevalent than punishment-centered bureaucracy? What conditions explain the variety of patterns that, according to Logan Wilson, organizations of academicians may display? Obviously, this problem is closely related to the problem of accounting for the differential impact that professional norms and values may have in shaping the organizational roles of professionals. Why, for instance, were professional pressures effective in the present instance and, apparently, not so effective in the Sick Fund of the General Federation of Labor in Israel? More generally, if it can be assumed that, by reason of their intensive training, professionals are equally motivated to live up to professional role prescriptions and to mold their organizational roles accordingly, what circumstances permit or prevent them from doing so?

Adequate answers to these questions are not yet at hand, unfortunately, partly because available studies of professionals in organizations do not focus to the same extent on possible explanatory factors that may be compared, and partly because the general problem itself is in only a rudimentary state of sociological analysis. That is, it seems highly likely that differences in such conditions as the relative number, formal power position, informal bargaining power, economic need, prestige, indispensability, degree of professionalization, and potential or actual alternative careers of professional persons may help account for observed differences in their organizational roles. But how these and other factors—such as organizational objectives, incentives, sanctions, and recruitment policies—may combine dynamically to produce specific role differences as well as particular types of bureaucratic patterns among professionals is not at all clear, even on the level of systematic speculation.

Lipset's incisive discussion of the analytic and methodological difficulties involved in accounting for differences in the structure of trade unions is equally applicable and instructive in the present context:

Clearly, it is impossible in the case of given organizations or individuals to abstract any one variable and make it the sole or even primary determinant of a given behavior pattern. The problem of how to deal with multi-factored determinants of specific behavior patterns is a basic one in the social sciences. When dealing with individuals, analysts may partially escape the difficulty by collecting data on a large number of cases, so that they can isolate the influence of specific factors through use of quantitative techniques. The analysis of organizations is hampered, however, by the fact that comparable data are rarely collected for more than a few cases. The cost of studying intensively even one large organization may be as much as that of gathering survey data from a large sample of individuals.

The usual procedure followed by most analysts in searching out the determinants of a given pattern of behavior, such as oligarchy or rank and file militancy within a given labor union, is to cite those factors present in the organization which seem to be related to the behavioral item in question. Such a procedure is essentially *post factum,* however, if the only cases in which the given pattern of significant variables is observed is the one under observation. The analyst rarely has the opportunity to establish any controls or comparisons. Often an attempt is made to escape this dilemma by citing illustrative materials from other cases, which appear to validate the hypothesis. Such illustrative data do not solve the methodological problem of validation, and usually only serve to give the reader a false sense of the general validity of the interpretation.

It is of crucial importance, therefore, that students of organizational behavior address themselves to the problem of verification of hypotheses. At the present time, one may spend a great deal of time examining the large number of studies of the individual trade unions or other large-scale organizations without being able to validate a single proposition about organizational behavior. The data collected in such case studies do not lend themselves to re-analysis to test hypotheses, since the researchers rarely focused their observations in terms of any set of explicit hypotheses.

Three methods may be tentatively suggested as ways through which greater progress can be made in this area: the gathering of quantitative data from a large number of organizations, clinical case studies, and deviant case analyses.[42]

All three of the research methods cited by Lipset could be used profitably by sociologists of the professions to explore systematically the factors that lead to various types of organization among professionals, as well as to investigate the nature and prevalence of the types themselves more thoroughly than has yet been done. Perhaps a measure of what remains to be accomplished is the fact that currently, with respect to physicians as well as other professionals who work in organized settings, it is impossible to indicate with any degree of *empirical* certainty what type of organization constitutes a "deviant case" and what type is modal.

ADDITIONAL DIRECTIONS FOR RESEARCH

In focusing on the formal structure of role relationships among physicians, this paper has essentially ignored the informal dimension: the network of interpersonal relationships

represented by friendship, enmity, or indifference that, as analysts of other organizational settings have shown, always arise
and frequently affect role behavior in work situations. How such
informal, affective ties condition the exercise and acceptance of
formal supervision among physicians, particularly with respect
to their professional work, must nevertheless eventually receive
investigative attention if control relationships among these professionals are to be fully understood.[43]

Moreover, although this paper has dealt exclusively with relatively explicit modes of control among physicians, the existence
of less explicit, more indirect, means must also be recognized
and their influence on professional behavior assessed. For example, some hospitals—and all medical schools—conduct regular clinical-pathological conferences, in which staff diagnoses
made on the basis of clinical evidence are compared with those
that emerge from post-mortem, laboratory examination of a
recently deceased patient. While such conferences are not formally viewed as a mechanism for controlling the professional
behavior of staff physicians, it seems exceedingly likely that,
through demonstrating areas of uncertainty, ignorance, and
error, they function ultimately in a control capacity. Likewise,
the academic milieu in general and the presence of medical
students in particular may serve as indirect control mechanisms.
In supervising the diagnostic and therapeutic work that students
do, staff physicians are sometimes challenged to justify their
opinions and advice by students who are otherwise convinced,
and their professional decisions are often subject to scrutiny of
students and staff alike. Physicians may, therefore, consciously
or unconsciously be somewhat more rigorous and careful in
their standards of patient care than would otherwise occur.
Even in nonteaching hospitals, adherence to acceptable standards of practice may be promoted by the sheer fact that the
hospital, unlike the private office, affords a place in which physicians can rather easily observe one another's work. To the
extent that the physician is psychologically and economically
dependent on the good opinion of his professional colleagues, he
will probably be motivated to live up to their expectations, at
least so far as his care of *hospitalized* patients is concerned.

Finally, apart from the matter of identifying various types of indirect organizational mechanisms for controlling professional conduct, there is the broad problem of delineating the socialization process through which physicians acquire their expectations concerning professional independence, supervision, and consultation.[44] The expectations of physicians in the advanced years of residency training and beyond have been of greatest concern in the present paper; what these expectations were at earlier stages of their training would, however, be worth knowing, since changes in expectations—and the experiences that produce them —constitute significant milestones in the socialization process.

Summary

Sociologists have held that bureaucratic and professional norms tend to be incompatible if not contradictory. It has therefore been assumed that professionals at work in apparently bureaucratic organizations experience strain and tension in living up to their diverse obligations. Yet it seems probable that professionals affect, as well as are affected by, bureaucratic forms of organization, so that, at least under certain conditions, strain is minimized. Study of the professional medical staff of a large teaching hospital suggests that in such a setting:

1. Professional norms and values set distinct limits to the ways in which organizational needs for policy-making, coordination, and supervision are met, and thus markedly affect the definition of organizational roles.

2. To reconcile professional norms and values with organizational needs, certain nonbureaucratic structural mechanisms are required. These include (a) a system of dual control (formal authority *and* formal advisory relations) within a single hierarchy of positions, where those with higher formal rank (b) have sufficient technical competence to qualify as expert consultants in the eyes of the professionals whose work they supervise, and (c) are assigned professional as well as administrative duties so that the latter occupy only part of their working time.

3. An organization with these characteristics can be classified

as a semibureaucracy; it is a combination of the pattern Gouldner has described as "representative" bureaucracy and the pattern identified in this paper as "advisory" bureaucracy. Systematic investigation of these propositions in formal organizations composed primarily of physicians or other professionals is recommended, as is further—and comparative—investigation of the antecedents, correlates, and consequences of the patterns of bureaucracy that have been outlined.

NOTES

1. Conducted intermittently over a period of five years by means of participant observation, and supplemented with a questionnaire survey of 507, or 84 per cent, of the physicians in the hospital (excluding interns) as well as by study of organizational documents. For details concerning research methods and findings, see Goss, *op. cit.* also "Influence and Authority among Physicians in an Outpatient Clinic," *American Sociological Review*, 26 (February, 1961), pp. 39-50; and "Administration and the Physician," *American Journal of Public Health* 52 (February, 1962), pp. 183-191.

2. H. H. Gerth and C. Wright Mills, trans., *From Max Weber: Essays in Sociology* (New York: Oxford University Press, 1946), pp. 196-264; A. M. Henderson and Talcott Parsons, trans., *Max Weber: The Theory of Social and Economic Organization* (New York: Oxford University Press, 1947), pp. 324-423.

3. This is Blau's capsule summary of the more detailed formulations advanced by Weber that are cited in the preceding note. See Peter M. Blau, *Bureaucracy in Modern Society* (New York: Random House, 1956), p. 19.

4. A. M. Carr-Saunders and P. A. Wilson, *The Professions* (Oxford: Clarendon Press, 1933), pp. 284-318; see also "Professions," *Encyclopedia of the Social Sciences*, Vol. XII, pp. 476-480.

5. Talcott Parsons, "Introduction," in Henderson and Parsons, *op. cit.*, pp. 58-60; Robert K. Merton, *Social Theory and Social Structure*, revised and enlarged ed. (New York: The Free Press of Glencoe, 1957), pp. 123-127, 207-224; Logan Wilson, *The Academic Man* (New York: Oxford University Press, 1942), pp. 71-93; Bernard Barber, *Science and the Social Order* (New York: The Free Press of Glencoe, 1952), pp. 144-146, 167-169; Mary Jean Huntington, "Sociology of Professions, 1945-55," in Hans L. Zetterberg, ed., *Sociology in the United States of America* (Paris: UNESCO, 1956), pp. 87-93; David N. Solomon, "Professional Persons in Bureaucratic Organizations," in *Symposium on Preventive and Social Psychiatry*, sponsored by Walter Reed Army Institute of Research *et. al.* (Washington, D.C.: U.S. Government Printing Office, 1958), pp. 253-266; Robert C. Stone, "The Sociology of Bureaucracy and Professions," in Joseph Rouček, ed., *Contemporary Sociology* (New York: Philosophical Library, 1958), pp. 491-506.

6. Philip Selznick, *TVA and the Grass Roots* (Berkeley: University of California Press, 1953); Alvin W. Gouldner, *Patterns of Industrial Bureaucracy* (New York: The Free Press of Glencoe, 1954); Peter M. Blau, *The Dynamics of Bureaucracy* (Chicago: University of Chicago Press, 1955); Roy G. Francis and Robert C. Stone, *Service and Procedure in Bureaucracy* (Minneapolis: University of Minnesota Press, 1956).

7. Gene N. Levine, Natalie Rogoff, and David Caplovitz, "Diversities in Role Conceptions," Bureau of Applied Social Research, Columbia University, 1955 (dittoed); Gene N. Levine, "The Good Physician," Bureau of Applied Social Research, Columbia University, 1957 (mimeographed); Harold L. Wilensky, *Intellectuals in Labor Unions* (New York: The Free Press of Glencoe, 1956), pp. 129-144; Renée C. Fox, *Experiment Perilous* (New York: The Free Press of Glencoe, 1959); Robert K. Merton, "Some Preliminaries to a Sociology of Medical Education," in Robert K. Merton, George G. Reader, and Patricia L. Kendall, eds., *The Student-Physician* (Cambridge: Harvard University Press, 1957), pp. 3-79, see especially pp. 71-79; Dennis C. McElrath, "Perspective and Participation of Physicians in Prepaid Group Practice," *American Sociological Review*, 26 (August, 1961), pp. 596-607.

8. Analyses that suggest the possibility are beginning to appear, however see, for example, Amitai Etzioni, "Authority Structure and Organizational Effectiveness," *Administrative Science Quarterly*, 4 (June, 1959), pp. 43-67, and "Interpersonal and Structural Factors in the Study of Mental Hospitals," *Psychiatry*, 23 (February, 1960), pp. 13-22; Eugene Litwak, "Models of Bureaucracy Which Permit Conflict," *American Journal of Sociology*, 67 (September, 1961), pp. 177-184.

9. Merton, "Role of the Intellectual in Public Bureaucracy," *op. cit.*, (1957), pp. 207-224.

10. Mark G. Field, *Doctor and Patient in Soviet Russia* (Cambridge: Harvard University Press, 1957).

11. Wilensky, *op. cit.*

12. Joseph Ben-David, "The Professional Role of the Physician in Bureaucratized Medicine: A Study in Role Conflict," *Human Relations*, 11 (No. 3, 1958), pp. 255-274; see also Simon Marcson, *The Scientist in American Industry* (Princeton, N. J.: Industrial Relations Section, Princeton University, 1960).

13. Talcott Parsons, "Suggestions for a Sociological Approach to the Theory of Organizations—II," *Administrative Science Quarterly*, 1 (September, 1956), pp. 225-239, especially pp. 235-237.

14. Logan Wilson, *op. cit.*

15. See the hospital studies cited in the following footnote; also, Etzioni, *op. cit.* (1959), and Erwin O. Smigel, "Professional Bureaucracy and the Large Wall Street Law Firms," paper presented at the 1961 meetings of the American Sociological Association, St. Louis, Mo.

16. A. H. Stanton and M. S. Schwartz, *The Mental Hospital* (New York: Basic Books, 1954); Harvey L. Smith, "The Sociological Study of Hospitals," unpublished Ph.D. dissertation, University of Chicago, 1949; Albert F. Wessen, "The Social Structure of a Modern Hospital," unpublished Ph.D. dissertation, Yale University, 1951; Temple Burling, Edith M. Lentz, and Robert N. Wilson, *The Give and Take in Hospitals* (New York: G. P. Putnam's Sons, 1956); Edith M. Lentz, "The American Voluntary

Hospital as an Example of Institutional Change," unpublished Ph.D. dissertation, Cornell University, 1956; Paul Barrabee, "A Study of a Mental Hospital," unpublished Ph.D. dissertation, Harvard University, 1951; George G. Reader and Mary E. W. Goss, "Medical Sociology with Particular Reference to the Study of Hospitals," *Transactions of the Fourth World Congress of Sociology* (London: International Sociological Association, 1959), Vol. II, pp. 139-152.

17. Harvey L. Smith, "Two Lines of Authority Are One Too Many," *Modern Hospital*, 84 (March, 1955), pp. 59-64.

18. For a case in which the reverse seems to be true, see Field, *op. cit.* For some impressionistic evidence that physicians in American hospitals are becoming more subject to bureaucratic controls than previously, see Edith Lentz, *op. cit.*

19. See, however, Oswald Hall, "Stages of a Medical Career," *American Journal of Sociology*, 53 (March, 1948), pp. 327-337, and "The Informal Organization of the Medical Profession," *Canadian Journal of Economics and Political Science*, 12 (February, 1946), pp. 30-44; also Rose Laub Coser, "Authority and Decision-Making in a Hospital," *American Sociological Review*, 23 (February, 1958), pp. 56-63.

20. Cf. Smigel, *op. cit.*

21. Logan Wilson, *op. cit.*, pp. 72-92. For a discussion of organizational pressures on professional roles in labor unions, see Wilensky, *op. cit.*; in a similar vein, Merton's analysis of the role of the intellectual in public bureaucracy stresses the significance of the organizational forces that impinge upon experts in social science and law who are employed by the government ("Role of the Intellectual . . . ," *loc. cit.*).

22. Field, *op. cit.*

23. Ben-David, *op. cit.*

24. *Ibid.*, p. 260.

25. *Ibid.*, p. 270.

26. As reported in Goss, "Physicians in Bureaucracy. . . ."

27. On the nature and prevalence of formal hierarchies within the professional medical staffs of hospitals, see Thomas Ritchie Ponton, *The Medical Staff in the Hospital*, 2nd Ed. (Chicago: Physicians' Record Company, 1955), especially Chap. IV, pp. 59-87; Malcolm T. MacEachern, *Hospital Organization and Management*, revised 3rd Ed. (Chicago: Physicians' Record Company, 1957), especially Chap. VI, pp. 157-312; Burling, Lentz, and Wilson, *op. cit.*, pp. 76-77.

28. Goss, *ibid.*, pp. 90-97.

29. Where careers can be effectively furthered or hindered by the prerogatives of rank, as would appear to be true in many European hospitals, rank may command more respect than competence; see Glaser, this volume.

30. Cf. Frederick L. Bates and Rodney F. White, "Differential Perceptions of Authority in Hospitals" (mimeographed MS, n.d.).

31. Cf. Wilensky, *op. cit.*, pp. 129-144.

32. *Op. cit.*, pp. 79-82.

33. Wilson was not, of course, alone in *recognizing* these factors; virtually everyone who has attended to the situation of professionals who work in organized settings has noted that control relationships with regard to professional work must differ from bureaucratic authority relationships. In specifying logical and feasible organizational alternatives, however, ana-

lyst appear to have been hampered by a tendency to see *all* aspects of the expert's work as professional, and to view individualism as the only alternative to bureaucratic authority.

34. Gouldner, *op. cit.*, pp. 181-228.

35. These descriptions represent slight paraphrases of those presented by Gouldner, *ibid.*, p. 217.

36. *Ibid.*, pp. 224-225.

37. Cf. Marcson, *op. cit.*, pp. 121-144, on "executive" versus "colleague" authority in relationship to representative bureaucracy among scientists.

38. Gouldner, *ibid.*, pp. 216-217.

39. In studying lawyers, Smigel arrived at a "fourth type of bureaucracy" that in some respects resembles the advisory pattern outlined here; see Smigel, *op. cit.*, on "professional bureaucracy."

40. Blau, *Bureaucracy in Modern Society*, p. 34.

41. Cf. Etzioni, "Authority Structure and Organizational Effectiveness," *loc. cit.*

42. Seymour Martin Lipset, "The Political Process in Trade Unions: A Theoretical Statement," in Morroe Berger, Theodore Abel, and Charles H. Page, eds., *Freedom and Control in Modern Society* (New York: Van Nostrand Co., 1954), pp. 122-123. Reprinted by permission of the author.

43. This is not to say that beginnings have not been made with respect to such research; see the studies by Hall (Note 19, above) and Eliot Freidson, "Client Control and Medical Practice," *American Journal of Sociology*, 65 (January, 1960), pp. 374-382.

44. The program of sociological research on medical education and professional socialization that is in progress at the Bureau of Applied Social Research Columbia University, may be expected to throw some light on the development of these expectations. For some preliminary reports, see Merton, Reader, and Kendall, *op. cit.* Also see Howard S. Becker, Blanche Geer, Everett C. Hughes and Anselm L. Strauss, *Boys in White* (Chicago: University of Chicago Press 1961), especially Chap. 17, pp. 341-363.

7

The Learning Environments
of Hospitals

PATRICIA L. KENDALL

This paper examines variations of hospital environments along several dimensions held to be significant in sociological theory. This is subject to two major restrictions. First, I do not characterize the entire hospital environment, but only the portion that constitutes the learning environment for interns and residents. Every hospital that offers training to house officers provides them with more or less routinized occasions for carrying out different activities, with a set of expectations about what they should get from their year of training, and with standards regarding the levels of performance they should achieve. These several and interrelated elements form the learning environment for the house staff.

The other restriction leads us to deal with only three dimensions of variability in these learning environments. The first of

This may be identified as publication number A-340 of the Bureau. I should like to thank Eliot Freidson, Paul F. Lazarsfeld, George G. Reader, and Mrs. Theresa Rogers for their helpful comments on an earlier version of this paper. I feel special gratitude toward Robert K. Merton for his generosity in reading successive drafts and for his cogent suggestions.

these is the *observability* of the house staff's performance by
its superiors in the hospital hierarchy. As Merton has pointed
out,[1] observability of a group's behavior is a precondition for
exercising social control over that group. To gain some impression of the extent to which a hospital exerts controls over its
house officers, we must therefore find out how visible their behavior is—and how much it is observed. Second, we examine one
part of the total *role-set* of interns and residents,[2] namely, their
relations with each other. These peer-group relations are assumed
to have various effects on the behavior of the house staff. For
example, they may affect the probability that house officers
select one another as reference individuals. Third is a focus on
the *local or cosmopolitan* orientation of different types of hospitals. This is assumed to be related to the kinds of men who are
attracted to the hospitals, and also to the kinds of doctors they
ultimately turn out.

Our interest in variations in the educational opportunities provided by different types of hospitals developed in several steps.
At the beginning, our studies in the sociology of medical education focused on the students in three medical schools, tracing
changes in their attitudes and orientations as they advanced
through medical school, and relating these changes to typical
experiences in the school.[3]

This was only a first step. We were of course aware that
medical education does not end abruptly with graduation from
medical school. Although he receives the M.D. degree at that
time, the graduate is required by law in most states to serve
an internship in an approved hospital before he can begin to
practice medicine. Furthermore, in this age of increasing specialization, most young physicians serve as residents for several years
beyond the internship.

The next step, therefore, took us to the period of graduate
medical education, as the years of hospital training are known.
We first returned to the nearly 1,500 graduates whose careers
as medical students had been followed, and examined their experiences as interns and residents, relating these to change—or
lack of it—in their attitudes.

This phase of the study of graduate medical education had

one obvious limitation: a relatively limited range of hospitals was covered in the survey. The three medical schools in the initial study are major institutions, and their graduates are usually able to obtain choice hospital assignments. Except for a few isolated cases, therefore, the follow-up study gave no clue to the kind of graduate training received in the many more small, and often obscure, hospitals in this country. We therefore proceeded to a nation-wide survey of graduate medical education. The findings of this will be clear only if we first outline the character of the survey.

Plan of the Study

The study was based on questionnaires and personal interviews in a sample of hospitals. To define the universe from which the sample could be selected, we chose from the list of over 800 nonfederal hospitals offering approved internships all those *general* hospitals that, in 1959–1960, filled *at least one* internship through the National Intern Matching Program.[4] About 450 hospitals remained on the list after screening by these two criteria.

We did not select a random sample from this universe of hospitals. Since the central hypothesis held that different kinds of hospitals provide different learning environments and that these, in turn, lead to predictable differences in the experiences of interns and residents, we wanted to make certain that the various types of hospitals were represented in sufficient numbers for analysis. Accordingly, we developed a system of stratification to differentiate the learning environments of hospitals. Preliminary field work suggested that both the size of the hospital and the degree of its affiliation with one or more medical schools greatly affected its educational program. We therefore decided to use these two variables—size and affiliation—as the basis for stratifying types of hospitals.

Available statistics showed that about half the hospitals in the universe have an average daily census of 300 or more inpatients. This figure of .300 was therefore taken to differentiate the "large" and the "small" hospitals. Three degrees of affiliation were distinguished. "Closely affiliated" hospitals were defined as those that are the major teaching units of a medical school;[5] "somewhat affiliated" hospitals are associated with a medical school but do not serve as its major teaching unit; the "unaffiliated" hospitals have no formal association with a medical school.

For each type, we then drew a random sample of hospitals. To obtain enough cases in the smaller hospitals, proportionately more of them were selected. Altogether, 167 hospitals were chosen; significantly, all but three agreed to take part in the study.[6] Each hospital sent us the names of house officers working on the four major services: medicine, obstetrics-gynecology, pediatrics, and surgery. Questionnaires could thus be sent directly to the interns and residents in the sample, helping to assure them that their anonymity would be preserved. Of the approximately 5,000 house officers to whom questionnaires were sent, 3,297, or about 65 per cent, returned usable schedules. The rate of response is not so high as we should have liked, but can be regarded as unusually high in view of the heavy schedules carried by interns and residents.[7]

Further, representatives of the Bureau visited about half the hospitals for several reasons. Published sources do not contain all the information we needed for each hospital. Such information—for example, the proportion of private beds in the hospital or the size of its staff of attending physicians—was obtained in an interview with the hospital administrator or director of medical education. We also wanted to know the positions taken by the chiefs directing the four major services on certain critical issues in graduate medical education. Each of them was therefore interviewed for 45 minutes to an hour. At that time, they also rated the performance of the house officers working under their direction.

Our data, then, are varied. From members of the house staff we have such information as their experiences in the hospital in which they are being trained, their work load, their attitudes toward patients, their standards of medical care, their plans for the future, and their satisfactions with the year of training.

From chiefs of service we have such information as the kind of behavior they expect of their house officers, the responsibilities and privileges they give interns and residents, their own standards of medical care, and their attitudes toward certain policies of medical education. From each hospital we have information on such matters as its success in filling house staff positions, the presence or absence of different residency programs, the kind of internship it offers (whether a rotating internship or straight internship), and, for the hospitals to which personal visits were made, a characterization of the patient clientele it serves.

Dimensions of Learning Environments in Hospitals

With this broad range of data, we could characterize the learning environments provided by different types of hospitals in many ways. We could, for example, focus on the kinds of available facilities. In how many and in which types of hospitals is there a library that is adequately stocked and open to qualified users at convenient times? In how many and, again, in which types of hospitals are there facilities for carrying out both laboratory and clinical investigations? Or, turning to the personnel available in different kinds of hospitals, we can ask in how many, and, once more, in which types of hospitals, the chiefs of service hold full-time or part-time appointments.

These learning environments of different types of hospitals can also be compared along other lines which are at once more subtle and less tangible than that of available facilities and personnel. We can study the kinds of "atmospheres" found in different hospital settings. As indicated earlier, we have elected to follow this approach.

RELATION OF HOUSE STAFF TO AUTHORITIES:
OBSERVABILITY AND SUPERVISION

Interns and residents are members of a hierarchy. As physicians, they occupy positions of authority over the so-called "ancillary personnel" in the hospital—nurses, aides, laboratory technicians, and so on. But the positions they occupy are definitely subordinate to those of chiefs of service, attending physicians, the director of medical education, and other senior physicians. And, as subordinates, the behavior of interns and residents is, to a greater or lesser extent, controlled by those in authority. This control, which takes the form of supervision in graduate medical training, presupposes the visibility of the house staff's performance. As Merton puts it: ". . . effective and stable authority involves the functional requirement of fairly full information about the actual (not the assumed) norms of the groups and the actual (not the assumed) role-performance of its members." [8]

Before studying variations in such visibility according to the type of hospital, we might consider briefly the reactions of interns and residents to supervision, or the exercise of controls over their behavior. In many fields of graduate education, notably the humanities and social sciences, the notion that a graduate student needs to be supervised in his daily activities is often viewed with disapproval. Independence in scholarship and research activities is the ideal, and acknowledgment of need for more than occasional supervision is taken as an admission that the student is incapable of such independence. This is not at all the case in graduate medical education. Most house officers welcome having their work closely supervised by accomplished physicians, for without this they cannot readily increase their knowledge or improve their skills. The comments made by a number of house officers strongly suggest that the extent of the supervision they received was an important criterion in evaluating their year of training. Consider, for example, the comments made by a third-year resident in obstetrics-gynecology in a small community hospital:

I am a spotted cow. I was never eligible to become chief resident. I fully expected, however, to be fully a part of the residency program and I expected the professors to see to it that I was well trained. This was not done. *None of them has ever watched me deliver a baby!* (#6580) [Emphasis supplied.]

Another man was also critical because he had not received enough supervision:

As a first-year resident in OB-Gyn, I am in charge of all ward deliveries when I am on duty. The intern *only* assists the attending for deliveries. This results in no advice or supervision of techniques. If all goes smoothly, all is well. If serious complications arise we only receive criticism and abuse, but never guidance as to how to avoid such a complication again (#5734). [Emphasis in original.]

Other comments underscore the importance attached to adequate supervision:

The house staff training program needs a lot of improvement. There is plenty of materials but supervision and teaching is inadequate (#5245).

The rotation here . . . is excellent in so far as county patients and responsibility, but supervision and formal training leaves much to be desired (#5227).

Clinical materials and opportunities for learning in the general surgical residency are great but the fine details of organization and supervision are haphazard (#7692).

House officers reporting that their work had been sufficiently supervised were more apt to judge the educational program favorably. They did not regard this as limiting their independence of action. For instance, a first-year resident in surgery wrote:

I feel the residency and internship program here is excellent with an advanced degree of responsibility *coupled with excellent supervision* especially in general surgery and medicine (#5777). [Emphasis supplied.]

And another surgical resident, working in a county hospital, reported the recent strengthening of the educational program:

There is an increase in supervision planned without intercepting the present high responsibility of the house staff. This seems to be an advantageous arrangement particularly with regard to surgery training where it is important for the resident physician [to] gain the personal experience of actually doing the surgery. Too much control only dampens initiative, but *an increase in helpful supervision is a good step forward* (#7807). [Emphasis supplied.]

It seems generally agreed that a good program in graduate medical education is one that, among other things, provides for "helpful supervision" of the house staff. But, as we have noted, effective supervision presupposes that the performance of the house staff is easily visible. We therefore want to find out whether there are systematic variations in visibility. With this in mind, we presented the house officers with two statements, and asked them to indicate "how much of the time, if ever" these applied to "this hospital." [9] The statements read as follows:

"Evaluation of the house staff goes on . . ."

"Work of the house staff is reviewed by other doctors . . ."

The interns and residents in the sample could answer "almost always," "fairly often," "occasionally," or "almost never."

Table 1 shows that constant evaluation of the house staff is more common in closely affiliated than in unaffiliated hospitals, particularly in the smaller hospitals: [10]

Table 1

Frequency of Evaluation of House Staff

DEGREE OF AFFILIATION WITH MEDICAL SCHOOL	PER CENT OF HOUSE OFFICERS SAYING EVALUATION TAKES PLACE "ALMOST ALWAYS"	
	Large	Small
Close	41	40
Some	39	31
None	35	20

The small, unaffiliated hospitals probably have fewer occasions on which the performance of house officers *could* be evaluated: the chiefs of service are almost all part-time men who spend only a limited part of their workday or work week directing their services, and the attending physicians are primarily practitioners who take time out from seeing their private patients to make brief visits to the hospital. And since, on the average, there are far fewer interns and residents in these small, unaffiliated institutions than in any other type of hospital,[11] each house officer is apt to work alone rather than in a group. Thus, even were the *motivation* to evaluate the house staff equally strong in all hospital types, the *opportunities* for doing so in small, unaffiliated hospitals are limited: the potential evaluators are not often on the scene, and, even when they are, it may be difficult to find the few house officers who are to be evaluated.

The second question—that concerned with reviews of the house staff's work—deals with a similar matter and might be expected to exhibit the same kinds of variations as were observed in Table 1. The extent to which this is the case is shown in Table 2:

Table 2

Frequency with Which Work of House Staff Is Reviewed

DEGREE OF AFFILIATION	PER CENT OF HOUSE OFFICERS SAYING WORK IS REVIEWED "ALMOST ALWAYS"	
	Large	Small
Close	32	36
Some	26	23
None	21	22

The atmospheres of the several hospital types differ in this matter as well: the work of the house staff is less often reviewed in the unaffiliated hospitals than in hospitals closely affiliated with a medical school. Unlike the findings of Table 1, however, size of the hospital does not play any role. The reasons for this are not immediately apparent. And yet, the explanation for the relatively greater freedom from review that house officers in the unaffiliated hospitals enjoy is probably very much the same as that offered previously: there are fewer staff resources for carrying out such reviews.

In sum, then, the work of house officers in closely affiliated hospitals tends to be supervised more fully than is the case in hospitals with some or no affiliation. The comments quoted earlier suggest that close supervision is welcomed. But the high degree of observability on which it is based can, of course, result in almost intolerable pressures. House officers may find it helpful to have their work watched rather closely; but the feeling that one is being evaluated without interruption and that one's work is subject to constant review may generate severe tensions. If this alone operated, we should expect the existence of pressures to parallel the existence of close supervision; in the light of our earlier findings, we should expect more tensions in closely affiliated than in unaffiliated hospitals. But we know, of course, that there are other sources of tensions for the house staff. For example, we can assume that the pressures experienced by interns and residents will be affected by such conditions as the ratio of patients to staff. The higher this ratio, the more probable it is that house officers will experience pressures. And, according to general information about the different types of hospitals, this ratio should be more favorable in closely affiliated than in unaffiliated hospitals. It is not entirely clear, therefore, just how the experience of pressures will be related to type of hospital.

To explore this, the respondents were presented with a third statement—"Demands are so great they're almost impossible to meet"—and were asked to indicate how generally this applied to their hospitals. The distribution of answers to this question is shown in Table 3.

The possible parallel between closeness of supervision and experience of pressures is not found. Do the data support the alternative possibility, that the existence of tensions is related to the work load of the house staff? To study this more directly, we used data pertaining to each of the participating hospitals —the average daily census of inpatients and the total number

Table 3

Experience of Pressures

DEGREE OF AFFILIATION	PER CENT OF HOUSE OFFICERS SAYING IT IS ALMOST IMPOSSIBLE TO MEET DEMANDS "ALMOST ALWAYS" OR "FAIRLY OFTEN"	
	Large	Small
Close	26	15
Some	18	19
None	26	28

of house officers working in the hospital. These two items of information made it possible to construct an index, based on the ratio of patients to interns and residents; for the sake of simplicity, we can call this an "index of work pressures" in the hospital.[12] Table 4 shows a fairly strong relationship between the work pressures present in the hospital and its characterization as a place in which it is difficult to fulfill all demands made on the house officers:

Table 4

Experience of Pressures According to Index of Work Pressures

Ratio of patients to house officers	Per cent of house officers saying it is impossible to meet demands "ALMOST ALWAYS" or "FAIRLY OFTEN"	Total Cases
1–5	17	(862)
6–10	20	(598)
11–20	27	(472)
21 or more	33	(104)

About a third of the straight interns and residents working in hospitals with the highest ratio of patients to house officers (twenty-one or more) reported frequent difficulties in meeting the demands made on them; this was true for only half as many of the men working in the hospitals with the lowest ratio of patients to house officers.

Up to this point we have been comparing different types of hospitals, each as a unitary whole. But this can be misleading. A general hospital is composed of several services and departments, and these may vary as much within a single hospital as different types of hospitals vary. Thus, a comparative study of learning environments should consider differences within hospitals as well as between hospitals. It is proverbial, for example, that departments of surgery generate more tension and pressure than do other departments. Is this actually the case? The rotating interns in our sample are in a particularly good position to answer this question. It will be recalled that these men were asked how generally each of the statements presented to them applied to their experience on the medical service, and how generally to the surgical service. By relying on their replies to the question about pressures, we can bypass all the methodological problems that would be encountered if we contrasted the characterizations given by the straight interns and residents assigned to the different departments:[13]

Table 5

Severity of Demands in Departments of Medicine and Surgery (Rotating interns)

DEGREE OF AFFILIATION	PER CENT SAYING THAT IT IS IMPOSSIBLE TO MEET DEMANDS "ALMOST ALWAYS" OR "FAIRLY OFTEN"		
	On Medicine	On Surgery	Total Cases
Close	21	46	(202)
Some	27	35	(423)
None	29	39	(393)

Table 5 shows differences in the extent to which the two departments make heavy demands on their house officers. As we look across each row, we see that, on every level of affiliation,[14] rotating interns reported having experienced greater demands from the department of surgery than from the department of medicine. To the extent that this one question can be relied on to indicate differences in atmosphere, traditional notions about levels of tension prevailing in different departments are confirmed.

RECIPROCAL RELATIONS OF HOUSE OFFICERS: GENERATING SOCIAL ATMOSPHERES

When we set out to study the relations house officers have with their superiors in their role-set, it seemed evident that we should think in terms of subordination-superordination. When we begin to examine the relations house officers have with their peers in their role-set, it seems equally evident to think in terms of competition-cooperation. We consider, then, this aspect of atmosphere prevailing in the several types of hospitals.

As before, the respondents were asked to serve as informants about their hospitals. But the procedure used in obtaining their judgments of competitiveness-cooperation differed somewhat from that used to elicit descriptions of typical modes of supervision. In the latter case, we were interested in the hospital as a whole. But in the case of competition-cooperation it was more useful to distinguish between the atmosphere prevailing among interns and among residents in the hospital. Accordingly, the straight interns and residents were given another set of descriptive statements, and were asked, first, to how many of the interns in the hospital each statement applied, and, then, to how many of the residents. Two of these statements dealt with professional cooperativeness:

[They] are open and free about exchanging information.
[They] are willing to help out when a fellow intern or resident has a lot of work to do.

It is not easy to guess how this sort of cooperativeness will vary by hospital type. From the previous section we know that the work of interns and residents is more frequently evaluated and reviewed in closely affiliated than in unaffiliated hospitals.

We might suppose that, because house officers in closely affiliated hospitals know that they are under fairly constant scrutiny and that, in some sense, their future careers depend on how well they perform, they will be "cagey" with each other. On this assumption, we should expect house officers in closely affiliated hospitals to be *less* open and free in the exchange of information and *less* willing to help each other out. This finds support in the words of a third-year resident in a hospital closely affiliated with a medical school; he wrote:

In teaching hospitals the residents are competing for hospital appointments and frequently sacrifice their opinions, integrity, and loyalty toward their subordinate house officers in order to gain favor with the attending staff and administration (#5413).

But we also know that many in the medical profession place high value on the "team approach" to patient care.[15] And we can assume that such teamwork, which obviously requires cooperation among house officers as well as with other members of the hospital staff, is more likely to be emphasized in closely affiliated hospitals where the larger numbers of full-time personnel make it more readily feasible.

In other words, there is reason to believe that the atmosphere in closely affiliated hospitals will be characterized by *less* cooperation than is the case in unaffiliated hospitals; and there is also reason to believe that the atmosphere of these university teaching centers will be characterized by *nore* cooperation. The net result may be a product of these countervailing forces. But the data suggest the greater effectiveness of the second tendency, although not with complete consistency. Let us review the questions one at a time.

The results in Table 6 are quite clear cut. From the closely affiliated to the unaffiliated hospitals, the proportion saying that almost all interns exchange information freely declines steadily. And, although the differences are not so large when residents are being described, they exhibit the same general trend.

Although size of the hospital is less important than degree of

Table 6

Freedom in Exchanging Information

	LARGE HOSPITALS			SMALL HOSPITALS		
	Close affil.	Some affil.	No affil.	Close affil.	Some affil.	No affil.
Per cent saying "almost all" INTERNS are open and free	80	73	66	81	63	60
Per cent saying "almost all" RESIDENTS are open and free	82	79	71	82	72	72

affiliation in producing differences in cooperativeness, it does play some slight role. In general, house officers in the larger institutions are more likely to say that almost all of their colleagues exchange information freely.

Furthermore, residents are more often described as being co-operative than are interns. This same tendency will be observed in the rest of the series of descriptive statements used to characterize different hospital atmospheres. In part, it is explained by the fact that most of the respondents providing the descriptions were themselves residents, and they seem to have indulged an understandable desire to depict themselves and each other in favorable terms.[16] But in this particular instance, the difference may perhaps be partially explained by the fact that interns have recently come from the sometimes competitive atmosphere of medical school, while residents have had a longer time to become socialized to the desirability of cooperation among members of the medical team.

Responses to the second statement show less clear-cut differences between hospital types. Closely affiliated hospitals appear to be more likely than unaffiliated hospitals to have almost all *interns* willing to help one another out; but there are no consistent differences when the cooperativeness of *residents* is examined.

In the first row of Table 7, we note that, as affiliation with a medical school declines, so does the proportion of house officers

Table 7

Willingness to Help Each Other

| | LARGE HOSPITALS | | | SMALL HOSPITALS | | |
	Close affil.	Some affil.	No affil.	Close affil.	Some affil.	No affil.
Per cent saying "almost all" INTERNS help each other	37	30	28	41	31	23
Per cent saying "almost all" RESIDENTS help each other	46	53	47	50	54	50

saying that almost all interns are willing to help a colleague when he is under pressure. The second row of the table shows the previously noted tendency of residents to provide more favorable descriptions of themselves than of interns. But the relationship of these descriptions to degree of affiliation is no longer apparent. (One interesting side light is that house officers describe one another as being considerably less willing to help out than to exchange information.)

Cooperativeness in professional activities is not the only kind of friendly behavior interns and residents manifest toward one another. They can also interact for noninstrumental purposes. To see whether some types of hospitals were characterized by a greater degree of sociability than others, we asked respondents how typical it was for members of the house staff to "get along together socially." The replies of straight interns and residents are shown in Table 8:

Table 8

Sociability

| | LARGE HOSPITALS | | | SMALL HOSPITALS | | |
	Close affil.	Some affil.	No affil.	Close affil.	Some affil.	No affil.
Per cent saying "almost all" INTERNS get along together	58	54	52	63	58	52
Per cent saying "almost all" RESIDENTS get along together	59	56	55	62	58	61

The small differences in Table 8 are neither statistically nor socially significant. In hospitals of every size and degree of affiliation, somewhat more than half of the house officers reported that almost all colleagues got along together.

Of course, there can be barriers to such interactions. One of these is imposed by the structure of the hospital. The division of the hospital into different departments, and the assignment of straight interns and residents to only one of these departments, may make it difficult for them to become acquainted with and to interact with men in other departments.

Another barrier may exist when members of the house staff come from different cultural backgrounds. This is especially apt to be the case when there are differences in their native languages. To study this, we separated the straight interns and residents who were citizens of the United States and then classified them according to the proportion of foreign-trained and generally, therefore, foreign-speaking house officers in their hospitals. Table 9 shows how the sociability of residents is related to the proportion of foreign-trained residents in the hospital.[17] The results suggest that cultural homogeneity affects close social interaction between members of the house staff. (Had there been enough cases, we could have made the corresponding comparison for foreign nationals. In that instance, we would have expected that, the larger the proportion of, say, Spanish-speaking residents, the *more* sociability there would be among them.)

Table 9

Sociability of Residents According to Proportion of Foreign-Trained Residents
(United States citizens)

Per cent of residents who are foreign-trained	Per cent saying "almost all" residents get along	Total cases
Less than 25	63	(1157)
25–50	57	(216)
51 or more	42	(59)

So far we have seen that relations between house officers
in closely affiliated hospitals are somewhat more friendly than
is true in unaffiliated institutions. But since the results are not
clear-cut, we look for other factors that might make for differences in the extent of friendly and cooperative relations
between members of the house staff. An obvious possibility,
again, is department. We have seen that departments of surgery
are more tense than departments of medicine. Do they also
have less amicability? To answer this, we shall once again call
on the rotating interns who, it will be remembered, were asked
to evaluate the relations between residents on the medical and
surgical services. Rather than consider their answers to the
separate questions, we have combined them into an index of
cooperativeness.[18] To do so, we counted the number of times
each rotating intern said that the medical residents in his hospital displayed friendly behavior; we repeated this count separately for the responses of rotating interns regarding residents
on the surgical service. The indices have values from 0 to 4,
and, the higher the value, the greater the amount of amicability
attributed to the residents. Table 10 shows the characterization
of medical and surgical residents by rotating interns. As we
look down each column of the table, we see that, quite consistently, the rotating interns report more friendliness among
medical residents than among surgical residents:

Table 10

Amicability of Medical and Surgical Residents
(Rotating interns)

	LARGE HOSPITALS			SMALL HOSPITALS		
	Close affil.	Some affil.	No affil.	Close affil.	Some affil.	No affil.
Average score for MEDICAL residents	2.54	2.42	2.34	2.45	2.58	2.28
Average score for SURGICAL residents	1.86	2.07	1.98	1.64	2.28	2.06
Total Cases	(135)	(221)	(188)	(76)	(214)	(216)

A structural factor also seems to make for differences in the degree of cooperative relations between members of the house staff. This is the "shape" of the residency system. Some residency programs offer the same number of positions in each year of residency training; for example, they may have three positions for first-year residents, three for second-year residents, and three for third-year residents. This kind of system we shall describe as a "parallelogram." Other hospitals (or other departments in the same hospital) may have what is called a "pyramidal" system, offering progressively fewer positions to the higher levels of residents. Such a pyramidal system, for example, may have six first-year positions, three second-year positions, and one third-year position.

It is generally recognized that pyramidal systems operate on the basis of competition among the advancing residents. Some look on such competition as promoting a high level of medical care. Thus, one prominent medical educator says: "Whatever the merits of the pyramidal system in terms of stimulating competition and developing a limited number of more highly trained men . . ." [19] Others are more critical of the competition a pyramidal system is assumed to create. Thus, we find the following comment in an article on the training of psychiatrists: "It seems unwise that residency training should be pointed toward having one or two people at the top of the residency heap in each department, the chief residents, who in a sense are victors in a competition." [20]

The residents in our sample who commented on pyramidal systems were uniformly critical of the competition engendered by them. Three first-year residents in general surgery, all of them working in university centers, had this to say:

The surgical house staff in general is quite disturbed about the competition in a pyramid plan and the very great uncertainty of completing the residency which it started. We feel that at the first-year resident level in our particular group the candidates are pretty evenly matched, yet some will suffer in the future 3 or 4 years (#0877).

Found what I expected here and am happy with my training, however have now developed some uncertainty because of recent increase
in competition for senior resident appointments in general surgery
(#8039).

There is a somewhat unhealthy competitive atmosphere among the
many senior assistant residents for the job of graduated responsibility with a chief residency at the summit in a pre-destined number
of years (#8630).

In other words, the competition created by a pyramidal system
can be seen as a healthy spur to excellence and as a source of
demoralization. But, in either case, a higher level of competitiveness is associated with the presence of pyramidal systems. To
examine the extent of this, we first classified each of the departments offering a residency program (of more than one year).
In the case of a pure parallelogram or a pure pyramid, this
classification did not offer any problems. But there were, as
there always are in empirical reality, intermediate cases that
did not conform to either of these polar types. For example,
some departments offer three first-year positions, three second-
year positions, and one third-year position. Others offer, let us
say, ten first-year positions, six second-year positions, six third-
year residencies, and two fourth-year positions. These intermediate cases, combining features of both the parallel and
pyramidal types, were designated "semipyramids."

The next step was to classify the respondents, in this case the
straight interns and residents, according to the "shape" of the
service on which they were working. Finally, using an index
similar to that constructed for rotating interns, we examined how
much cooperativeness these several groups attributed to the
residents in their hospital. The results are shown in Table 11.[21]

Bearing in mind that the higher the score-value of the index,
the greater the degree of cooperativeness, we find that interns
and residents working on services organized as pyramidal systems perceive more competitiveness among their colleagues than
do those working in departments with an equal number of positions on each level of residency training. The single exception is

Table 11

Cooperativeness of Residents According to "Shape" of Residency Programs

DEPARTMENT	AVERAGE SCORE ON INDEX*		
	Pyramid	Semi-pyramid	Parallel-ogram
Medicine	2.66	2.78	2.86
Obstetrics-gynecology	2.36	2.50	2.55
Pediatrics	2.47	2.55	2.51
Surgery	2.03	2.44	2.57

* The totals on which these average score values are based are as follows:

Department	Pyramid	Semi-pyramid	Parallel-ogram
Medicine	387	202	160
Obstetrics-gynecology	22	100	211
Pediatrics	108	49	83
Surgery	86	488	164

in departments of pediatrics; but this is only a slight deviation from the basic tendency.

RELATIONS OF HOUSE STAFF WITH PRACTITIONERS AND THE SCIENTIFIC COMMUNITY: LOCAL AND COSMOPOLITAN ORIENTATIONS

We have dealt so far with the relations of house officers to their superiors and to each other. In this final section, we consider the relations of the house staff in different types of hospitals to the broader medical community. We now take them out of the hospital, but we do so only to characterize the learning environments within different kinds of hospitals. In describing these relations of house officers to the larger medical community, we shall draw on concepts of "local" and "cosmopolitan" orientations that had their origin in a quite different context.

The distinction was originally developed in a community study of people who influenced the decisions, tastes, and behavior of others.[22] These influentials were found to be of two types, depending on their orientation to the community. The "local influentials" were found to be primarily oriented to the community, to be more concerned about its problems than about national or international situations, to have a wide network of friends and acquaintances in the community, to belong to a variety of local organizations, and so on. The "cosmopolitan influentials," in contrast, were found to be more interested in what was going on outside the community, to be less loyal and devoted to the community, to have fewer friends among their neighbors, and the like.

Subsequently, other investigators have extended the concepts to apply to other types of situations. Thus, for example, Gouldner has made use of the distinction in an analysis of the orientation of a college faculty.[23]

The concepts can be extended to the field of medicine. Here the equivalent of a local influential is the physician who is primarily concerned with what is going on *within* his immediate environment: with his relations with patients and other doctors in the community, with developments in the county medical society rather than in national organizations, and so on. In contrast, the medical equivalent of the cosmopolitan influential is the physician primarily oriented to what is taking place *outside* his immediate environment: he wants to know what is going on in other hospitals and medical centers; he wants to find out about the latest developments in research; he probably prefers membership in national medical organizations to active participation in the county medical society; and so on. To put it most succinctly, we define a local orientation as one in which the physician is primarily concerned with patients and problems of practice, and a cosmopolitan orientation as one in which he is primarily concerned with scientific medicine and research. From all this, we should of course expect that closely affiliated hospitals are characterized by greater cosmopolitanism than unaffiliated hospitals.

Here, as in previous sections, we are not interested in finding out *which* interns and residents in our sample have a local and which a cosmopolitan orientation. Rather, as before, we want to determine how the climates or atmospheres of different hospitals vary. Once more, therefore, we asked our respondents to serve as informants about the hospitals in which they were working. We did so in several ways.

A first indicator of whether a hospital is primarily cosmopolitan or local is the orientation of the attending physicians with whom house officers work most closely. With this in mind, we asked a direct question:

During this year, have you actually worked mostly with attending physicians who are scientifically oriented, or who are patient and practice oriented?

The great majority of the house officers in our sample reported that they had worked mostly with attendings who, according to our definition, were locally oriented. But, as Table 12 makes clear, the size of these majorities depends greatly on the extent to which a hospital is or is not affiliated with a medical school:

Table 12

Orientation of Attending Physicians

DEGREE OF AFFILIATION	PER CENT OF HOUSE OFFICERS SAYING MOST ATTENDINGS ARE "PATIENT AND PRACTICE ORIENTED" *	
	Large	Small
Close	63	59
Some	89	90
None	94	95

* This question was asked of the entire sample; the base figures are as follows:

Degree of affiliation	Large	Small
Close	961	591
Some	515	443
None	427	360

Almost two-thirds of the interns and residents in closely affiliated hospitals reported that most of the attending physicians who supervised their work were primarily oriented to patients and problems of practice; the other third told us that their attendings were scientifically oriented. However, in hospitals with some, but not close, affiliation, nine out of every ten respondents said that their attendings were primarily patient-oriented; and in hospitals with no affiliation this is almost universal, with such reports being given by 95 per cent of the house staff. In this respect, then, expectations are borne out: university teaching hospitals are more cosmopolitan in their orientation.

A second measure of this orientation was based on a semi-projective question. With the help of a medical educator, we devised a list of six titles of lectures. Two of these dealt quite obviously with questions about the practice of medicine: "Group Practice—Pros and Cons" and "How to Avoid Malpractice Suits"; these were intended as measures of a local orientation. Two others dealt with topics in basic medical science: "Lipid Metabolism" and "The Role of Serotonin in Disorders of the Gut"; they were intended to indicate a cosmopolitan orientation. The two remaining titles were meant to suggest practical applications of medical knowledge: "Office Treatment of Thyroid Disorders" and "Stimulants and Sedatives."

The titles were arranged so that these pairs were not grouped. The respondents were then asked: "Suppose the following lectures were offered in your hospital. In your opinion, which two lectures would bring out the largest audience in this hospital?" [24] We expected, first of all, that interns and residents in unaffiliated community hospitals would more often say that lectures dealing with problems of practice would be popular in their institutions, thereby indicating the primarily local orientation of these hospitals. Table 13 indicates that this is the case, especially in connection with the question of how to avoid malpractice suits.

Conversely, we expected that when lectures dealing with topics of basic medical science were considered, they would be selected more frequently by interns and residents in closely affiliated hospitals, indicating the more cosmopolitan orientation

Table 13

Selection of Practice-Oriented Lecture Titles

	LARGE HOSPITALS			SMALL HOSPITALS		
	Close affil.	Some affil.	No affil.	Close affil.	Some affil.	No affil.
Per cent selecting "How to Avoid Malpractice Suits"	43	57	68	43	62	66
Per cent selecting "Group Practice—Pros and Cons"	31	38	39	31	39	37

of such hospitals. As Table 14 shows, neither of these lectures seems likely to attract a large audience. But, according to the interns and residents in our sample, they would be considerably more popular in closely affiliated than in unaffiliated hospitals:

Table 14

Selection of Basic Science Lecture Titles

	LARGE HOSPITALS			SMALL HOSPITALS		
	Close affil.	Some affil.	No affil.	Close affil.	Some affil.	No affil.
Per cent selecting "Lipid Metabolism"	38	21	13	38	25	10
Per cent selecting "The Role of Serotonin in Disorders of the Gut"	30	23	8	32	11	10

The local or cosmopolitan orientation of a hospital will also be affected by the orientations of its house staff. How are they characterized in this regard? As in previous sections, straight interns and residents were presented with descriptive statements, and were asked to how many of the interns and residents in their hospitals these applied.[25] The first of these questions asked, "How many house officers make an effort to keep up with current medical literature?" Such behavior, it will be recalled, is an essential element in our definition of cosmopolitanism. In Table 15 we find once again that the house staffs of closely affiliated hospitals are more cosmopolitan, although differences between hospitals with some and with no affiliation are barely perceptible. And, except in closely affiliated hospitals, residents in large institutions are more often described as being diligent in their reading than are their counterparts in small hospitals:

Table 15

Keeping Informed of Current Medical Literature

	LARGE HOSPITALS			SMALL HOSPITALS		
	Close affil.	Some affil.	No affil.	Close affil.	Some affil.	No affil.
Per cent saying "almost all" INTERNS keep up with literature	12	8	4	16	7	4
Per cent saying "almost all" RESIDENTS keep up with literature	43	37	34	43	28	26

An interesting aspect of Table 15 is the markedly different way in which the behavior of interns and residents is described. Far fewer said that almost all interns in their hospitals kept up with literature than reported this about their colleagues serving residencies. This is not explained entirely by the previously noted tendency of the respondents, most of whom were themselves residents, to describe residents more favorably than interns. Beyond this tendency, which is involved here to some extent, is the fact that different behavior is *expected* of interns and residents. This is seen most clearly in the responses of the approximately 350 chiefs of service whom we were able to interview. They were asked how important it was for interns and residents to keep up with the "latest medical literature." Their replies suggest that they discriminate sharply in their definitions of appropriate behavior for the two groups of house officers:

while about 50 per cent said that it was "very important" for interns to keep up with their reading, about 90 per cent attached this degree of importance to reading by residents. And the impressive fact is that such differences in role expectations can produce radical shifts in behavior in the space of only one year.

Another statement enabling the respondents to describe the cosmopolitan or local orientations of house officers in their hospitals dealt with arrangements made by interns and residents to set up a practice while they were still serving on the house staff. It asked how many house officers "are primarily interested in lining up a practice." In terms of our definition an interest in such arrangements is indicative of a local orientation. This was quite clear in some of the reasons advanced for decisions to accept particular house staff positions. For example, a rotating intern in a small, unaffiliated hospital volunteered the following comment at the end of his questionnaire:

My internship is at a private hospital and I feel it was very good in that *I learned much about how medicine is practiced in the community*. However, it was somewhat *lacking in the scientific and teaching aspect* of medicine, which I feel is more important. I went to this hospital knowing this, *mainly because it is in the city where I want to practice some day and I felt it was important to get to know the other MD's in the area and to let them know me*. I hope my residency, which I plan to take at a university hospital will make up for what my internship lacked (#1039). [Emphasis supplied.]

This states quite explicitly that, in so far as membership on the house staff of the small hospital selected by this man will help him establish a practice in the local community, he is willing to isolate himself temporarily from the scientific (cosmopolitan) orientation that he considers more important.

A first-year resident in another small, community hospital, was somewhat less explicit. He implies that, in order to line up a practice, one must be prepared to forego the scientific orientation characteristic of a major teaching center:

It could be excellent training, but at present [it] is poor. [The hospital is] not located in a teaching center. I had an excellent internship. [My] main reason for taking one year residency here was to facilitate going into practice in this area (#5683).

Since we want to find out the types of hospitals most likely to be cosmopolitan, our interest is in the response that "almost none" of the house staff is primarily concerned with lining up a practice. Table 16 shows once more that there is a higher level of cosmopolitanism in the closely affiliated hospitals. In general, also, large hospitals are more cosmopolitan than are small hospitals:[26]

Table 16

Interest in Lining Up a Practice

	LARGE HOSPITALS			SMALL HOSPITALS		
	Close affil.	Some affil.	No affil.	Close affil.	Some affil.	No affil.
Per cent saying "almost no" INTERNS want to line up practice	66	64	46	65	52	41
Per cent saying "almost no" RESIDENTS want to line up practice	48	47	35	50	39	45

All the findings reviewed in this section point to the conclusion that a cosmopolitan orientation is typical of closely affiliated hospitals, while a local orientation is typical of those institutions that do not have any formal association with a medical school.

It is not clear whether a hospital with a cosmopolitan orientation offers an environment more favorable to learning medicine than does one with a local orientation. A first assumption might hold that, almost by definition, a cosmopolitan hospital, with its emphasis on science and research, would provide more and better learning opportunities. This assumption is supported by two house officers training in major teaching centers. One of these was enthusiastic about his residency precisely because of its emphasis on scientific and academic medicine:

Residency and internship at this hospital are excellent opportunity for scientific and medical advancement. Most people trained at this hospital enter some academic career. We would all like to be excellent doctors, scientists, teachers, and socially acceptable human beings. I am not certain all of the goals are possible with the rapid advances taking place. My training has been such that [it] acquaints me with any future that can be foreseen in medicine (#5954).

Another, an intern in internal medicine, was more critical, because he felt that scientific and academic medicine had not received sufficient emphasis during his year of training:

The X Division of Y Hospital is a controversial place where many feel there is too little teaching, as do I, and where the spirit this year has been less than desirable. *Better, i.e. more academic attendings are necessary* at a place which has the reputation of Y Hospital. The assistant residency is worthwhile more than the internship; but one always has the feeling that keeping up thoroughly with the journals here is a job, although worth it. The house staff in general are highly competent. In short, for my purposes, there is simply *too little house staff reading, too little emphasis on academic medicine,* i.e., the thorough and scientific study of disease (#8928). [Emphasis supplied.]

In spite of his criticism, he would undoubtedly agree that the learning opportunities are greater in hospitals with a scientific orientation.

But more careful reflection suggests that this need not always be the case. It is probably true that a cosmopolitan atmosphere is more conducive to learning *of a certain kind*. This would be the learning of those matters that, by definition, form its primary concern: basic sciences, recent research findings, and the like. But there may be other areas of learning, perhaps those generally encompassed in the "art of medicine," which might be learned more easily and more effectively in an environment more concerned with problems of practice. Current discussions of graduate medical education abound with comments about what is called the "gap" between hospital training and private practice. Consider the following, for example:

"I could fill a handbook with practical information they didn't teach me during my residency."

This, or some similar complaint, is too often voiced by the newly established private physician. It betrays a serious, often-observed, but seldom corrected gap between residency training and private practice.

Simply stated, the problem is how to outfit a resident with perspicacity and technic on both the academic and practical levels.

In retrospect it seems the former is stressed to the detriment of the latter.[27]

In a similar vein, a medical educator writes:

The medical schools must devise some means, not only of teaching clinical procedures and moral and ethical standards to students, but also the means of teaching them how to translate these into community practice. The last mentioned is the great missing link in contemporary medical education.[28]

Another physician calls on personal experience to support his judgment that medical education—on all levels—should be more practical:

As a senior in medical school, I was on externe duty one day when I was assigned to a patient with a simple nail-puncture wound. Should I cleanse it? Let it bleed? Stitch it up? Give a tetanus shot? I simply didn't know. This experience confirmed my growing suspicion that my medical education had not been much help in preparing me to handle many of the common problems I'd find in my chosen field, family practice. . . .

If, as I've found, the family doctor could profitably have more instruction in handling routine problems, might not this be true of the specialist also? There are indications that men in some specialized fields do feel the need for more down-to-earth training.[29]

There is some opinion that community hospitals can be more successful than university teaching centers in offering this kind of training. As one physician has put it:

Are these teachers [professors in medical schools and full-time attendings] isolated as they are in their ivory tower, qualified to do this [deal effectively with people]? . . . Such training falls naturally to the staff of a community hospital. They know people. They know the family history (a most seriously neglected facet of good diagnosis). They regularly bring some of the economics of medicine to their house staff not only from the point of view of the physicians, but even more important, from that of the patient. They bring heart as well as mind to the bedside.[30]

This somewhat impassioned plea is echoed in a more subdued way by the comments of several of the house officers in this study. Thus, one resident in an unaffiliated hospital had this to say about his training in obstetrics-gynecology:

I feel that the training at this hospital is the best available in the U.S. for the *active practice* of Ob-Gyn. Those primarily interested in teaching or doing research would not like this type of training. However, for a "doing" doctor as opposed to a "talking" doctor or a "lab" doctor I am thoroughly satisfied with this whole system for Ob-Gyn residency training (#8567). [Emphasis in the original.]

A rotating intern in an unaffiliated hospital was less enthusiastic about his experiences but advanced a somewhat similar argument:

I feel that this hospital offers adequate training for general practice. This type of internship is particularly valuable in demonstrating how medicine is practiced in communities other than large medical centers (#1891).

Conversely, two house officers in major teaching centers criticized these hospitals because of their lack of concern with "practical" problems. A rotating intern wrote:

A good internship; however, not quite enough instruction (so far as teaching hospitals go) on technical procedures such as minor surgical and medical procedures. . . . *Too much emphasis on furtherment of science and research* rather than clinical medicine (#3103). [Emphasis supplied.]

And a fourth-year resident in surgery at an important teaching
hospital had this to say:

There is a growing trend at my hospital for educating researchers
and less emphasis on the training of practitioners of medicine. *A
certain amount of research orientation is important; however, the
skills and arts are important to master* (#7845). [Emphasis supplied.]

From comments such as these we must conclude that the
seemingly obvious assumption that a cosmopolitan orientation
automatically means a more favorable learning environment is
premature. It still needs to be investigated.

Summary

Hospitals that offer graduate training programs for interns
and residents differ in the kinds of learning environments they
provide. These can be variously described. They can be characterized in terms of the physical facilities or the categories of
personnel that are available, and in terms of the atmospheres that
prevail. For the present purposes, we adopted the second
approach.

To describe the learning environments found in different types
of hospitals, we selected three sociological variables bearing on
the relations of house officers to others in their role-set and to
the broader medical community. We saw, first of all, that the
visibility of the house staff's performance significantly affects
their relations with superiors in the hospital structure. Only
when the behavior of interns and residents is observable can
they receive the kind of supervision they generally report as
helpful. Conditions making for such observability were more
often found in closely affiliated than in unaffiliated hospitals,
and, therefore, adequate supervision is more general in the former
rather than the latter. We did not find that such observability
resulted in tensions or pressures on the house staff. Instead, the
degree of tension seems to follow departmental lines, and to
be more directly related to the work load of the house officers.

Next we investigated how the relations that interns and residents have with their colleagues vary from one kind of hospital to another. House officers tend to have more amicable relations with their peers in closely affiliated rather than in unaffiliated hospitals. But the absence of clear-cut differences by size of hospital or degree of affiliation led us to look for other structural factors that might account for variations in these interpersonal relations. Cultural homogeneity was found to be a condition for close interaction between house officers; in the eyes of rotating interns, at least, there is more cooperativeness among medical than among surgical residents; and the degree to which residents cooperate with one another is influenced by structural arrangements of the residency program in their hospital.

A final section examined the local-cosmopolitan orientation of different types of hospitals, and considered the implications this might have for the adequacy of educational programs in these hospitals. It was found, as we expected, that closely affiliated hospitals have more of a cosmopolitan orientation than do hospitals of other types. There are some who assume that such an orientation, with its emphasis on scientifically based medicine and research findings, automatically makes for a superior learning environment. To clarify this assumption, we examined opposing arguments set forth by medical educators, as well as by the house staff in the study. These generally stated that what is missing in the scientifically and research-oriented (cosmopolitan) hospital is a proper concern for the practical problems of medical practice.

NOTES

1. Robert K. Merton, *Social Theory and Social Structure* (New York: The Free Press of Glencoe, 1957), p. 321.

2. Merton defines role-set as that "complement of role relationships which persons have by virtue of occupying a particular social status." He illustrates this by pointing out that "the single status of medical student entails not only the role of a student in relation to his teachers, but also an array of other roles relating the occupant of that status to other students, nurses, physicians, social workers, medical technicians, etc." (*ibid.*, p. 369).

3. See Robert K. Merton, George G. Reader, and Patricia Kendall, eds., *The Student-Physician* (Cambridge: Harvard University Press, 1957). These studies in the sociology of medical education have been supported by grants from The Commonwealth Fund.

4. At the present time, there are in the hospitals of this country approximately twice as many internship positions available each year as there are graduates of American medical schools to fill them. As a result, some hospitals are unable to fill all—or even any—of their internship positions with American graduates. (Graduates of American schools are matched to the hospitals of their choice through the National Intern Matching Program.) Sometimes these hospitals are able to attract graduates of foreign medical schools to fill their internships. In 1959–1960, the year during which the field work for our study was carried out, American graduates filled 53 per cent of the somewhat more than 12,000 internship positions available; an additional 29 per cent were filled by foreign graduates; 18 per cent remained unfilled. See John C. Nunemaker, John Hinman, Willard V. Thompson, and Rose Tracy, "Graduate Medical Education in the United States," *Journal of the American Medical Association*, 174: 6 (October 8, 1960), pp. 574-576.

5. Two criteria were used to decide whether or not a hospital was a major teaching unit. One was whether medical students were regularly assigned to the wards and clinics of the hospital. The second was whether the chiefs of service in the hospital also held appointments on the faculty of the medical school.

6. The three hospitals that declined to participate in the study were replaced by three comparable hospitals, selected at random from the appropriate types.

7. We had some information about the nonrespondents that permitted us to compare them with the house officers who did respond to our questionnaire. By and large, there are no important or consistent differences between the two groups. There is some indication that the nonrespondents contained a somewhat higher proportion of graduates from foreign medical schools. But, significantly, scores received on examinations given by the National Board of Medical Examiners were virtually identical in both the respondent and nonrespondent groups. (In order to ascertain this, the names of 300 respondents and 300 nonrespondents were drawn, and, with the cooperation of the National Board of Medical Examiners, their examination scores compared.) Examination of the other characteristics supports the conclusion that the two groups do not differ in any consistent or important ways.

8. Merton, *op. cit.*, p. 341.

9. Rotating interns, who divide their time between the four major services, were asked to indicate how much of the time each statement applied to the medical service and how much to the surgical service. Because their answers referred to particular services rather than to the hospital as a whole, they will be excluded from the tables that follow unless otherwise indicated. In other words, most tables will be based only on the responses of straight interns and residents.

10. The distribution of straight interns and residents in the several hospital types is as follows:

Degree of affiliation	Large	Small
Close	826	515
Some	294	229
No	239	144

Except for minor variations due to occasional no answers, all tables making use of the responses of straight interns and residents have these totals as their bases.

11. The average numbers of house officers in different hospital types are as follows:

	AVERAGE NUMBER OF INTERNS		AVERAGE NUMBER OF RESIDENTS	
Degree of affiliation	*Large*	*Small*	*Large*	*Small*
Close	34.9	20.9	137.8	78.3
Some	18.6	10.1	40.0	17.6
No	14.7	7.1	22.7	11.4

12. Of course, this ratio is an average, pertaining to the hospital as a whole. But within individual hospitals there are likely to be variations from one service to another. On some services the ratio of patients to house officers is likely to be higher than the average; on others it is likely to be lower. Had it been possible to construct this type of index for each service, individually, findings of the kind reported in Table 4 might have been even more clear cut.

13. One problem in using the responses of straight interns and residents to study the atmospheres of different departments is that they were asked how much of the time each statement applied to "this hospital." While it is quite probable that, for many of the respondents, efforts to characterize the total hospital were influenced by experiences within a particular department, it is also undoubtedly the case that many of the straight interns and residents did try to comply with our request that they describe the hospital as a whole, and, in doing so, did try to see beyond the limits of the department with which they were associated. In other words, we might underestimate departmental differences if we relied on the reports of these straight interns and residents. A second methodological problem that might become involved in a comparison of the reports given by men working in different departments is that the very qualities that attracted them to the departments in which they were working might also be associated with differences in perceptual acuity. At least this would have to be explored. But both these problems can be circumvented by giving voice to the hitherto muted rotating interns. In their case, the same people were asked to describe their experiences in two settings.

14. Because size of hospital made no difference in the replies of rotating interns, it is not considered here. We control only by degree of affiliation.

15. See, for example, James Bordley, III, "Effect of House Staff Training Programs on Patient Care," *Journal of the American Medical Association,* 173: 12 (July 23, 1960).

16. In hospitals throughout the country there are approximately twice

as many residents as interns. This is reflected in our data: our total sample included 1,300 interns and about 2,000 residents. When the somewhat more than 1,000 rotating interns are excluded, as they have been here, the preponderance of residents becomes even more marked. The possibility of comparing directly the responses of interns and residents is limited by the fact that, outside closely affiliated hospitals, there are virtually no straight interns. However, in that type of hospital the tendency we have noted does exist.

17. The same sort of relationship is found when the sociability of interns and the proportion of foreign-trained interns are considered. For the sake of brevity we do not show that table here.

18. In constructing this index, we added a fourth descriptive statement —how often do members of the house staff try "to beat the other fellow out?"—which has not been previously considered. In other words, the index is based on four, not three, questions.

19. Edward Leveroos, "Current Problems in Residency Training," *Conference on Graduate Medical Education* (February, 1956), pp. 4-5.

20. Maurice Levine, "The Education of the Psychiatrist," *Resident Physician*, 5: 8 (August, 1959), p. 171.

21. Although we shall not try to explain why this is so, there are marked variations in the shapes of the residency programs offered by different departments. Because of this, it has been necessary to control by department in Table 11.

22. See Robert K. Merton, "Patterns of Influence: A Study of Interpersonal Influence and of Communications Behavior in a Local Community," in P. F. Lazarsfeld and F. N. Stanton, eds., *Communications Research, 1948–1949* (New York: Harper & Brothers, 1949).

23. Alvin W. Gouldner, "Cosmopolitans and Locals: Toward an Analysis of Latent Social Roles," *Administrative Science Quarterly*, 2 (1957-1958), Part I, pp. 281-306; Part II, pp. 444-480.

24. Respondents were also asked which two lectures would interest them most personally. Their replies to this part of the question will not be considered here.

25. As before, rotating interns, who were asked about the behavior of residents on the medical and surgical services, are not included in the analysis that follows.

26. Table 15 seemed to indicate that interns have a less cosmopolitan orientation than do residents; Table 16 suggests exactly the opposite. This apparent discrepancy must be explained in terms of the specific content of the two questions. As we have already indicated, chiefs of service expect their interns to read less than residents. At the same time, however, problems of arranging for a practice are more remote in time for most of them than they are for residents.

27. Carson Cochran, "Bridging the Gap between Residency and Private Practice," *Resident Physician*, 6: 12 (December, 1960), p. 58.

28. Joseph S. Collings, "The Need for a New Educational Approach," *Journal of Medical Education*, 28: 9 (September, 1953), p. 23.

29. Jack L. Gibbs, "Medical Training Should Be More Practical," *RISS*, 3: 10 (October, 1960), pp. 37-40.

30. Herbert Berger, "The Intern Shortage Isn't Hopeless," *New York State Journal of Medicine*, 57 (1957), p. 3357.

8

Alienation and
the Social Structure

CASE ANALYSIS

OF A HOSPITAL

Rose Laub Coser

In his by now famous paper "Social Structure and Anomie," [1]
Merton examines several types of adaptation that individuals
may make to culturally approved goals and to the culturally

This paper is one report of research conducted under a grant by
the National Institute of Mental Health No. 2325, with additional
support from the then National Foundation for Infantile Paralysis.
My sincere thanks go to Dr. Leon Lewis for his cooperation and
encouragement in this research, as well as to the physicians, administrators, and nurses of Sunnydale Hospital and of the Rehabilitation
Center where the study was conducted; among them, Mrs. Frances
Brown showed active interest in the study. Mrs. N. McClellan was
most helpful as my assistant during the field work. For a critical
reading of earlier versions of this paper, I am grateful to Professor
Robert K. Merton and Dr. Natalie Rogoff. My thanks go also to
Miss Rachel Kahn-Hut for her assistance in editing the present
version.

approved means for achieving these goals. He examines, among others, two types of adaptations in which the lofty cultural goal has been abandoned or scaled down: *ritualism,* that is, a type of behavior in which active striving has been given up though "one continues to abide almost compulsively by institutional norms." An alternative to this type of behavior in the absence of a culturally approved goal is the abandonment of the culturally approved means as well—that is, *retreatism,* an escape from active involvement in either goals or means.

This paper sets out to specify some mechanisms through which "the social structure operates to exert pressure upon individuals for one or another of these alternative modes of behavior." It will appear that some of the mechanisms that Merton describes in his theory of reference-group behavior [2] as leading to the articulation of roles between interacting members of a social system also lead to the integration of goals and means.

The case described here is not one in which goals are abandoned by individuals, but rather one where the organization itself has little of a culturally valued goal orientation. As a result, its members have only culturally approved means at their disposal; in so far as they conform to these, they are engaged in *ritualistic* behavior. Owing to their previous professional training, however, it can be assumed that one condition that Merton singles out as fostering *retreatism* is present here, namely, "both the cultural goals and the institutional practices were roughly assimilated and imbued with affect and high value," but in the present setting "accessible institutional avenues are not productive of success." The measure of retreatism that will be discussed here consists not in a privatized but in a collective adaptation.[3]

Whether ritualistic or retreatist, the deviant adaptation, as will be shown, is not limited to behavior only; it is part of a broader outlook on self as working in social isolation. It therefore tends to be associated with alienation from work and from self.

Generally, in our culture, the explicit goal of medical treatment is that of partial or complete recovery of the patient. This tends to be the most valued goal in an achievement-oriented society; it not only is unquestioned by the public but also is implicitly assumed or stated explicitly in much sociological writing about health and illness. Thus Parsons points out that "traditionally the emphasis [of medical practice] has been on 'treatment' or 'therapy,'" and that the culturally defined obligation of the patient is "to want to get well." [4] This assumption must, however, be qualified: not all patients can get well. A physician's task is not only to help get the patients better but also to help those unable to improve to maintain at least as much as possible of what is left of their health. Similarly, the task of the hospital's personnel is not only to cooperate with the medical staff to make patients better but also to care for them if their disability is irreversible.

In Catholic cultures, taking care of suffering tends itself to be considered a "good deed," and nuns who engage in this activity are highly esteemed in the community. By contrast, in our achievement-oriented culture not much prestige is associated with the task per se of caring for patients. As a result, if the hospital is defined as one that "only" cares for patients who cannot get better, its abandonment of the culturally approved goal of "curing the sick" has several significant consequences. The scaled-down goal has a direct effect on its members by encouraging either ritualistic or retreatist behavior. And by its definition of organizational needs, the organization evolves a social structure that also contributes to converting ritualistic and retreatist behavior into a socially established pattern.

Sunnydale Hospital, a community hospital on the outskirts of the industrial center of Maplewood in the western United States, provides a good opportunity for studying the relation between selected kinds of behavior and social structure. Sunnydale's 650 beds, occupied by patients who are said not to be capable of improvement, are distributed over five buildings. One hundred additional beds are located in a sixth building, which is the Rehabilitation Center for patients with polio, respiratory, muscular, rheumatic, and other diseases requiring intensive rehabilitation programs.[5] The social structure of the Center and the attitudes of its staff will be compared with the structure and attitudes of Sunnydale proper.[6] The data are derived from structured interviews with twenty-seven registered nurses (out of a total of thirty registered nurses of the day shift),[7] focused interviews with ten interns, participant observation, and from systematic observation in all wards of the interaction between staff and patients and of staff members among themselves.

Alienation

THE DEFINITION OF THE SITUATION

The different goal orientations of the two types of wards are recognized by all the registered nurses interviewed. At least once during the interview, all Center nurses mention the goal of restoring patients to the community, whereas none of the Sunnydale nurses ever do so. The different orientations are based in large part on the nature of the illness of the patients. Three of Sunnydale's buildings are assigned to "custodial" cases; these give the "stamp" to the hospital in spite of the fact that two of its buildings are said to consist of "active treatment" wards, one for acute and one for long-term patients. Moreover, in the opinion of physicians both at Sunnydale and at the Center— though generally Sunnydale's patients are defined as "terminal" or "custodial"—a number of Sunnydale's patients could be rehabilitated. In spite of the fact that Sunnydale's patient population is not homogeneous in regard to prognosis, the nurses refer to their hospital in such terms as, "This is only an old people's home as far as I am concerned," or, "This is considered the end of the road, and people here talk of them as vegetables." On the other hand, the Center, whose patients are being prepared for return to the community, also has patients whose illness is irreversible. For example, in a discussion about a terminal case at the Center, a physician impatiently retorted to the objection that the patient knew she had at most five years to live, "We all have to die." He remarked that if we let the therapy program be guided by such considerations, we "may as well have a concentration camp instead of a hospital." [8] Thus, despite differences between wards as well as individual differences within the wards, in both environments all patients tend to be regarded *as if* they fit the respective goal, whether or not they actually do.

The stated goal, then, provides the definition of the situation. What is considered disruptive in one situation is considered rewarding in the other. If patients are defined as "terminal and custodial," plans to discharge them can be seen as disrupting activities. Several Sunnydale nurses say that they prefer a low turnover of patients "because of the type of help we have" or because "there's too much desk work" involved in discharging and admitting patients. One nurse explains that "the doctor will listen to me" if she feels that the patient should not be discharged because "if they do get discharged and come back in a week or two, it's more trouble in work and time." She adds: "You like the same patients in the same beds instead of having all the book work that is necessitated by changes."

Center nurses do not make such comments. Where the goal is to restore patients to the community, discharge becomes gratifying, as indicated by the following: "On this unit we have the satisfaction of getting patients discharged out of the hospital; nurses really get satisfaction if a patient comes in hemoplegic and then is discharged home walking within a few months." Discharge of patients at the Center is seen as reward for achievement. When such rewards cannot be expected, work is not seen as a means of achievement but as "a job to be done."

Further evidence concerning the differing orientations of Sunnydale and Center nurses comes from the responses to two questions that were asked in the interview: the first asked the nurses' judgment about their site of work, the other, their perception of needs for the future. In their answers to both questions, Sunnydale nurses are means-oriented in contrast to Center nurses, who are goal-oriented.

In answer to the question "How would you describe a ward when it's looking at its best?" Sunnydale nurses are more likely than Center nurses to stress the physical appearance of the ward (Table 1), indicating that housekeeping problems stand in the foreground of attention. The following is a typical Sunnydale description of "a ward at its best": "When it is finished and you stand at the head of the ward and look in, it is beautifully done, everything is clean." Almost all Center nurses, on the other hand, respond by referring to the behavior of patients, a concern to be expected among those who pursue the goal of restoring patients to the community. The following is a typical answer from the Center: "I like to see everybody out of bed and as active as possible. I like a certain amount of, not humor, but at least cheerful informal ward setting." [9]

Table 1

Nurses' Conceptions about "Ward at Its Best"

Answers to the question, "How would you describe a ward when its looking its best?"

In Terms of:	Center	Sunnydale
Patients' activity and social relations	9	1
Housekeeping	1	16

The emphasis by Sunnydale nurses on physical aspects in contrast to the emphasis on human achievement in the Center is consistent with their perceptions of future needs. Asked "What are the most important things needed in your ward?" Sunnydale nurses emphasize physical improvements to facilitate work and efficiency; some of the Center nurses who want physical improvements explain that their purpose is to benefit patients. Center nurses are also more likely to stress the need for better personal relations among the staff or between staff and patients (Table 2).

Table 2

Nurses' Conceptions of Needed Improvements

Answers to the question, "What are the most important things needed in the ward?"

In Terms of:	Center	Sunnydale
Better social relations or better care of patients	5	1
Physical improvements for personnel or "nothing" *	4	15
No answer	1	1

* One Sunnydale nurse says that no improvements are needed.

Responses to both questions suggest that goal orientation is associated with a focus on things. The answers about "needed improvements" are consistent with the answers about sources of satisfaction and dissatisfaction. In response to both sets of questions, Center nurses, in expressing professional concerns, usually emphasize staff relations or achievements with patients, while Sunnydale nurses, concerned with the "job" aspects of their work, usually refer to the physical aspects of labor.

Clearly, work has a different meaning at Sunnydale, where attention is focused on shortage of personnel, paper work, or other routine. In contrast to the *organic* conception of work, in which concern is with human implications, is the *ritualistic* concept of work, where focus is on "dead matter" and work is *mechanical*. As one nurse so cogently explained: "Well, my dear, I don't know. There isn't anything that I find unpleasant. *I have done it so long, I just automatically do it.*" (Emphasis supplied.)

INVOLVEMENT IN WORK

Sunnydale nurses are not deeply involved in their work. Although they don't dislike it much, neither do they have important reasons for liking it. When asked about their feelings, they reply by referring to routine matters. But Center nurses seem to have strong feelings about the sources of gratification as well as of frustration.

Asked "What do you like least in your work?" most Sunnydale nurses mention some routine as a source of dissatisfaction, such as "I don't like removing impactions." Furthermore, their references to sources of dissatisfaction are not expressed with much affect. The first impression upon interviewing Sunnydale nurses is that if there are any dissatisfactions, they do not concern professional issues. The example given by the nurses' director of Sunnydale illustrates this point: "There are not a great many grievances. A year ago they had complaints about the parking situation; they had to park the cars too far from the buildings. So now we've changed that."

Table 3

Nurses' Focus of Concern

Answers to the question, "What do you like least about your work?"

Concern Is with:	Center	Sunnydale
Professional relations or professional goals	8	0
Job performance	2	13
No dislike	0	3
No answer	0	1

In contrast, the complaints of Center nurses show concern with professional relations and professional issues (Table 3). These nurses tend to "dislike most" conflicts among the staff or certain conditions of the patients: "The thing I like least is the stress I feel when we have such a tremendous working organization and we can't communicate to get the job done." Or again, when "some patients get exasperated." These typical statements also suggest both presence and awareness of strong feelings—"The stress I feel" or "patients get exasperated."

Sources of satifaction of work also differ between the two groups. Sunnydale nurses less frequently see either professional achievement or professional relationships with other people as a source of gratification (Table 4):

Table 4

Sources of Main Satisfaction

Answers to the question, "What do you like best in your work?"

Satisfaction Derives from:	Center	Sunnydale
Professional achievement	6	3
Professional relations	4	4
General care	0	9
No answer	0	1

They tend to answer in general rather than in concrete terms; they like "the care of humanity" or "nursing care." One Sunny-dale nurse implies that her gratification stems from being able to get away from work: "It's a well-rounded day. . . . The employees can put in requests for vacation." In contrast, the majority of Center nurses derive satisfaction from professional achievements, and express their feelings about them. One nurse, typical of the others, says that she likes best "taking someone who is crippled or injured and showing them the means so that they can be self-sufficient, and seeing them accomplish it. It's a tremendous challenge."

Sources both of dissatisfaction and satisfaction in work tend to be a matter of little consequence to Sunnydale nurses. The different attitudes toward work in the two settings are revealed also in the images nurses hold of themselves in regard to their work.

SELF-IMAGE

Everett Hughes has called attention to the importance of a person's work for his experience of self: "A man's work is one of the more important parts of his social identity, of his self; indeed, of his fate in the one life he has to live, for there is something almost as irrevocable about the choice of occupation as there is about choice of a mate." [10] So much is this the case, Hughes suggests, that when you ask people what work they do, they are likely to answer in terms of "who they are"; that is, they attempt to establish and validate their own identity by referring to the identity of their work in a publicly recognized and preferably esteemed occupational or professional category. Our interviews with nurses, however, suggest that not all of them give such self-enhancing descriptions of "who they are" when asked "What is the most important thing you do?" Although many of them give a broad, inclusive description of the nature of their work, such as "problem-solving" or "helping patients reach their goal," others give simple concrete descriptions of tasks such as "keep patients clean" or "watch for symptoms." This suggests two different types of orientation to work. Some nurses refer to some concrete part of what they do; others develop a more inclusive conception of their occupational roles.

Table 5

Nurses' Views of Their Tasks

Answers to the question, "What is the most important thing you do?"

In Terms of:	Center	Sunnydale
Inclusive role	9	2
Specific task	1	13
No answer	0	2

As we see in Table 5, most Center nurses refer to their inclusive role (almost half of them use nouns rather than verbs to describe their tasks), while most Sunnydale nurses refer to some specific task.[11] This would suggest that when Hughes says work is one of the most important parts of a person's social identity, he refers to one type of work and one type of person; he speaks of relatively unalienated work and relatively unalienated people. But in industrial society many types of work and work situations do not lend themselves to the formation of a sense of identity through work. The prototype of such an alienated work situation is the assembly line. Alienation, in Marx's sense, means that "the work is external to the worker, that it is not part of his nature, that he consequently does not fulfill himself in his work but denies himself. . . . It is not the satisfaction of a need, but only a *means* for satisfying other needs" (emphasis in the original).[12] This seems to describe fairly well the meaning of work for Sunnydale nurses.[13] Work does not contribute substantially to their sense of social identity. For them, it is mainly a task-oriented routine. To the extent, then, that they see work as a mechanical type of activity, they see it as divorced from the self.

This leads to the question whether a routinized mechanical view of tasks and alienation of self in the work situation is associated with a different perception of the social field. Marx had something to say about the relation between fragmented labor, alienation of self, and estrangement from others:

Each man has a particular, exclusive sphere of activity. . . . Labor is separated from its object; *i.e.*, what he *does* is separated from *what* he does. He works next to others, but not with others. This is, in the last analysis the alienation of man from man; individuals are isolated from and set against each other. . . . Man's alienation from himself is simultaneously an estrangement from his fellow men.[14] [Emphasis in the original.]

Table 6 shows that nurses who express their identity by defining their role inclusively are more likely to describe a "good-looking ward" in terms of the people who occupy it, while nurses who give a restricted description of their work tend to see the ward in terms of routine tasks of housekeeping:

Table 6

Nurses' Views of Their Tasks by Conceptions of Ideal Ward

GOOD-LOOKING WARD IS DESCRIBED IN TERMS OF:	NURSES ANSWER IN TERMS OF		
	Inclusive Role	Specific Task	N. A.
Patients and social relations	9	1	0
Housekeeping	2	13	2

The connection between conception of work role and the perception of the social field is highlighted in the drawings the nurses were asked to make of "a nurse at work."[15] Eight nurses drew a picture of a nurse without a patient; one of these nurses was at the Center, the seven others were at Sunnydale (Table 7).

Table 7

Drawings of "Nurse at Work"

Drawings Show:	Center	Sunnydale
Nurse and patient	9	4
Patient only	0	1
Nurse only	1	7
No answer	0	5 *

* Respondents refused to draw a picture, claiming inability to do so.

This graphic presentation of "the nurse at work" gains significance when it is compared with the nurses' conceptions of their
"most important task" (Table 8). This exhibits an association

Table 8

Nurses' Views of Tasks and Drawings of "Nurse at Work"

	NURSES ANSWER IN TERMS OF		
	Inclusive Role	Specific Task	No Answer
Drawing shows patient *	10	3	1
Drawing does not show patient	1	7	0
No answer	0	4	1

* One nurse, who drew a picture of a patient only, answered in terms of her inclusive role.

between the way they conceive of their work and the way they
perceive themselves in relation to others. Most of the nurses
with task-specific images of their work drew pictures of the
nurse at work as unrelated to others, or claimed that they cannot
portray the role at all. The nurses with inclusive images have
almost always the role-partner, the patient, in mind when con-
ceiving of "the nurse at work." This illustrates the thesis of
George Herbert Mead that our selves exist and enter into our
experience only so far as the selves of others exist and enter
into our experience.[16]

These differences add relevance to the differing reports on
sources of work satisfaction that we have examined. It will be
remembered that Center nurses showed more professional involvement than Sunnydale nurses (Table 4). And now we find
that these differences in professional involvement are associated
with differences in self-image (Table 9).

All nurses deriving their work satisfaction from achievement
who drew a picture make the patient a part of their image of
"a nurse at work," and so do most nurses who derive their
satisfaction from professional relations. But none of the nurses
who speak of their satisfaction in terms of general care have
their drawings depict work as part of a social arrangement.
This is also consistent with the conceptions of improvements

Table 9

Source of Satisfaction in Work by Graphic Presentation of "Nurse at Work"

| | WORK SATISFACTION DERIVES FROM | | | |
	Professional Achievement	Professional Relations	General Care	N. A.
Drawing shows patient *	9	5	0	0
Drawing does not show patient	0	1	7	0
No drawing	0	2	2	1

* One nurse, who drew a picture of a patient only, derived satisfaction from achievement.

needed in the ward. As will be remembered from Table 2, six nurses, one from Sunnydale and five from the Center, focus their attention on better staff relations or on better care of patients when describing needed improvements: all these include a patient in their drawings of a "nurse at work." The data support the hypothesis that a worker's alienation from his work is associated with his alienation from those with whom he is associated in his occupational role.

Melvin Seeman [17] has identified five alternative uses of alienation in sociological writings. He distinguishes between powerlessness, meaninglessness, normlessness, self-estrangement, and isolation. Although these are indeed distinct dimensions, they do not seem to offer alternative meanings of the concept. Rather the concept refers to a condition in which all these elements are present and interrelated. The Sunnydale syndrome provides a case in point: Sunnydale nurses are alienated because they are *powerless* to implement a significant goal. Unable to obtain gratifying results from their work, they find it *meaningless* and so cannot use it to fashion a meaningful self-image. Not being able to express their social identity in their work, they are *self-estranged* in the work situation. Consequently, they become estranged from their social field and see themselves as *isolated* individuals. It will become clear in what follows that Sunnydale nurses work under conditions that also isolate them physically from other professional groups—a condition that contributes to the *normlessness* of behavior in the form of retreatism. *Alienation*, it seems, is a *syndrome* composed of all the elements that Seeman has carefully defined.[18]

Interactive Processes and Social Control

DEVIATION FROM PROFESSIONAL NORMS

As can be expected from the preceding findings, a much higher proportion of all the observed interactions consists of staff-patient interactions in the Center than in Sunnydale.[19] The interaction pattern at Sunnydale becomes more significant, however, if we compare its different wards. In Sunnydale's custodial wards, more than half of the patients suffer from a complete mental or physical deterioration that either makes for complete helplessness or for other disturbances such as incontinence, aggressive behavior, and so on. In view of the shortage of personnel, one would expect that staff would have to act more frequently "on" the patients, without being able or motivated to elicit responses from them. At the same time one would expect staff to spend more time in interaction with those patients in these custodial wards who are ambulatory or in wheel chairs (about one-third of the patients), since these are very well able to communicate. But, in fact, as Table 10 shows, while the proportion of "acting on" patients is hardly higher than in the treatment wards, the proportion of staff-patient interactions is significantly lower. Instead, staff-staff interaction is higher here than in any other wards.[20]

This apparently paradoxical finding can become understandable. Because of the excessive demands imposed by the helplessness and mental disturbance of patients upon an exceedingly small staff, professional activity seems almost pointless. Rather than attempting to deal with patients, nurses as well as orderlies and aides often withdraw from the ward and seek support from one another in the nurses' office, over a cup of coffee or a cigarette.

Table 10

Type of Interaction Observed by Type of Ward

Type of Interaction	Center	Active Treatment	Long-Term Treatment	Custodial	Total No. of Interactions Observed
Staff acting on patient (without eliciting response)	11.2%	32.0%	30.4%	33.5%	105
Staff-patient interaction	57.5	34.0	30.4	20.8	126
Staff-staff interaction	31.3	34.0	39.2	45.7	147
Total Number of observed interactions	80	85	69	144	378
Total number of minutes observed per ward	72.5	54.0	71.3	81.7	
Number of wards	6	8	8	12	

This observed interaction usually did not deal with professional concerns. Therefore it should not be confused with interprofessional relations centered on tasks at hand, about which more will be said later. For example, the observer often noted scenes such as the following: "When I left the ward (at 3:55 P.M.) only one aide was still on the floor, reading a magazine in the linen room. I relayed a request by a patient for a bedpan. She thanked me, but five minutes later had not come out. Janitor joined her and they were chatting as I left." There is further evidence of withdrawal, as the head nurse of one of the custodial buildings testifies: "We have so much absenteeism and tardiness. Today two people were supposed to be on duty, but they didn't show up. It's unfair to their co-workers; it doesn't bother me. That is the most irksome quality here. . . . So many of them feel that the hospital work is the last work; if they have something to do downtown, that comes first."

Conditions in the custodial wards are extreme; so is the rate of staff-staff interaction. However, they seem to illustrate a general trend. As a comparison of all types of wards confirms, the frequency of interaction among staff is correlated with patient-nurse ratio (Table 11), a seemingly unexpected

Table 11

Comparison between Staff-Staff Interaction Rate and Patient-Nurse Ratio

Type of Ward	S/S Interaction Observed (% of All Int.) N = 147	P/N Ratio on a Typical Winter day *	P/N Ratio at Maximum Bed Capacity	Number of Patients on a Typical Winter Day *	Number of Patients at Maximum Bed Capacity
Center	31.3	7.2	8.9	88	107
Active-Treatment Wards	34.0	19.3	19.8	135	139
Long-Term-Treatment Wards	39.2	27.4	28.0	137	140
Custodial Wards	45.7	53.8	59.3	323	356

* According to census taken on February 11, 1958.

result: the greater the number of patients in relation to nurses in a ward, the more staff tend to spend time among themselves.

There is not only this tendency for *ad hoc* withdrawal from professional tasks at Sunnydale; there are also mechanisms associated with the structure of interprofessional relations on the wards for the *systematic* withdrawal of professional staff. Most staff activities that were observed were those of nurses and aides, in part because there are relatively few physicians to cover the large number of wards. There is one full-time staff physician in charge of Sunnydale (though for a short while there were two). He is assisted by four or five interns who are sent out from Maplewood for a period of from six to thirteen weeks. The interns rotate between the five wards and the emergency room, so that they are in charge of the same 100 to 150 patients for only two or three weeks. An intern explained how he handles this situation: "I try to let the nurses keep me up on everything and then I try to weed out those that can wait a couple of days; after they have been let go, in a fair majority of cases, it will clear up by itself. . . . The cases that are more interesting to me, I spend more time on and let the other ones go." Faced with the situation of not being able to take care of that many patients during the two-week charge of the building (in some cases an intern is in charge of two buildings), they cease to feel harassed and do not even feel called upon to be active. As was revealed in several conversations with interns, they look forward while still at Maplewood to the time they can spend at Sunnydale, because they expect it to be an opportunity for some rest.

An acute shortage of personnel does not necessarily increase each person's load; it may get so bad that it legitimizes withdrawal from the task. At Sunnydale, abandoning the prestigeful goal of recovery results also in abandoning some professionally prescribed means of medical practice. A nurses' supervisor illustrates this point: "The intern would go through the charts on his day and never change the prescriptions; sometimes he would just add to the old prescriptions, and *we* can't change them." At Sunnydale, interns as well as nurses engage in retreatist behavior. This fact derives from the circumstances that (1) only few professional groups actually encounter each other, and the frequency of such encounters decreases from active treatment to long-term treatment to custodial wards, and (2) mechanisms are at work that make for the mutual avoidance of the few professionals who are on the premises. Thus, the almost linear correlation between the rate of staff-staff interaction and patient-nurse ratio (see Figure 8-1) is not to be understood only in terms of shortage of nursing staff. Rather it is to be seen within the structural context of professional life at Sunnydale.

1. There are not many professional groups at Sunnydale, the main ones being the nurses and physicians. There is a social service, but the social workers deal almost exclusively with the administration; their main task concerns the eligibility of patients and the collection of old-age and other types of insurance. The following comment by the nurses' supervisor who reported that interns do not change prescriptions illustrates how interprofessional relationships could be a source of social control: ["When the new staff physician came] *we told him,* and he went over all the prescriptions and took the old ones off the list" (emphasis supplied). Such social control by nurses over physicians (or for that matter vice versa) is relatively rare at Sunnydale; in this case it had to wait for a change at the top of the medical hierarchy.

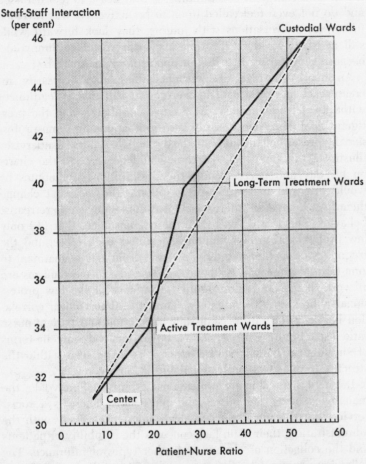

Staff-Staff Interaction (per cent)

Patient-Nurse Ratio

Figure 8-1

Staff-staff interaction rate by patient-nurse ratio on one typical winter day (see Table 11).

2. Not only do interns withdraw from the wards; more important still, nurses and interns help each other to maintain this type of withdrawal. Physicians do not interfere in the active-treatment ward when the buzzers at the beds of patients are disconnected and the electric cord tied up so that patients cannot connect it themselves.[21] In turn, nurses know that if they "call

[a doctor] without too much need he doesn't like it," and consequently they are, in the praiseful words of one intern, "outstanding [since they are] ultraconservative in calling the doctor." Another intern thinks that the nurses are not always reliable since, as he explains, "they sometimes call for minor things." In this case it seems that the competence of the nurse is measured not so much by her achievements as by her willingness to help the doctor to stand aside. Thus, where sanctions are at work at Sunnydale, they often press for the evasion of norms. It is partly on this basis that some consensus between doctors and nurses is established. "I have nothing but pleasant experiences," one nurse says. "They know that I won't ask them to come unless I need them. . . . They know I'm only trying to help them, keep them from coming over here."

Consequently, Sunnydale is characterized by a lack of those interprofessional conflicts described by observers in other hospitals. But lack of conflict is not necessarily functional for an organization. As in this case, it may be a result of relative withdrawal from the task. One nurse in an active-treatment ward explains that she has little difficulty with doctors: "[I have] very little contact with interns. They go their own way." Not only are there too few physicians to be "underfoot"—a frequent accusation in other hospitals—and not only do they stay too short a time for strong sentiments, either positive or negative, to develop, but the interaction between nurses and physicians is greatly curbed by both professional groups encouraging mutual avoidance. It appears that avoidance is a means for adapting to tasks that seem to be deprived of a meaningful goal. It also serves to deal with latent hostilities that cannot be dealt with openly; in case of tensions arising between nurses and interns there is no ulterior goal that can be referred to as a normative guide of behavior. To be sure there are hostilities, as illustrated by the following words of a nurse who says that she "never had any trouble getting along with doctors": "I feel sorry for an intern who thinks he knows it all before he leaves. He's in for a rude awakening." Hostility is handled by another nurse who says she experiences "no difficulties" with doctors: "The nicest thing is that they don't stay with us forever." [22]

For readers of George Homans' analysis of Hilltown—a New

England town in which the normative system had become weak indeed—Sunnydale may touch a familiar cord. As in Hilltown, at Sunnydale *the number of activities that members of the group carry on together is small.* As in Hilltown, this does not mean that individuals have nothing to do. Like the Hilltowners who have little to do *with* other Hilltowners, in Sunnydale nurses have little to do *with* other professionals. As a consequence, *the low frequency of interaction is associated with weakness of interpersonal sentiments.* The indifference noted in regard to satisfaction and dissatisfaction in work as well as the reported lack of difficulties with doctors, provide cases in point.

Low frequency of interaction and weakness of interpersonal sentiment have a mutual effect on each other so that, in turn, sentiments are not strong enough to motivate the members of the professions to collaborate with each other.[23]

The low frequency of interaction and the lack of involvement of professionals with each other are related to the stated goal of the organization. As will become clear in what follows, they are also rooted in the social structure.

AFFIRMATION OF PROFESSIONAL NORMS

The social structure of the Center offers a contrast sufficient to highlight some structural determinants of alienation. The staff there is characterized by its multiple professional affiliations, and mechanisms have evolved that assure a large measure of social control. The various professional groups work next to each other, with each other, and often in competition with each other. The staff includes ten physicians (including a psychiatrist) in part-time capacity, several physical and occupational therapists, two psychologists, two social workers, and twelve registered nurses, supplemented by practical nurses who take an active part in treatment. There is also a part-time speech therapist, and there are occasional visits from outside social workers as representatives of a foundation or of the vocational services of the community.

As we have known ever since Durkheim, the interdependence of various occupations resulting from the division of labor brings about the "organic solidarity" that helps hold modern society together. Organic solidarity consists of involvement with one another of interdependent status-occupants. They are bound by common interests, though they may be in conflict regarding the means for implementing these interests. In some settings, such as the Center, they can observe one another at close quarters, and each one is under pressure to orient himself to differential expectations in these complex crisscrossing circles. Persons of various status positions and different professional orientations and expectations are held together by their common commitment to the concrete goal of returning patients to the community; there is strong concern on everyone's part with achievement and failure. And precisely because of such zeal, conflicts do arise. As we see in Table 12, all nurses in the Center report difficulties with doctors, whereas only a third of the nurses at Sunnydale do so. As one nurse explains: "Everybody feels that they like to be in charge of the situation. Everybody says, 'This is my business,' and nobody gets an over-all picture."

Table 12

Nurses' Statements about Difficulties with Doctors

Answers to the question, "Do you find that some doctors are difficult to work with?"

	Center	Sunnydale
Yes	10	5
No	0	11
No Answer	0	1

The greater frequency with which Center nurses report difficulties with doctors is not merely the result of some difficult relations between professional groups that exist in the Center, difficulties that in part arise from the complexities of having many diverse groups there. The contrasting reports of Center and Sunnydale nurses also reflect the fact that, at the Center, conflicts are freely described to the interviewer precisely because they are carried out openly in ward life. Fighting over controversial issues is considered legitimate. Differences of opinion and expectation are dealt with at regular and frequent all-staff meetings or smaller conferences. These provide a patterned opportunity for the carrying out of conflicts between the different professional groups, which continuously recall the goal to be pursued and the norms that should govern behavior.[24] The following interchange at an all-staff conference is an example of the usually, but not always, friendly discussion of issues:

Physician (addressing himself to physical therapist): How come this patient hasn't been going on with her program?
Physical therapist: She says she doesn't like it.
Physician: Is that a reason for stopping it?
Psychologist: Doctor, you forget that this patient knows that she has less than five years to live.
Physician: If you see it that way, we may as well have a concentration camp instead of a hospital.
Psychologist: But don't you see that there is a reality-situation here?
Physician: What's the reality? That we all have to die?

Here the staff is being reminded by the physician of the professional norm that as long as there is life, efforts have to be directed at prolonging it. In another case, it is a physician who is the object of normative control:

Psychologist to physician-in-chief: May I remind you, before this patient comes in, that he is very anxious, and that much of his response at this conference will depend on how he is being talked to.
Nurse: I would like to add that this morning the patient was very upset about [description follows of upsetting situation]. (Patient is brought in, interviewed, and led out again.)
Physician-in-chief to psychologist: How did I do, teacher?
Psychologist: Go to the head of the class.
Physician-in-chief, addressing the conference of about thirty people: In this place, if I look over one shoulder, there stands a psychologist; if I look over the other shoulder, there stands a sociologist (smiling): This is some way of practicing medicine! [25]

These examples may illustrate the way in which the meetings provide an occasion for reaffirming the goal and formulating norms, and also bring onto the level of rational discourse and instrumental behavior feelings that without such a forum might become laden with affect. The open expressions of opinions and judgments give a professional definition to personal involvement.[26] This is especially important in an atmosphere of deep involvements since these could give rise to a clash of personalities; but since antagonisms are recognized, conflicts at the Center tend to be limited to the functionally specific task at hand. Instead of being a sign of social disorganization they are expressions of, as well as means for, social control among various professional groups and individuals.

Social control is reinforced by the fact that the meetings provide institutionalized settings for *observability* among persons of various fields of specialization and in various positions in the hierarchy. At the same time, they largely limit the time and place of observability, thus assuring a patterned measure of insulation. We need not belabor the point that if persons variously located in the social structure are to evaluate the behavior of others, they must at regular intervals either see one another behave or at least be in a position to obtain information about their behavior.[27] If such information is lacking, status-occupants become exempted from the judgment of competent colleagues, and role performance may sink below tolerable standards.[28] But some insulation from observability is also needed so that persons can go about their work without unpredicted interference by role-partners with whom they stand in an authority relationship. A social mechanism that serves these double requirements can be formulated as follows:

PROPOSITION 1: *Some measure of observability of role performance by members of the role-set is required, if the social requirement of accountability is to be met. This statement obviously does not contradict the fact that some measure of insulation from observability is also required for the effective operation of social structures. Instead, the two statements, taken in conjunction, hold that there is some optimum of observability, difficult as yet to identify in measurable terms and doubtless varying for different social statuses, that will simultaneously make for ac-*

countability of role-performance and for autonomy of role-performance.[29]

The conferences and meetings do more than provide information about the professional behavior of those in the social system. They also make status-occupants aware of the differing expectations held by role-partners significant to them. As a result, persons in different positions are helped to articulate their roles and to formulate a professional self-image.[30] The following example shows how a nurse facing differing expectations is forced to think about her obligations: "Miss R. has battled with Dr. B. and some of the others because they all said they knew what the nurses' responsibilities were. He wants the nurse to carry on procedures that, according to Miss R., are physical therapy procedures. True, it's a mistake to make jacks-of-all-trades of us." She continues thinking about the role of the nurse. "This doesn't mean that we don't have to know what the other person does. In a rehabilitation service where there are no physical therapists, it's surprising what the nursing service can accomplish." Again, a nurse reacts to conflicting expectations in this fashion: "We have been taught by Dr. X. that [this patient] must always catheterize himself. On the unit another doctor said we have to get away from these catheterizations." She adds: "I have two days to clear up the matter." In the process of coping with contradictions derived from such significant role-partners, the nurse is likely to form an image of herself as a significant actor in the social system. It is not surprising, then, that this nurse, when asked to describe the most important thing she does, says: "Along the lines of a tremendous teaching service and continuity of responsibilities . . . that go over and beyond the patient-care aspects." The circumstance that status-occupants are under pressure to resolve the contradictory demands of different role-partners leads to the operation of another mechanism:

Proposition 2: *Confronted with contradictory demands by members of his role-set, each of whom assures that the legitimacy of his demands is beyond dispute, the occupant of a status can act to make these contradictions manifest. To some extent . . . this redirects the conflict so that it is one between members*

*of the role-set rather than, as was at first the case, between them
and the occupant of the status. . . . At the very least, this serves
to make evident that it is no willful malfeasance on the part of
the status-occupant that keeps him from conforming to all the
contradictory expectations imposed upon him. . . . The replacing
of pluralistic ignorance by common knowledge serves to make
for a redefinition of what can properly be expected of the status-
occupant.*[31]

A further property of social structure that facilitates articulation of the nurses' roles at the Center is the presence of a sufficiently large number of registered nurses in one unit. Every
nurse knows that she is not alone in facing contradictory
expectations of many role-partners.[32] They can therefore articulate their roles *collectively,* as they did in the following inci-
dent: Several nurses reported complaints coming from patients
about the "doctors' manners" in violating privacy. "Doctors and
other staff charged into their cubicles when they had their curtains drawn without knocking or warning or anything, or maybe
knock and walk in at the same time." Another nurse: "[The
patients] know that they have a right to their integrity and their
privacy." She adds: "The patients have a right to expect *me* to
do something about the problem they bring to me because this
is *my job.*" Yet, as everyone who is acquainted with hospital etiquette knows, a particular nurse cannot call a particular doctor
to task. In most hospitals, she will have to "go through channels"; a complaint about a physician will in all likelihood be
brought to his attention through the intermediary of the nurses'
director and the chief of service. But at the Center, nurses do
not find it useful to appeal to the nurses' director, since, being
associated with Sunnydale proper, she is considered an "outsider" by the Center personnel. Center nurses, bound to the
Center staff by the common therapeutic goal, are more loyal to
Center physicians than to Sunnydale nurses of whatever rank.
They therefore use their own initiative in dealing with physicians. One nurse explains how this can be done. (She is the one
who describes doctors as "charging into the patients' cubicles.")
This problem, as well as others such as "one doctor telling one
thing and another doctor telling another one," led her to call a

meeting: "I said, why don't we have a meeting with the doctors? . . . We [that is, the registered nurses] all went. . . . We told them and of course then their annoyance came up too, but they were very accepting." The opportunity for persons who occupy the same status position to engage in collective action is described in the following mechanism:

PROPOSITION 3: *The mechanism of social support by others in similar social statuses with similar difficulties of coping with an unintegrated role-set . . . presupposes the not unusual structural situation that others occupying the same social status have much the same problem of dealing with their role-sets. . . . The individual subject to conflicts need not meet them as a wholly private problem which must be handled in a wholly private fashion. . . . Conflicts of role-expectations become patterned and shared by occupants of the same social status.*[33]

Both the fact that all nurses share the same difficulties and that there are avenues for verbalizing them make it possible for these issues to be removed from the level of "personal problems" to that of social organization. The nurses are in a position not so much to discuss their "personal problems" as to articulate their *professional* role. Thus, the nurse who called the meeting says that "teaching" is her most important task, and adds, "This puts me in the position of a staff counselor." At another point in the interview she implies the ways in which relations among nurses help to articulate roles: "I have to go to informal staff conferences every morning and ask for their report, and this again is nice too because the supervisor and the head nurse can *use me as a sounding board* just as well as can the staff." (Emphasis supplied.)

At the Center, then, the very conditions and mechanisms that provide a source of social control—multiplicity of role-partners, conflicts among professional groups, mutual observability, as well as its limitation, and the regular meetings to deal with these—also provide the conditions for the articulation of roles and formation of professional self-images.

These conditions do not prevail at Sunnydale, where the mechanisms covered by propositions 1, 2, and 3, above, are not operative. This is so because (1) the goal of caring for patients, as it is understood, restricts the staff's task primarily to problems of housekeeping, and (2) social arrangements are such that status-occupants suffer from a restricted role-set, that is, from a restriction of the number of significant role-partners.

1. With too much work to do, everyone is more concerned with specific problems of housekeeping than with problems concerning either staff relations or more remote goals. The understaffing of Sunnydale's wards is, to a large extent, a result of the definition of "custodial care": given this goal orientation, the composition of the population—patients as well as staff—is geared to the definition of this goal.

Under these conditions, a goal that does not seem "worthy" (interns tend to say that it isn't "worthwhile" to spend much energy on "these" patients) and an overwhelming work load, the few people who are in potentially responsible positions tend to withdraw. This keeps them from being informed about the norms and behavior of others. Also, they are not motivated to seek information about it, since prevailing conditions seem to make it impossible for them to use the information effectively.

2. With too few professional persons available, few professions represented, and the tendency of the few available persons to withdraw, status-occupants at Sunnydale suffer from a *restricted role-set*, that is, from a restriction of the number of role-partners. This has the following consequences: (*a*) Sunnydale nurses (as well as all other status-occupants at Sunnydale) work under conditions of *low exposure to observability*—a condition that results in the reduction of social control; (*b*) since there are few persons *differentially* located in the social structure, there are hardly any conflicting expectations faced by status-occupants; therefore they are not required to be *continuously engaged in articulating their roles in relation to the members of their role-sets* and consequently forming a professional self-image. (*c*) Given their scarcity, registered nurses are relatively deprived of role-partners occupying the *same* status position as themselves, so that there is little opportunity for them to articulate collectively, as professionals, the responsibilities and limitations of the relationships they share.

The scaling down of the goal of recovery of the sick not only has the direct consequence of inducing the staff to adopt ritualistic or retreatist behavior. By restricting the number of role-partners for status-occupants in responsible positions—an organizational restriction that is a further consequence of the scaling down of the goal—it provides the structural setting for patterned nonconformity as well as institutionalization of the alienation syndrome.

Discussion

This inquiry suggests that the complexity of the role-sets of status-occupants in an organization seems to contribute to the avoidance of alienation. The social mechanisms that operate in resolving contradictions in expectations provide the opportunity for continual articulation of roles. This requires deliberate consideration by the person of his relation with his work and with his various role-partners. This process seems to be similar to the development of self-consciousness in the *game* as described by Mead in contrast to mere *play:*

If we contrast play with an organized game . . . , we note the essential difference that the child who plays in a game must be ready to take the attitude of everyone else involved in that game, and that these different roles must have a definite relationship to each other. . . . In a game where a number of individuals are involved . . . the child taking one role must be ready to take the role of everyone else. . . . The attitudes of the other players which the participant assumes organize into a sort of unit and it is that organization which controls the response of the individual. . . . [This] is essential to self-consciousness in the full sense of the term.

If the role-set consists of many role-partners of different outlook and status, the status-occupant finds himself in the situation of a *game* in which, as at the Center, he becomes conscious of his own role. In a restricted role-set, however, his condition is more nearly similar to that of the actor in *play,* in which, as in

Sunnydale, "there is just a set of responses that follow on each other indefinitely" and in which "he does not organize his life as a whole. . . . He is not a whole self." [34]

Further evidence supports the assumption that complex role-sets are important for the formation of personal identity. One method used with mental patients in therapeutic settings is the "psychodrama," which is, in effect, an attempt to create an artificial role-set for the person who experiences severe disturbances in his interpersonal relations. By facing several role-partners simultaneously on the stage, he learns to perceive his own role in relation to these partners. [35]

It would be a mistake to conclude that the existence of many departments and status groups in an organization by itself provides complex role-sets for its members. The question is, rather, with how many members in these departments and subgroups status-occupants are engaged in formal transactions. Although complex organizations may afford some members the opportunity for complex role-sets, there is differential access to role-partners variously located in the social structure for different status-occupants. In large industrial organizations, for example, where complex role-sets may exist for some status-occupants, assembly-line workers have a restricted one since they have few role-partners in social positions other than their own. The assembly-line worker tends to find himself in this respect, as well as in regard to his alienation from work, in a situation similar to that of Sunnydale's registered nurses. [36]

Moreover, some principles of bureaucratic organization, aimed at maximizing efficiency, rationality, and discipline by reducing the possibility of conflicting orders and expectations, may, when they are too rigidly applied, have the dysfunctional consequence of so restricting the role-sets for some status-occupants as to alienate them from work and from colleagues as well. It would be worth investigating whether ritualistic behavior (for example, emphasis on rules) or retreatist behavior (such as "passing the buck") in bureaucratic structures is associated with a strong emphasis on "going through channels," a procedure in which each status-occupant can deal in his formal transactions with only one or two members in the organization and, conversely, is approached by only one or two persons who seek communication with him. Such structurally built-in restriction of communication between members of an organization tends to isolate its members from the goals of the organization and encourages ritualistic attention to work. Furthermore, narrow channels restrict the number of role-partners differentially located in the structure with concomitantly different expectations of the status-occupant, and hence put him in a position in which he does not have to articulate his own role and become conscious of it. This was illustrated in my earlier case study [37] of two hospital wards. On the medical ward, authority was consistently delegated down the line; only the intern gave orders to the nurse, and he was the only physician with whom she discussed patients. When interprofessional grievances turned up, nurses would take theirs up the ladder of the nurses' hierarchy, and the complaints would then come down the medical ladder again till they reached the physician concerned. In this narrow hierarchy, nurses tended to be ritualistic in their behavior. In contrast was the surgical ward, where authority was not rigidly delegated at all, where all physicians passed on orders to the nurse, and she herself took her problems to whomever they concerned; nobody objected if she dealt directly with other services in the hospital, such as social service. As a result, nurses on the surgical ward showed initiative, worked their way around the rules when necessary, and considered themselves important agents of the postoperative improvement of patients.

Seen in the light of the theory of the role-set, Whyte's observation that "long, narrow hierarchies . . . are relatively low both in economic efficiency and in employees' morale" raises the problem whether "low morale" is not in part a function of the restricted role-sets in such hierarchical arrangements. Whyte says that in such organizations people are prevented from "discovering what their strengths and weaknesses are" and from "feeling that they themselves have really mastered their jobs." [38] This is what is meant in this paper by inability to form a conception of one's identity in relation to work.

In developing the concept of role-set, Merton sees the fact that "anyone occupying a particular status has role-partners who are differently located in the social structure," a "basic source of disturbance." [39] He proceeds to specify a number of mechanisms through which some reasonable degree of articulation among the roles of the role-set is secured. We can now add to his thought one functional consequence of the relationships with differently located role-partners: to the extent that such relationships call into operation mechanisms that help to overcome the stresses and strains of differing expectations, to that extent a complex role-set is functional for the formation of self-image. In the absence of such mechanisms, of course, complex role-sets may be a source of serious social instability and may result in the withdrawal altogether of some status-occupants from their positions.[40] But because complex role-sets tend to encourage the development of social mechanisms for articulating roles, they are important for the status-occupant's active involvement in work and in the social relationships required for the formation and maintenance of an occupational self-image.

NOTES

1. Robert K. Merton, "Social Structure and Anomie," in *Social Theory and Social Structure* (New York: The Free Press of Glencoe, 1957), pp. 131–194.

2. *Ibid.*, pp. 371–379.

3. In his first definition of retreatism from both culturally approved goals and culturally approved means, Merton sees this as a form of adaptation of people who, "strictly speaking, are *in* the society but not *of* it," and sees it as a "privatized rather than a collective mode of adaptation" (*ibid.*, p. 153). However, in the "Continuities" to this paper (*ibid.*, pp. 187–190), he speaks about apathy as a form of retreatism, found among some workers, or among the elderly. This is the type of retreatism dealt with in this paper.

4. Talcott Parsons, *The Social System* (New York: The Free Press of Glencoe, 1951), pp. 429 and 437 respectively. I have also stated elsewhere that the goal of medical practice is recovery: "In the hospital, where the physician is endeavoring to be 'more of a physician' and a nurse is trying to be 'more of a nurse,' a patient is expected as time goes on to be 'less of a patient'" (Rose Laub Coser, *Life in the Ward* [East Lansing: Michigan State University Press, 1962], p. 11). The case of patients whose physical condition does not permit them even to try to be "less of a patient" has rarely been considered in sociological investigations.

5. The Rehabilitation Center is under the administrative jurisdiction of Sunnydale, but has its own director and largely recruits its own personnel, who are under the administrative authority of Sunnydale. Its financial

support comes partly from the same sources as does Sunnydale's and partly from foundation funds that are administered by the medical school in the area. In this paper, the rehabilitation ward will be called the "Center," and the other five buildings of the hospital will be called "Sunnydale."

6. Sunnydale Hospital is run efficiently; the standard of care is higher there than in most hospitals with a similar function. Therefore, any short-comings in staff performance that may be noted in this paper would apply *a fortiori* to other hospitals with the same goal orientation. The syndrome is not the result of characteristics of its personnel, but exists in spite of their good intentions; as will be seen, it is rooted in the social structure of the organization.

7. SAMPLE OF REGISTERED NURSES INTERVIEWED

	Total No. of Reg. Nurses Day Shift	No. of Reg. Nurses Interviewed
Rehabilitation wards	12	10
All other wards	18	17
Total	30	27

8. For a verbatim account of this discussion, see p. 252.

9. The following response by a Sunnydale nurse, although less specific in its references than the response of Center nurses, was coded as an example of social relations: "Everybody cooperates to help each other; a happy ward."

One Sunnydale nurse finds the "ward at its best" when the patients are away. Her housekeeper's description, "When the patients are fed and resting and the janitor has been around to clean up," is preceded by the sentences: "Yesterday all the patients were out on the porch. It looked pretty nice then."

10. Everett C. Hughes, *Men and Their Work* (New York: The Free Press of Glencoe, 1958), p. 43.

11. Examples of the "inclusive" role description are: "I am a team leader. . . ." "I think setting sort of an example, . . ." "Well, teaching. . . . This puts me in the kind of a position of a staff counselor. . . ." "The RN is . . . a go-between the supervisor and the team . . . a diplomat that's what it is, politician. . . ."

Examples of the "task-specific" description: "Carrying out doctors' orders"; "Seeing that the patients are fed and cared for"; "Medicines and bedside care."

12. Karl Marx, *Economic and Philosophical Manuscripts*, in T. B. Bottomore and Maximilien Rubel, eds., *Karl Marx: Selected Writings in Sociology and Social Philosophy* (London: Watts & Co., 1956), p. 169.

13. Sunnydale nurses seem to be, in this respect, similar to the industrial workers studied by Robert Dubin, in which it was found that only 24 per cent of the interviewed workers found their central life interest in their work ("Industrial Workers' Worlds: A Study of the 'Central Life Interests' of Industrial Workers," *Social Problems*, 3 [January, 1956] pp. 131-142). In contrast, Louis H. Orzack, in a similar study of registered nurses, found that for 79 per cent of these professional persons work was a central life interest ("Work as a 'Central Life Interest' of Professionals," *Social Problems*, 7 [Fall, 1959], pp. 125-132).

14. Quoted by Herbert Marcuse, *Reason and Revolution* (New York: Oxford University Press, 1941), p. 279.

15. This method was suggested to me by Hans Mauksch.

16. George H. Mead, *Mind, Self and Society* (Chicago: University of Chicago Press, 1946), p. 164.

17. Melvin Seeman, "On the Meaning of Alienation," *American Sociological Review*, 24 (December, 1959), pp. 783-791.

18. After this paper went to press, Dwight G. Dean's article on "Alienation, Its Meaning and Measurement" came to my attention. Dean finds that powerlessness, normlessness, and social isolation indeed correlate significantly with one another, and hence belong to the same general concept of alienation. He comes to the same conclusion as I do, namely, that alienation "may be considered a general syndrome" (*American Sociological Review*, 26 [October, 1961], pp. 753-758).

I also tend to agree with the communication in the same issue of the *Review* (p. 780) by Browning, Farmer, Kirk, and Mitchell who see in the various aspects of alienation, as defined by Seeman, stages of a process rather than disparate phenomena. While my data do not provide evidence about the order of the stages of this process—only a longitudinal study could do that—my study supports the hypothesis of these authors that the collective attitudes of powerlessness, meaninglessness, social isolation, and normlessness are part of a logical sequence in the process of adaptation to a social structure in which "the actor's means-ends scheme is no longer meaningful."

19. Systematic observations were made twice in each building. For two weeks, an observer went from ward to ward, spending thirty minutes in each and rotating in such a way as to alternate observations mornings (busy times) and afternoons (quiet times). The following activities were observed: staff-patient interaction, staff-staff interaction, and staff occupied with patients without eliciting response.

20. These figures refer to interactions inside or outside the wards, and do not include meetings and conferences, which are very frequent at the Center. In regard to staff-patient interaction in the Center, this was even more frequent than the figures of Table 10 indicate, because many patients in the Rehabilitation Center are busy in the physical therapy room and the occupational therapy room, and these places were not included in the observations. Moreover, whether it consisted in a brief greeting or whether a nurse was occupied with one patient for a longer stretch of time, every interaction that was observed was counted as 1. In the Center, a nurse was often seen working with a patient for some time; if a stopwatch had been used to time interactions, the rate of staff-patient interaction at the Center would be higher still.

21. An employee in the administration building had this to say about this one type of deviant behavior: "The patients can't reach the bell to call the nurse; they can't reach the water. . . . When the nurse walks out the patient can't call for help. . . . I go up to a patient and he says, 'I'm sorry, my bed is wet, but I couldn't call for the bedpan.' They encourage incontinence here. . . ."

22. That lack of conflict may be a sign of a weak rather than of a strong relationship has been shown by Lewis A. Coser in *The Functions of Social Conflict* (New York: The Free Press of Glencoe, 1956) pp. 83-85.

23. The preceding paragraphs are chiefly based on George Homans' formulation. (See George C. Homans, *The Human Group* [London: Routledge & Kegan Paul Ltd., 1951], pp. 356 ff.)

24. On the function of conflict for the strengthening of norms, see Lewis A. Coser, *op. cit.*, *passim*, esp. Chap. 6.

25. This was said in a jocular tone because this physician, the director of the Center, is himself responsible for the condition he laughingly criticizes. As a *sociologue qui s'ignore*, he repeatedly stressed, privately and publicly, that the best way to practice medicine is within an interdisciplinary framework and that staff meetings and conferences are essential for good medical practice.

26. Cf. Lewis A. Coser's distinction between realistic and nonrealistic conflict, *ibid.*, pp. 48 ff.

27. The concept of "observability" has been dealt with by Merton in various contexts. See especially *Social Theory and Social Structure, op. cit.*, pp. 247, 319-322, 336-357, 374-377. See also Rose Laub Coser, "Insulation from Observability and Types of Social Conformity," *American Sociological Review,* 26 (February, 1961), pp. 28-39.

28. Cf. Merton, *op. cit.*, p. 376.

29. Cf. *ibid.*, p. 351.

30. On social mechanisms for the articulation of roles, see Merton, *ibid.*, pp. 371-379.

31. *Ibid.*, p. 377.

32. Cf. Merton, *ibid.*, pp. 377-379.

33. *Ibid.*, pp. 377-378.

34. George H. Mead, *op. cit.*, pp. 151-154.

35. Maxwell Jones, in his *Therapeutic Community*—a center for the treatment of desocialized patients" who were "unable to hold jobs and prone to cause disturbances"—used this method extensively.

In one case described by Jones, the "actor" was, in the beginning, capable only of performing purely mechanical activities—such as drawing the curtains—in which he had to face neither role-partner nor audience. Through repeated rehearsals he learned to interact with his role-partners, but still refused to face the audience. Later, he became capable of presenting himself to the audience also. See *The Therapeutic Community* (New York: Basic Books, Inc., 1953), p. viii.

It is worth considering whether the degree of complexity of role-sets for hospital patients is not one important distinction between a "therapeutic" and a "nontherapeutic" milieu. The theory advanced here seems to specify what many writers on the subject have called the nontherapeutic effects of a simplified social milieu. It also sheds light on an important problem in geriatrics: older people generally move in a much more restricted role-set than members of younger generations; if those who have an impaired sense of identity are hospitalized, it is to be expected that the further restriction of the number of role-partners that hospitalization implies accentuates their loss of identity. In many cases, it would seem, the deterioration of geriatric patients is social in the strictest sense of the word; it operates as a social process, no matter how hygienic, well equipped and antiseptic the hospital and no matter how well intentioned its personnel.

36. Of course, role-partners are also "differentially" distributed at the Center. A complete analysis of the Center would specify these statuses. For

example, if we take the graphic representation of a "nurse at work" as a projection of a person's relation to his work, we find that on the lower rungs of the nursing hierarchy, in contrast to the registered nurses, as we have seen, almost one-half (46 per cent) of the drawings represent a nurse only. Of course, this figure does not present sufficient evidence for, but is only suggestive of, the fact that at the Center those who have low positions in the hierarchy may be alienated from their work. Indeed, practical nurses and aides usually have only two-role partners—patients and registered nurses; moreover, they do not participate in the meetings and conferences where role-partners of different position and professional outlook get together. In view of the close interaction among professionals at the Center, those on the lower rungs of the hierarchy may suffer from more *relative deprivation* of role-partners and be even more alienated from work and from one another than in a milieu in which they are not made to feel "outsiders."

37. Rose Laub Coser, "Authority and Decision-Making in a Hospital: A Comparative Analysis," *American Sociological Review*, 23 (February, 1958), pp. 57-63.

38. William Foote Whyte, "Small Groups and Large Organizations," in J. Rohrer and M. Sherif, eds., *Social Psychology at the Crossroads* (New York: Harper & Brothers, 1951), pp. 297-312.

39. *Op. cit.*, p. 370.

40. *Ibid.*, p. 329.

9

The Sociology of Time and Space
in an Obstetrical Hospital

WILLIAM R. ROSENGREN

SPENCER DEVAULT

Duncan and Schnore recently argued that studies of social organization seem increasingly to stem from either a cultural or a behavioral perspective, with a corresponding dearth of investigations from a distinctly ecological or morphological point of view.[1] This trend appears to be true not only of studies of the organization of communities but of investigations of particular social establishments as well. In this sense, therefore, there are numerous reports of the behavioral and cultural aspects of general and mental hospitals, of various industrial organizations, of government agencies, and so forth. Furthermore, sociological studies of the organization of social establishments seem increasingly to focus upon informal patterns of behavior in so far as clique structures, differences in channels of communications, incongruous and unmet role expectancies, and differences in values and meanings converge or fail to converge with the officially prescribed goals and procedures of the establishment. This suggests that in many ways the "cultural" and "behavioral" perspectives typically are joined to form an interpersonal model from which the analysis of organizational activity then proceeds.

(266)

Implied here is that investigators are forced to choose between *either* an ecological *or* a culture-behavior approach to social organization.

In his discussion of cultural ecology, Steward eschews such an "either-or" point of view. He suggests that although the cultural system may in many ways affect the manner in which the ecological environment acquires meaning and is put to use, the environment does itself limit the uses to which it can be put.[2] Just as a "rice culture" is not feasible in a geography of timberline, so too one might suspect that norms of subordination-superordination are contingent upon compatible physical settings.

We suggest, then, three possible general models for the analysis of either a community or a social establishment. A model in which: (1) the ecological or physical setting is regarded as the prime factor in the social behavior taking place in it; (2) the behavior system of a community or an organization manipulates the environment to conform to the norms of the participants; (3) the normative patterns are only compatible with— limiting and limited by—the facts of the physical setting. In other words, in model (1) persons are "used" by the setting; in (2) the environment is "used" by the persons acting in it; in (3) neither personal conduct is changed substantially because of the setting, nor is the setting and its existing limits circumvented to any great extent by the participants. Rather, each exists in a condition of unstable equilibrium or minimal accommodation. In urban ecology, for example, luxury apartments (and their attendant way of life) are seldom found in the light-industry region of the city. Also, the persons involved in such a way of life often do not wish to live there. Similarly, the suburbs are seldom dominated by steel mills, and industrialists often do not want to set up factories in such an environment. In both instances, therefore, not only is the way of life dependent upon the ecology of the place but the stability of the ecological pattern is dependent upon the presence of a compatible way of life as well. Each adapts to, and is adapted by, the other. In yet another sense, however, certain places are less clearly defined in their relation to ecological and normative compati-

bility. We might refer to the "rurban fringe" in which we sometimes find a condition of accommodation between urbanism and
ruralism as ways of life. Here the relations between the ecology
and the social organization are less precise. Neither the environment fully articulates the normative system, nor does the
normative system fully adapt the environment. We may look here
for a condition of unstable equilibrium inasmuch as the culture-
behavioral system exists within the context of a relatively un-
friendly ecological setting, and under which the environment is
continually being insulted by the normative pattern.

By way of introduction, we persist in our conviction that
one need not make a choice between *either* an ecological approach *or* a behavioral approach. Rather, we think that observations might best proceed jointly from three perspectives: the
possible independence of the ecological complex, the possible
independence of the normative system, and the possibility of a
state of unstable adjustment between the two. The last, we suggest, is a major contributing factor to the emergence of "informal organization" and "patterned deviations" in social
establishments as well as in communities.

The term "ecology" has thus far remained undefined. Hawley
regards ecology as "the study of the morphology of collective
life in both its static and dynamic aspects" [3]—an approach that
points to the basic and cogent nature of viewing social behavior in terms of both spatial and temporal dimensions. From
such a perspective a few studies have emerged showing a concern with ecological processes in organizational life. Rose Laub
Coser, for example, studied spatial patterns in relation to decision-making processes in two wards of a general hospital.[4]
Freidson has discussed the location of patients in different referral systems in relation to practitioner controls.[5] Wilson has
illustrated the importance of tempo and timing in the organization of the surgical team,[6] and Mack has pointed out that the
patterns of ethnic segregation characteristic of the larger community tended to be duplicated within a specific industrial establishment.[7] As we have suggested, none the less, the study of
social establishments has focused more upon the adaptation of

the environment to the norms shared by the participants than upon mutual interactions.

Our purpose is to describe some aspects of the social organization of an obstetrical hospital from an ecological viewpoint rather than from an interpersonal model. More specifically, our aim is to suggest the ways in which both the cultural and the behavioral processes in one social establishment seem to be, in part at least, functionally associated with its social morphology.

The Hospital Setting

The observations that formed the basis for this essay were made in a large lying-in hospital in an eastern metropolitan area. In addition to providing obstetrical services for the patients of privately practicing obstetricians, the hospital also has an active clinic service with its own staff. In 1958 the hospital ranked fifth in the nation for the number of deliveries that took place in it—more than 8,000. As might well be expected, the clinic service clientele is drawn mainly from the lower socioeconomic groups in the community, with an overrepresentation of ethnically distinct persons—chiefly Italian and Portuguese. Prenatal care of the clinic patients takes place in the hospital. The private patients are seen in the obstetricians' offices in the city, but both clinic and private patients share a common delivery service.

In a four-month period we spent some 150 hours observing in this delivery service. This was done in connection with two independent studies of social psychological factors in pregnancy.[8] We had numerous contacts with the interns and residents in the service for more than a year before we began to make our observations. As a result of these earlier meetings, an adequate rapport seemed to exist. Our procedures were simple. On the days (or nights) on which we came to the hospital, we were provided with a room in the residents' quarters, and supplied with hospital uniforms, caps, masks, and insulated shoes. We then observed all the activities of the service, talked in-

formally with the staff during coffee breaks, while relaxing in
the lounges, and in the work situations. During the first two or
three evenings, the most pronounced obstacle to both accurate
observation and acceptance by the personnel was the fact that
from their point of view we had neither legitimate status nor
meaningful roles in the hospital. Simply, people wondered what
we were doing there and how they should relate themselves to
us. Initially, many of the personnel—particularly the staff nurses
—seemed to think that we were new externs (medical students).
And perhaps because of this we were occasionally called upon
by the nurses to assist in a subordinate fashion with some of the
minor tasks preparatory to delivery. Others seemed to feel that
we were "inspectors" from the National Institute of Neurological
Diseases and Blindness.[9] For ourselves, we remained mum on the
issue. The first definition of us by the staff gave us meaningful
roles but no status. The second gave us legitimate status but no
meaningful role. As observers, therefore, we were caught up in
an almost ideal contradiction of status and role. The dilemma
was gradually resolved: First we were given a kind of status,
primarily by being allowed to observe high-status private obstetricians and their patients. We were then provided with a
meaningful role, from the point of view of the obstetrical team,
by helping them with some of the observations and recordings
required by the National Collaborative Study which the team
members found burdensome to do themselves.

All our observations were independently recorded when time
permitted, with both of us working from a general outline of
factors for which to search. We both recorded the typical field-
note type of material, and we compared them after each observational experience. Our original purpose was not that of
posing questions about the social organization of the delivery
service. As time went on, however, we were increasingly impressed that the behavior of the personnel seemed to differ
markedly, depending upon where it took place and in what
sequence. Although we did not set out to make an informal study
of the social morphology of the obstetrical hospital, we were
eventually convinced that the ecological organization we observed was intimately in exchange with many of the salient

social processes of the hospital. For example, the structures of both time and space appeared more and more to serve to delineate status and define roles. Whereas most studies of medical settings persist at the level of status and role, we became more interested in the relations between status and role and the morphological structures that underlay the conduct we observed. We found it improper, for example, to speak only of the "doctor-nurse" relationship without specifying where those two persons interacted and when. Inadvertently, as it were, the notion of the importance of the physical setting was in some sense thrust upon us. We began, therefore, to focus what we saw and heard more specifically in terms of time and space associations.

Spatial and Temporal Aspects

Following these initial leads, we found it useful to consider our experiences under these general rubrics:

1. The *spatial* distribution of activities in the delivery service in so far as certain regions appeared to be set aside for particular modes of behavior and attitudes—staff to staff and staff to patients. That is, it became increasingly clear that both attitudes and overt behavior of the several functionaries in the service—patients, nurses, and doctors—varied, depending upon the particular place in which they might be found.

2. The *segregation* of behaviors, one from the other, in so far as persons occupying the same status appeared to behave differently in different places, depending upon the ecological factors involved in each place—its position in temporal sequences, its physical symbols, and the ways in which each place was physically separated from other places. In other words, the differences in behavior that were noted to be dependent upon particular areas were not fully a function of purposive choice on the part of either the personnel or the patients, but they were both sanctioned by the normative system and elicited by the nature of the physical settings themselves. In addition, what was actually at stake here was the association between the morphol-

ogy of the service and the patterning of status relationships among the personnel.

3. The *rhythm* of activities—the periodicity with which events took place to the extent that the behavior of the personnel was organized and patterned in terms of regularities of occurrence.

4. The *tempo* of activities—the number of events, both social and physiological, that occurred within any given unit of time. Important here is the fact that the temporal organization of the hospital was, in part, a function of the continual imperfect balance between the physiological and functional organization of activities.

5. The *timing* of activities—the coordination of separate and diverse pulsations—both physiological and functional—in so far as different rhythms and tempos were taking place at the same time. It was by means of timing sequences, therefore, that temporal organization could actually take place.[10]

Although these were the main ecological factors guiding our observations, their importance is not that they constituted a kind of taxonomy, but rather that they provided a kind of base line from which to look for interrelationships.

DISTRIBUTION AND SEGREGATION OF ACTIVITIES: BARRIERS AND ATMOSPHERES

The obstetrical service is schematically represented in Figure 9-1. The two places of greatest spatial segregation are the clinic examination rooms and the delivery service itself. The clinic is located in a wing completely separate from the delivery service. Thus, the patient has no contact with the delivery service until the day of delivery arrives, except in the case of some private patients who are given a "tour" of the service during their prenatal care. For most patients, however, the transition from the prenatal area to that of the delivery service represents—both spatially and symbolically—their retirement from one world and their entrance into a totally new and different world, with a corresponding spatially enforced change in self-image.

More than that, each region in the service is itself set apart in several ways from the others. This segregation appears to be

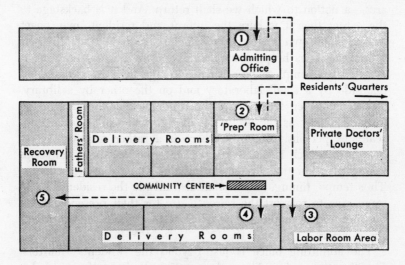

Figure 9-1
**Map of the obstetrical service. Arrows indicate
route taken by patients.**

accomplished not only by space but also by rules of dress, of expected behavior, and of decorum—all of which serve to indicate the dissimilarity of each place, as well as to present an image of the place that might cast both patients and staff into desired roles with respect to one another.

First, the residents' quarters are separated from the other parts of the service by a long corridor and heavy doors. The general atmosphere here is not unlike that of a modern motel—comfortable but austere and suggestive of the fact that people never really settle down here, as indeed the residents do not. This region is the temporary retreat for the residents and interns, but allows little means by which those who have gone before may be remembered by those currently in residence. By the very spatial location and physical trappings of the place, the occupants are in some sense depersonalized, and this fact is generally in keeping with both the residents' comparatively low status and the rather diffuse roles that they enact. In large part, the residents' quarters serve, in Goffman's terms,[11] as their backstage

area—a notion to which we shall return. And it is backstage to
the extent that it is here the interns and residents may enact
among their own kind the informal roles that attach to their
formal status as hospital staff members. As a backstage area it
is less than complete because the lounge area is bordered on
one side by a small laboratory and on the other by a library.
These rooms serve to remind the residents that they are in the
hospital chiefly as the occupants of a formal work-role and not
really as persons. Moreover, there is a rather massive "scoreboard" on which is noted essential information about deliveries
taking place in the service during the past twenty-four hours.
Thus tempo, timing, and rhythm also invade the residents' backstage area to reassert the *raison d'être* for their presence at the
hospital and to modulate the effect of the spatial segregation of
the quarters.

The admitting office is just beyond the residents' quarters.
Significantly, perhaps, here there are no barriers of any kind—
not even doors—almost as a symbol of welcome to the incoming
patient. A mood of friendly casualness characterizes the behavior of the admitting room staff, and it is here where the
staff is most casual in regard to decorum in both attitudes and
dress. This is consistent with the function of the admitting office
as the intermediary stage in the hospitalization of the patient,
for the physical setting, its spatial location, and the behavior of
personnel in it serve as a gradual introduction of the patient to
the new world of the service.

Directly opposite the admitting room is the preparation or
"prep" room where the incoming patient is stripped of her self-
image as "person," and cast most effectively and promptly into
her new status of "medical phenomenon." Of interest to us as
observers and corresponding to Hughes's observation,[12] we were
invited into the prep room only when it was occupied by an un-
married, lower-class Negro prostitute. Until that time we were
told almost nothing of what took place in "prepping," nor were
we told the names of those who worked there or their occupational status. Segregation of the prep room was accomplished
not only by physical and symbolic barriers but also by an
atmosphere of anonymity exceeded nowhere else in the service.

This aura of *mystique* surrounding the prep room does not seem to conform to the popular image of childbirth. Ordinarily modern hospital childbirth calls forth an image of immaculate lying-in rooms, urgently attentive doctors and nurses, the drama of birth, and subsequent visits by a proud father, friends, and relatives. The total reality is, of course, considerably more mundane. The organizational stages of delivery involve situations and tasks that must be performed and that do not conform to the common image. Indeed, every social establishment is faced with the need to accomplish certain tasks and to fulfill certain functions that are at odds with, inconsistent with, or otherwise in greater or lesser conflict with both the ultimate goals of the establishment and its own image and ideology. And it may well not be unique to this one obstetrical hospital that the distribution of such "deviant" functions occurs in the context not only of the status system of the organization but within the ecological system as well. It is true, in any event, that it is in keeping with the professional image of the modern obstetrical hospital, as well as the folklore of childbirth, that the "climax" of the human career in the hospital should take place in the delivery room in which the miraculous and often dramatic birth takes place. But it is equally obvious that much else takes place—both before and after this single climax time and place—that is essential to the operation of the organization. In a larger sense, these other activities—prepping, labor, and recovery in particular—are the deviant but necessary functions of this particular establishment. It is fitting, we think, that these deviant activities should be accomplished in regions segregated both physically and symbolically from the rest of the service and that the overseers of these activities should be the lower-status personnel—nurses and student nurses in particular.

In the area of the labor rooms, one is isolated from the nurses in charge, and from the patients, by a sturdy shoulder-high and seemingly nonfunctional barricade. This not only segregates the patients from those who pass by but also symbolically segregates the attending nurses from others in the hospital. Perhaps implicit in this mode of segregation is the notion that the nurses are definitely "in charge" and that others in service have no authority beyond that point. Moreover, the area of the labor rooms in some sense corresponds to the residents' quarters in so far as it serves as the nurses' backstage area. Also, the physical barrier—serving to maintain status differences—seemed to us to be reinforced symbolically by the dim lighting and drab decor of the interior of the labor rooms. The staff was in agreement that the patients seemed to "behave better" while in labor under the quieting effect of the gray decor of the rooms. At the same time, here the nurse was most likely to conduct herself with most confidence in the role of the nurse in the presence of other personnel, and perhaps least like a nurse when interacting only with other nurses. From a slightly different perspective, both the physical and the symbolic segregation of the labor rooms may be understood to be a function of labor as a kind of "deviant" activity in the service. That is, there is none of the "highlighting" of the place or of the patients here to suggest that what takes place in the region is actually germane to the entire process.

Thus far we have discussed some of the regions of the service in terms of spatial and segregational aspects as if they had distinct boundaries. Of course, this is not true; if it were, it would suggest that moods, attitudes, and behaviors had discrete boundaries as well. It is more proper to speak of the overlapping of regional boundaries—a frame of reference that may account for the periodic times and occasional places where the behavior patterns among the staff are less clear and distinct than they are when one is observing well within a bounded area. This overlapping of boundaries could be seen most clearly in the hallways, where the regions of the labor rooms, the doctors' lounge, and the delivery rooms converge. For this area was ambiguous not only as to its spatial relationship to the several other distinct regions of which we have talked, but also with regard to the relationships between the functionaries in the service who interacted there. Doctors and nurses appeared to know quite clearly what the appropriate modes of interaction were between them when they were within one of the distinct regions, but this was less true in overlapping areas. The formalized aspects of doctor-nurse interaction seemed to break down here, and those persons tended to interact in a more spontaneous and less formalized fashion.

On one occasion, for example, an attending nurse rushed into this "interstitial" area, announced to a private obstetrician that a patient who had recently been ordered to the delivery room by the doctor should not have been so ordered, and insisted that the doctor return the patient to the labor room. A heated discussion ensued between the nurse and the doctor, and the outcome was that the patient was returned to the labor rooms. The tenor of the encounter was not that of a subordinate-superordinate relation, but rather that of a dispute between professional equals with a disregard for the possible impact the exchange might have upon the surrounding audience. The stresses and conflicts among and between the doctors and nurses that were less manifest within a specific region became considerably more apparent in such "interstitial" areas. Whereas each particular functionary group in the service had, to a greater or lesser extent, its own backstage region, areas of overlap between distinct regions served more as the backstage place for interaction between functionaries.

The administrative nurses hold forth in the area of the delivery rooms. At this point—which is really the "community center" and the point of both physiological and social climax—we found it interesting to note that the projected image of the hospital and, consequently, the expected roles and attitudes of both staff and patient are cast most effectively by symbols—uniforms, stainless steel, medicines with their odors, brilliant lighting, and so forth.

The operating arena is just beyond the delivery room; it is segregated from the rest of the service by a wide red line painted wall to wall and ceiling to floor. No one without surgical cap, face mask, and insulated shoes is allowed beyond that point. During our first conducted tour of the service we entered that region without the required accoutrements—perhaps because we were not yet really considered a "part" of the scene.

Farther along this corridor, and perhaps significantly farthest from the community center, is the recovery room. This is a large, dimly lit room attended by one nurse. The functions here are also of the "deviant" variety. The mother is relegated here after delivery of the child, while the newborn is retained in the community center where much attention is paid to it by high-status personnel—obstetricians and pediatricians. This spatial indication of the importance of the child is reinforced by timing sequences, and the value placed on the child may, in fact, account for the emphasis that is placed upon administering anesthesia. Without anesthesia the patient may become troublesome to the obstetrical team, and their reassuring and comforting gestures toward the patient often give way to irritability.

A further mode of segregation indicative of status differences seemed to relate to having delivery-room doors open or closed. Never in our experience was a delivery-room door closed when a clinic patient was there, but this frequently happened with private patients, thus limiting access to the place of climax.

The "fathers' room" is adjacent to the recovery room—unattended and suggestive that the father is regarded as the least important person in the process. By its sparseness of furnishing, its physical isolation, and its small size, this room seemed to communicate symbolically the idea that the fathers are unnecessary and functionally peripheral.

The lounge for the private obstetricians is immediately adjacent to the labor rooms and near the center of communication. It is segregated from the rest of the service both by soundproofing and by doors without windows. The lounge is tastefully and discretely decorated and suggests many personal touches left by some of the private obstetricians. The anonymity of the residents' quarters is absent, and in further contrast the work-role symbols of library, laboratory, and scoreboard are absent. Lastly, and consistent with the comparative high status of the private doctors, this lounge permits the doctors to come and go with little chance of being observed by others in the service. The interns and externs from the clinic service are free to use the private lounge whenever they desire, but they seldom do so unless they are called "to scrub" with a private obstetrician. Implied here is the question of relations between normative and ecological systems. One might say that the failure of the interns to use the lounge is a function of the understood status differences between themselves and the "pros." On the other hand, such a pattern may be a function of the spatial and symbolic separation of the lounge from other parts of the service. More likely, perhaps, it is a mutual effect of both, inasmuch as the interns use it under certain specified conditions and not under others.

In general, it would appear that the behavior in each of the several regions in the service is at least partially a function of the kinds of spatial, symbolic, and physical segregation that set each region apart from others. Each functionary in the establishment has, to a greater or lesser degree, an area of "front-staging" and "back-staging." But the extent of available backstage area appears to be related to status. The higher the status of the personnel (the private doctors), the greater is the availability of a "pure" backstage area; the lower the status (the student nurses), the least available is the backstage region. Although the spatial distribution and segregation do not actually determine the formal and informal status systems in the service, they do lend a distinctive idiom to relationships among the staff and to their demeanor toward the patients.

In terms of spatial patterns, it would appear that the extent of spatial segregation relates to the value placed upon the activities in the region relative to the "business" or "goals" of the establishment. That is, those areas that are most dispensable with regard to the delivery of babies are those that are spatially most apart from the community center. Physical segregation, on the other hand, seemed to be most related to status differences among the staff members—doors, walls, counters, and the like. Finally, symbolic forms of segregation between regions appeared to us to be most related to the communication of organizationally appropriate attitudes and values—colors, odors, lighting, signs, and so forth. Whereas physical segregation served in some sense to declare gradations in status, symbolic forms of segregation appeared more to articulate roles. Such associations may appear quite clear in most instances, but they are less clear in others. This is consistent with our earlier position that mutually interdependent contingencies exist between the dominance of ecology on the one hand, and the dominance of the behavior norms on the other.

For example, the relation of status to anonymity is exemplified by the fact that the staff, when talking among themselves about patients, most often refer to the clinic patients by name. With the private patients, however, a perhaps implicit shield of anonymity is erected, for they are referred to by room number.

From a similar perspective, differential behavior of the nurses toward the doctors, interns, and student externs was noted by place—generally depending upon whether the patient could hear what was being said. In the presence of the wakeful patient, the nurses tended to refer to the student externs respectfully as "Dr." even though they do not hold the M.D. degree. This form of address functions not only to maintain patient confidence in those who are caring for her but also to maintain the self-image of the nurse as one who "takes orders only from superiors." In the delivery room, with the patient under anesthesia, the demeanor of the nurses toward the younger interns and externs frequently changed to giving orders and calling by last name only.

Differential expression of humor seemed also to be graded by status. The doctor heading the obstetrical team expressed the greatest amount of tension release through humor, going gradually down to the student nurses who were the most sober and serious members of the team. In some sense, therefore, the higher-status personnel could "backstage" in regions where low-status personnel could not. This seemed to be less true, however, with patients of extremely low social status. Here the expression of humor was more often diffused through the entire team.

RHYTHM: THE CONTINGENT NATURE OF THE ROLE OF THE PATIENT

An important factor in establishing rhythmic patterns of behavior in the hospital is the fact that the patient is potentially both "ill" and "not ill." Pregnancy does not necessarily entail abnormal complications, but that possibility always exists. Because of this the demeanor of the doctors and nurses takes on a studied casualness about childbirth—but always with a watchful eye toward unforseen difficulties. This was most pronounced when the team included student externs. The students were always more oriented toward complications and pathology in labor and delivery than were the resident doctors. As a consequence, perhaps, a modulated kind of crisis seemed always to exist on the service. In cases where no complications were medically indicated, an atmosphere of general apprehension pervaded the team—particularly during delivery. In cases with possible imminent complications, the members of the team seemed to be considerably more at ease, tension lessened, and they appeared more able to set about their tasks in a more relaxed and workmanlike fashion. To the students, the latter situations were those in which they were actually "learning something."

As in most hospitals, the nurses and doctors refer to the complaining and excitable patients as "crocks." This most frequently meant that the patient was demanding too much sedation while in labor. The term "crock" was often applied by the residents to the patients of private obstetricians, but it was also used to refer to clinic patients under their care as well. The clinic-patient "crock" was regarded as a drug addict. The private-patient "crock," on the other hand, was usually regarded as having been "pampered." In terms of rhythm, however, the clinic crock is simply disturbing the usual periodicity with which medication is ordinarily offered—she is upsetting the rhythmic expectations to which the team members have become accustomed. The disturbance of rhythm by the private-patient crock, however, relates to other rhythms in the social morphology of the service. In such cases, the residents are usually reluctant to administer medication over and beyond what the private doctor might have ordered—a case not only of status differences but of the sacredness of private clientele as well. Thus, the "crock" label was most frequently applied to private patients during the late evening and nighttime hours when the private obstetrician was least likely to be on the service to minister to his complaining lady. The former, then, related to the rhythm of medication, while the latter was associated with the work rhythms of the establishment.

TEMPO: CONCEPTIONS OF THE "NORMAL" IN THE HOSPITAL

The number of deliveries taking place in a given period of time particularly relates to the tempo of the service. In the clinic service, the number of births in a twenty-four-hour period may range from as few as one or two to as many as fifteen or twenty. This lack of a natural tempo seemed to be handled in a number of ways in order to impose a "functional" tempo where a "physiological" tempo did not exist. For example, when deliveries were occurring at a naturally slow pace, the residents showed much anxiety and concern over the one or two women who might have been holding up the tempo of events in labor—constantly checking and rechecking for signs of change. Similarly, in the delivery room itself, there seemed to be an attempt to impose a tempo—to adhere to a pace of scrubbing, of administering anesthesia, and so forth. There was also an emphasis upon keeping track of the length of time involved in each delivery. In terms of tempo, the unusually prolonged delivery was as upsetting to the team as was an unusually rapid delivery—even though both might be equally normal or abnormal from a medical point of view. As one resident put it, "Our [the residents'] average length of delivery is about 50 minutes, and the Pros [the private doctors] is about 40 minutes." Thus, the "correct" tempo becomes a matter of status competition and a measure of professional adeptness. The use of forceps is also a means by which the tempo is maintained in the delivery room, and they are so often used that the procedure is regarded as normal.

The student externs showed particular reluctance about admitting patients to the service because of the possibility that the patient might be in "false labor." This would upset both the rhythm and the tempo. It may not be unrelated to the fact that such a "mistake" on the part of low-status personnel is much more crucial than a similar mistake on the part of higher-status personnel. In addition, the potential high tempo for the obstetrician is necessarily limited; he can be in attendance for just one case at a time. When the physiological tempo begins to outrun the functional tempo, the margin of safety can be partially maintained by the anesthetist, who can hurry cases along or delay them, depending upon the kind and amount of anesthesia he administers. As one anesthetist joyously announced one night when the physiological tempo was very high, "I've got five going [ready for delivery but delayed] at once now."

TIMING: EXPECTATIONS OF THE NORMAL COURSE OF EVENTS

In the naturally expected sequences of events, it is of interest to note how the coming together of the team members for delivery differs from the situation in the regular surgical setting. Ordinarily the high-status personnel—the surgeons—arrive last.[13] In the obstetrical service, however, it is difficult to know whether the patient can actually wait for the doctor. Frequently, therefore, the doctors arrive on the scene before the subordinates do, and not infrequently before the patient herself. This disturbance in timing usually leaves the doctors either making "busy-work" with the administrative nurses or leaving the region to check another patient in labor whom minutes before they may have referred to as a "crock."

The normal circuit: admitting office, to prep room, to labor room, to delivery room, to recovery room, and finally to the lying-in room is adhered to scrupulously. The physiological tempo would often indicate that at least one or more room might better be forgotten, but the patient must adhere to this timing of movements from region to region, even if it means at a fast trot.

Timing may also be disturbed if key personnel happen to be absent from one of the places in the timing sequence. One evening, for example, a man rushed into the service claiming that his wife was about to have her child and that no one was in the admitting office. The doctors' advice—in all candor and sincerity—was that she was probably in false labor, and they encouraged the man to return to the admitting room. In a second instance, a woman who had previously given birth to seven children appeared in the last stages of labor. There was not enough time to administer the usual anesthesia, even though it seemed obvious that she could bear her child easily without it. The obstetrical team, however, was in a state of much agitation until the baby suddenly appeared. These inroads upon the timing of events are highly disturbing to the service personnel. And, in general, it may be said that there appeared to be a kind of gradient of the temporal organization of the hospital, with the greater emphasis upon rhythm, tempo, and timing, the closer one got to the community center.

A SUBSTANTIVE EXAMPLE: THE ECOLOGY OF PAIN

Thus far, we have discussed the social morphology of the obstetrical service strictly from the view of the flow of work in both time and space, threading into our discussion appropriate substantive examples. To express more fully the interrelationships between time, space, and social behavior, we turn now to a specific substantive area: the ways in which the hospital is organized to define, legitimatize, sanction, and handle the expression of pain by patients.

As Parsons [14] has pointed out in his theoretical analysis of the doctor-patient relationship, a requisite for the maintenance of the professional self-image and, therefore, professional behavior toward patients, is the maintenance of an affectively neutral orientation toward the patient. The patient must be regarded as a clinical phenomenon rather than as a person in order for the doctor to behave as doctor. It may well be that an important function of the "prepping" process in the flow of work is to reassert both the clinical nature of the patient and the professional self-images of the personnel. Certainly the expression of pain by a patient as well as the recognition of painfulness, as such, by the doctor is a salient means by which the affectively neutral orientation may be changed to that of an emotionally involved or affective orientation. Such a contingency is handled in a variety of ways.

There are, first of all, certain places in the service where pain is legitimatized and defined as such, and others in which it is not. By and large, pain is not sanctioned in any place other than the delivery room, for it is only here that the hospital provides the means to handle pain in an affectively neutral fashion—namely, anesthesia. The acceptance or sanctioning of pain in any other regions—the admitting room, the prep room, and even the labor rooms—would necessitate a more personalized orientation toward the patient by the staff, rather than the technical, mechanical, and personally neutral means that are so characteristic of the delivery room. This is not to say that women are in pain only in the delivery room, but merely that it is neither accepted nor dealt with as such by the staff—particularly high-status staff. And not only does the staff segregate pain in this spatial sense, but this meaning appears to be shared by the patients as well—many patients seem a bit apologetic about having pain when in these other regions. In places not sanctioning pain, when the patient's discomfort intrudes itself upon the staff, various means are employed to cope with it in an affectively neutral fashion. In the prep room it is handled by the use of humor and comparatively low-status personnel; in the labor room, not only by the more intimate contact taking place between patient and low-status personnel but also by defining the phenomenon as something other than pain—complaining, pampering, nervousness, or what have you; and in the recovery room by its spatial and symbolic segregation as well as by defining it as unconscious behavior of one who is still under the effects of anesthesia.

The symbolism of lighting, individual segregation of patients, and perhaps even the mood and attitudes of the nurses on duty, serve to minimize the patient's attempts to legitimatize her discomfort as genuine pain. Spatially there appeared to be a kind of gradient as to the legitimation of pain, with the greater sanctioning of pain found the closer the "place" is to the delivery rooms, and a corresponding decrease as one moves away from the community center. Significantly, it is in this "climax" region of the delivery room, where pain is most fully sanctioned and accepted by the staff, that the affectively neutral orientation is most likely to break down. For here—perhaps for the first time—the entire obstetrical team is confronted, and at close quarters, with the patient and her discomfort. She is high-lighted not only in a physical and interactional sense but in an organizational sense as well. An important relation between status and "place" is clearly evident here because the anesthetist has no part to play in the labor room, even though the manifestation of pain there may actually be as great as, or even greater than, that shown in the delivery room. Once pain is accepted as such —in the delivery room—there is then a special functionary to handle it in an affectively neutral fashion: the anesthetist. Pain is not only sanctioned in the delivery room; it is expected, too. If there is no pain, this would mean that the anesthetist, who occupies a position of considerable prestige, would be superfluous. Moreover, the legitimation of pain is also organized temporally. There are patterns according to which pain is sanctioned and expected—only so often and for only so long. To show pain either too frequently or too infrequently or, indeed, not at all, is disrupting to the obstetrical team.

On one occasion, for example, the team was preparing for the delivery of a patient, a mother of several children. The chief resident was heading the team and he was assisted by an intern, a staff nurse, and a student nurse. The anesthetist, of course, was on the service should he be needed. All phases of the preparatory stage were going according to schedule until the staff nurse attempted to administer anesthesia by means of a nose mask. Apparently for technical reasons, the apparatus failed to operate. There are three masks in each delivery room—each containing a different form of anesthesia—and the nurse tried the other two; neither one worked. Although the patient did not appear to be suffering undue pain, with each failure of the apparatus the team members—particularly the chief resident—became increasingly agitated, excited, and alarmed. This pattern of deprofessionalization of the doctor continued until he excitedly hurried from the room in search of the anesthetist who hopefully could somehow handle the situation. What was apparently happening in this instance, and according to our frame of reference, was first that pain was sanctioned and accepted as such by the physician in the delivery room—it was expected as well. Second, the delivery room was the place where the hospital was organized to maintain affective neutrality in the face of pain by means of the anesthesia apparatus. When this apparatus did not function properly, an important mechanism by which affective neutrality is maintained broke down. With it the affective neutrality of the obstetrical team also broke down.

SOME IMPLICATIONS FOR THE STUDY OF SOCIAL ESTABLISHMENTS

We said at the outset that three possible approaches to the relations between the ecological setting and the normative system would be pursued. First was that which regarded the ecological system as dominant and determining the nature of the normative patterns between the participants. Second was that which viewed the normative patterns as determinants of the uses to which the ecological system would be put. Third was that in which a condition of unstable accommodation existed between the "givens" of the physical setting and the requirements of the normative system. We shall now consider our observations in the light of these perspectives.

The first approach would suggest that the patterns of normative behavior we observed would have been dramatically different in the context of a different physical setting. For example, would the relatively blasé attitudes toward the period of postpartum recovery have persisted without the presence of a defined place in which such attitudes might be elicited and distinguished (the recovery room)? Or would the demeanor of the interns vis-à-vis the privately practicing "pros" have been what it was without the spatial segregation of the residents' quarters and the physical and symbolic segregation of the private lounge? In all candor we must confess that, on the basis of a field study of this type, such questions cannot easily be answered with any degree of confidence. It was impossible, in the context of our observations, to manipulate such "givens" and then to derive indicators of their relative importance. We suspect, however, that the dominance of the ecological setting, through spatial segregation, symbolic segregation, and temporal organization, might qualify normative patterns, the forms in which they might be expressed, and their relative importance in the conduct of the participants. Although a pattern of subordination-superordination is commonly found in relations between doctors, interns, and nurses, it would have greater or lesser saliency depending upon the time and space structures of the environment.

A further aspect of the dominance of ecology is related to the association between status and place and what Hughes has

referred to as professional mistakes.[15] In large part, the lower
the status of the functionary (nurse, intern, or student nurse),
the less is the likelihood that he will risk the possibility of committing either an interpersonal or a technical mistake. The reverse seems to be true of high-status personnel. The physician
in the delivery room need not fear such errors—his status is
sufficiently high that he may correct it—or not correct it—
without loss of the esteem of the team. The staff nurse may
sometimes point out a mistake to the doctor, but ordinarily in
only indirect ways—by mood, attitude, and other forms of non-
verbal communication. Her danger lies not in failing to point
out a mistake but in pointing it out incorrectly. The student
nurse is seldom to be found either making a mistake or pointing
out the errors of others. However, in the interstitial areas of the
service—the hallways, the community center, and even in the
cafeteria—normative taboos against pointing out errors made by
high-status personnel are less in evidence. Here the doctor, nurse,
intern, and student nurse may be found speaking together in the
most candid fashion. In the interstitial areas the most blunt
questions can be asked without prestige and esteem becoming
serious considerations. In Homans' terms,[16] the behavior of the
participants is contingent upon the interpersonal costs involved
in relation to the interpersonal profits. The ecological system is
crucial in so far as both the costs and the returns are highly
associated with where the behavior takes place. For the nurses,
the cost of risking an error in the delivery room is quite high
—with the potential returns at a minimum. In the interstitial
areas, on the other hand, costs are reduced and potential returns are increased.

Our second approach—that which views the normative system
as dominant—raises different questions: Would the patterns of
behavior that we observed have remained substantially the same
in the context of a thoroughly different physical setting? Perhaps most crucial in the normative system between functionaries
are the clients—the patients. It would appear that in some
sense the ecological structures seemed to be least salient when
there was no significant audience before which the participants
acted. This raises the question whether the pattern of subor-

dination-superordination between doctors and nurses is strictly a consequence of the "shoulder-high" barrier in front of the labor rooms, or whether the counter comes to have symbolic meaning only in relation to an already existing pattern of professional prerogatives. We would suppose that the "physical barrier" of the counter would tend to have less significance in the relations between doctors and nurses if the labor rooms were empty of patients. By and large, it would seem that the posture the functionaries took toward each other in the clearly defined places of the service was contingent upon the presence of the patient, who always stood in need of having her role articulated for her by others in the establishment. One might say, then, that where there are lacunae in the behavioral expectations among persons acting in a physical setting, the physical setting itself—spatially and symbolically—will provide symbolic cues to fill such lacunae. On the other hand, where the physical setting itself is less than complete in boundaries and barriers, the normative system will define such barriers to conform with itself.

Often, however, neither the physical setting nor the normative system is fully adapted one to the other. This is the third approach, in which a condition of unstable equilibrium exists between the normative system and the ecology. This may well be the most typical condition not only in our single hospital but in most social establishments. This is merely to say that there is no such thing as a "social psychology of architecture."

There are, then, numerous contingencies in the tasks that occur in the hospital in which the normative system is endangered by events that might take place in certain places, and certain aspects of the physical setting that lend a kind of ludicrousness to some aspects of the normative system. It is in the light of such contingencies that interstitial areas become places where the normative system changes, to some extent, and the dominance of "place" becomes less pronounced. The hallways, the community center, and the like appear to be ill-defined areas in which incongruities between the physical setting and the normative system are resolved. It is here that informal social organization becomes most apparent, where candor between doctors, interns, and nurses is expressed most fully. These contingency situations also appear to arise in the face of crises—the break-down of technical equipment, the deviation of a patient from the normally expected series of physiological stages, and the like. Such crisis situations are seldom fully resolved within the confines of a clearly defined ecological area in the service, per-haps because their resolution would alter the normative pat-terns regarded as appropriate for that *place*. Rather, resolution of crises is more often found in the interstitial areas where roles may be transcended, where the usual rights and obligations of status need not be adhered to, and where esteem and prestige are less at stake. In short, it is here where the costs of "mis-takes" are decreased. Moreover, in the interstitial areas com-munication between the functionaries is less stereotyped and more spontaneous. There, the resolution of a problem can be of more significance than the distribution of roles among the members of the obstetrical team because both normative and ecological systems are ill defined and emergent.

In general, it appeared to us that both the spatial and the temporal organization of the service seemed to be geared to cast the incoming patient into a role and mood that would allow the personnel of the service to behave in the ways which they had learned to expect that they should. The staff members them-selves—residents, interns, and so on—seemed to be subject to the same proscriptions that stemmed from the morphology of the hospital. In the case of both staff and patients this process was accomplished apparently less by verbal instruction, or even by informal socialization processes, than by the erection of both physical and symbolic barriers to the undesired behaviors and attitudes.

It is perhaps gratuitous to point out that all social establish-ments, as well as communities, are organized within and around distinctive physical settings. These physical settings may be con-sidered as consisting of many interrelated parts spatially separate from each other. None the less, the basis of social organization and social establishments consists of the integration of those parts into time and space. We suggest that the behaviors that might otherwise legitimately be viewed from a cultural-behavioral perspective are importantly related to the spatial and temporal aspects of the hospital. Although many social psychologists may tend to be particularly enamored of an approach that focuses exclusively upon the normative system, we might well profit by becoming increasingly sensitive to the major role played by ecological factors.[17]

It would be audacious not to make a necessary caveat at this point. Our observations stemmed from experiences in a single setting. It is not possible to assert certitude as to the validity and reliability of these observations and remarks, or to suggest generalizability to other social establishments—particularly hospitals. We suspect that the ecological structure of this one hospital is in many ways unique. Very likely the normative patterns among the staff are in many ways unlike those found in other settings. Our purpose has been to suggest an approach and a perspective that may have future meaning for the study not only of social establishments but of communities as well. The rigid "either-or" choice between a morphological approach on the one hand, and a "culture-behavior" approach on the other, appears to us to be unduly constraining.

NOTES

1. Otis Dudley Duncan and Leo Schnore, "Cultural, Behavioral, and Ecological Perspectives in the Study of Social Organization," *American Journal of Sociology* 65 (September, 1959), pp. 132-146.

2. Julian Steward, *Theory of Culture Change: The Methodology of Multilinear Evolution* (Urbana: University of Illinois Press, 1955).

3. Amos H. Hawley, *Human Ecology: A Theory of Community Structure* (New York: Ronald Press, 1950).

4. Rose Laub Coser, "Authority and Decision-Making in a Hospital," *American Sociological Review*, 23 (February, 1958), pp. 56-63.

5. Eliot Freidson, "Client Control and Medical Practice," *American Journal of Sociology*, 65 (January, 1960), pp. 374-382.

6. Robert N. Wilson, "Teamwork in the Operating Room," *Human Organization*, 12 (Winter, 1954), pp. 9-14.

7. Raymond W. Mack, "Ecological Patterns in an Industrial Shop," *Social Forces*, 32 (May, 1954), pp. 351-356.

8. One is a study entitled "Socio-Cultural Factors Affecting the Behavior of Expectant Mothers," under a grant from the Association for the Aid of Crippled Children, New York. The other is entitled "A Psychological Study of Emotional Factors in Pregnancy," under a grant from the U.S.

Public Health Service. It is under the direction of Dr. Anthony Davids of Brown University and the E. P. Bradley Hospital.

9. The hospital in which these observations were made is one of sixteen throughout the country that are participating in a long-range medical investigation of birth defects. Part of the research procedure involves maintaining detailed accounts of each delivery as it takes place. We helped in the completion of these records.

10. These conceptions of ecological processes are from Hawley, *op. cit.*

11. Erving Goffman, *The Presentation of Self in Everyday Life* (New York: Doubleday Anchor, 1959).

12. During an informal colloquium at the Department of Sociology and Anthropology at Brown University in December, 1957, Professor Hughes pointed out that the extent of both physical and symbolic "closeness" between staff and patients was related to the social status of the patient.

13. R. N. Wilson, *op. cit.*

14. Talcott Parsons, *The Social System* (New York: The Free Press of Glencoe, 1953).

15. Everett C. Hughes, *Men and Their Work* (Chicago: University of Chicago Press, 1958).

16. George C. Homans, *Social Behavior: Its Elementary Forms* (New York: Harcourt, Brace and World, 1961).

17. Studies from a nonecological perspective stemming from this same research are found in William R. Rosengren, "Social Sources of Pregnancy as Illness or Disease," *Social Forces,* 39 (March, 1961), pp. 260-267; and by the same author, "Social-Psychological Aspects of Delivery Room Difficulties," *Journal of Nervous and Mental Disease,* 132 (June, 1961), pp. 515-521; "Social Instability and Attitudes Toward Pregnancy as a Social Role," *Social Problems,* 9 (Spring, 1962), pp. 371-378.

10

Information and
the Control of Treatment
in Tuberculosis Hospitals

JULIUS A. ROTH

Discussions of the exchange and use of information in a treatment setting commonly make the following assumptions:

1. The medical staff has reliable techniques for finding out what they need to know about patients, and the patients should help them out by providing information the staff requests of them so that the staff can take better care of them.

2. The staff should provide to the patients the information necessary to enable the patient to cooperate in his treatment, and the patients will accept this information from experts who are working for the patients' welfare.

This paper is based on a study that was supported in part by Public Health Service Research Grant E-1477 from the National Institute of Allergy and Infectious Diseases, Public Health Service.

The total study concerns itself with relevant social-psychological aspects of the hospital treatment of tuberculosis. Information was gathered by the author by long-term observation in five public tuberculosis hospitals and ward units—in two as a patient, in two as a sociological observer, and in one as a ward employee.

(293)

It is my thesis that these assumptions taken by themselves do not come close to describing what happens in a hospital-treatment situation and, furthermore, that there is no compelling reason to expect them to. In the following discussion of the discovery, manipulation, and use of information in the hospital treatment of tuberculosis, I have tried to balance the picture by placing my emphasis on the other side of the story, namely:

1. Patients are never satisfied with the information they receive from official hospital sources, and with some degree of success work at getting information that they use for their own purposes, which are sometimes in conflict with the purposes of the staff.

2. The staff often has difficulty obtaining reliable information about the patient, partly because some kinds of information by their very nature resist definition and measurement, and partly because of manipulation of information by patients and various staff groups.

The use of information in the tuberculosis-treatment situation is an illustration of the function served by information in any professional-client or tradesman-customer relationship. The professional or tradesman uses his generally superior knowledge and specialized language and viewpoint to assert his right to make decisions for his clients or customers. However, all professionals and tradesmen run into some degree of resistance from clients or customers who are not willing to have the decisions for the service taken entirely out of their hands. Generally speaking, the more closely a client's experience and knowledge approach those of the professional (or perhaps more correctly, the more closely the client *believes* his experience is comparable to that of the professional), the greater and the more effective will be the resistance to giving up control of the service to the professional.

The tuberculosis hospital is an example of one fairly narrow range in this continuum of client knowledge. The patients have the same disease and receive much the same kinds of treatment. They remain in the hospital for months, sometimes years, and for the most part are mentally intact and alert. Thus, they have both the time and ability to develop highly communicative social interaction. The prolonged disabilities their disease imposes upon them encourages them to search constantly for ways out of their predicament. This search includes learning about their disease, its diagnosis and treatment, and the decision-making behavior of physicians, nurses, and others who have some control over them. They find that they need not rely on official sources of information about themselves and their hospital situation. They learn that information that the staff obtains about them is sometimes used in a way that is not in the patients' interest (from the viewpoint of the patients). They come to see themselves to some degree as "experts" on treatment and hospital living.

The staff, however, does not accept the patients as colleagues in carrying out treatment. Rather, the patients are objects of a professional service to be manipulated for their own good—that is, for the success of the treatment. Furthermore, the patients (from the viewpoint of the staff) are often not cooperative either in providing information about themselves or in making appropriate use of information given to them by the staff.

In such a situation, bits of information about diagnosis, treatment, and hospital life often become counters in a struggle for control over the behavior and treatment of the patients.

How Staff Gets and Uses Information

WHAT THE STAFF LEARNS FROM THE PATIENT

A patient is most likely to tell the staff those things about himself that he thinks it important for the staff to know to protect his health. But how does he know what is important? One task of the physician is to educate the patient to report his symptoms properly. The physician does not want the patient telling him everything under the sun. However, he *does* want the patient to tell him the significant things. The difficult part is to get the patient to learn which things are significant and which are not.

The physician can discourage the patient from taking up too

much of his time by making himself unavailable, or by simply walking away from the patient or by indicating by tone of voice or disparaging remarks that the patient's information is not important or that the patient worries or complains too much. A physician who discourages patients from giving him many unimportant symptoms in an indiscriminate manner may end by discouraging patients from reporting any symptoms at all. Thus, toxic reactions to therapeutic drugs are sometimes missed because the patient believes the doctor would be annoyed if he was told about the patient's dizziness, skin rash, upset stomach, numbness in the extremities, and so on. Complications following surgery may not be picked up in their early stages because the patient's complaints are dismissed as the "normal" discomfort associated with surgical trauma.

Even the most searching effort to obtain information from the patient is unlikely to elicit

. . . the most elusive symptoms of all—those the patient has accepted as part of his existence. Indeed, these symptoms tend not even to be defined as symptoms by the patient, but as idiosyncrasies or annoying but tolerable facts of life. Chronic indigestion, persistent colds, headaches, backaches, and nervousness are often accepted by the patient in this fashion, particularly after their significance has been shrugged off or deprecated by a physician or two in the past.[1]

Such elusive symptoms are common among tuberculosis patients —the long-persistent cough, abnormal sputum production, shortness of breath, tiredness. A patient who has gradually become shorter of breath over a period of years may not have noticed the change because of its very gradualness. He may not think of himself as short of breath unless at some time he has an opportunity to compare himself with a "healthy" person of about the same age on some activity such as running or stair climbing. He may therefore answer "No" to the doctor's question of whether he is short of breath. The patient who has been "hawking and spitting" most of his life may deny that his sputum production is abnormal because to him it is indeed "normal" simply because he has been used to it so long. Objective tests can now check on the matter of shortness of breath, although these tests are not often used. The frequency of coughing can be checked by very close observation of a patient over a long period of time, but nursing personnel are seldom able to give the time for prolonged observation of a single patient. Other symptoms, such as tiredness, are almost wholly subjective, and the physician must rely entirely on the patient's report.

Patients often do not consider it appropriate to discuss with staff members their personal problems and their negative feelings about the treatment, the staff, and the hospital. They are likely to reserve these matters for the more sympathetic audience of their fellow patients, and their family and friends. The staff may thus be caught by surprise by patients' reactions to staff decisions and actions. The staff may assume that a patient does not care when he is discharged simply because they have not heard him say anything about it. They do not realize how upset a patient gets when information on his treatment conference is delayed for a few days, because the patient does not make a deliberate effort to bring his irritation to the attention of the staff. The staff's first knowledge of a patient's emotional crisis is often an eruption which cannot be ignored—a threat to leave the hospital against advice, a threat or attempt to commit suicide, an outright refusal to accept some treatment procedure, a fight with another patient or with an employee, a tantrum or psychotic episode.

Physicians and nurses make very little use of patients as sources of information about other patients. This is consistent with the notion that treating patients as colleagues in treatment poses a threat to the medical authority's control of that treatment. Of course, in the case of rule violations, such information would be regarded as "squealing." However, even when the issue of squealing is clearly not involved, this source of information is seldom tapped. In surgical recovery areas, patients several days past surgery are never questioned about the behavior of the new post-surgery cases even though the "older" surgery case spends more time observing the "newer" case than do all staff members combined. In one case, when a patient went into a coma after receiving some medicine, the physician questioned every nurse and aide on the ward in a vain effort to learn pre-

cisely how the patient had behaved just before becoming coma-
tose, but he never questioned the patient's roommate who had
been present throughout the entire affair. The comment of this
roommate typifies the attitude of the patient who has been
around for a while and has learned the patient's place in a
medical treatment system:

I could have told him [the physician] everything she did before
she went into a coma, but why should I say anything when he
doesn't even bother to ask me? Every time you try to tell these
people anything around here they act as if you're trying to run their
business. I've learned to keep my mouth shut.

The unreliability of staff information sometimes results from
deliberate distortion and withholding of information by a patient.
Patients believe that information the staff gets about them may
be used against them in the sense of denying privileges or
passes, keeping the patient in the hospital longer, prescribing
further treatment that the patient does not want, or simply
restricting the patient's life more narrowly in the hospital. The
patient may therefore consider it to be in his own interest to
deny certain information to the staff.

Patients sometimes suppress the fact that they have a fever [2]
because they are afraid the doctor will cancel a promised pass
or postpone their discharge if he finds out about it. They may
also suppress information about a cough, sputum production,
or subjective feelings of ill health if they are anxious to get
a pass, promotion, or discharge. Patients on outpatient status
who want to return to work may make a job look much easier
than it is in an effort to get the physician to approve their
resumption of work. A patient who is anxious to be taken off
PAS [3] may exaggerate the stomach upset he suffers (and perhaps
even stage vomiting spells) in order to convince the physician
that the medicine should be discontinued. On the other hand,
a patient who is convinced that PAS is vital to his recovery
from tuberculosis may minimize his stomach upset so that the
physician does not discontinue his medication.

In some cases sputum specimens may be faked. A patient

who wants to prove that his sputum is negative can have another patient whose sputum is consistently negative spit into his specimen cup for him.[4] On the other hand, if a patient wants to prove that he has active tuberculosis in order to get a disability award or some other compensation, he may have a patient who is consistently positive spit into his sputum cup. More rarely used tricks are squeezing blood from a pricked finger into one's sputum specimen to simulate a pulmonary hemorrhage (if the patient wants to stay in the hospital), or swallowing a large dose of ground-up Isoniazid[5] tablets just before a gastric-juice specimen is drawn for laboratory cultures (if the patient wants to get out of the hospital).

Thus, the physician and nurse can never be sure whether the patient is cooperating in some parts of the diagnosis or treatment. They usually deal with such doubts by assuming that things are going right unless they have evidence to the contrary. Thus, they will assume that a patient is taking all his medicine unless they find some pills in his bedside stand or unless his roommate tips them off that he is throwing his pills into the toilet.

In addition to such more obvious tricks, the patient makes an effort to control the information the staff receives about him so that he can project what he believes is a desirable image. Although the tubercular patient does not have the problem of hiding neurotic symptoms as the psychiatric patient often does,[6] he realizes that the reputation he has with the staff may make a difference in the way they will treat him. For example, most patients want to appear fairly cooperative with the demands of the treatment and management program if for no other reason than their belief that such a reputation will cause the staff to trust them with more information about themselves, with more freedom of action while in the hospital, and perhaps with an earlier discharge. They will make an effort to keep their violations of rules and treatment procedures hidden from those in authority. If they sharply reject some aspect of the treatment, they may disguise their feelings about it if possible. If they argue for a favor or concession, they try to keep their argument within the framework of the staff's principles of treatment as

well as our middle-class conceptions of fairness and proper behavior. Patients, of course, vary in ability to project the desired
image. From this viewpoint, a successful patient may be defined
as one who correctly gauges the kind of behavior those in
authority want from a patient and who is able to maintain a
close approximation of this behavior outwardly while at the
same time he is able to obtain a maximum of information and
concessions to his own preferences from the staff.

THE CHART

The staff does not rely on the reports of the patient to
accumulate and distribute information about him. Physicians
lean heavily on X-rays, laboratory procedures, and direct anatom-
ical and functional observations that—while often crude and
subject to considerable error—at least are not subject to the
conscious or unconscious manipulation of the patient.[7] Nurses,
too, make systematic observations of given aspects of a patient's
behavior or condition, some routinely—for example, the daily
temperature and pulse, the weekly weighing—and some on
special order of the physician.

A record of such observations and reports on diagnostic and
treatment procedures is kept in the patient's chart—a collection
of documents that the nurses (or ward clerks) maintain for
each patient. The chart also contains physicians' and nurses'
notes on their impressions and less systematic observations of
the patient's condition and behavior. Often it contains reports
and statements from hospitals, clinics, and physicians that examined and treated the patient at an earlier time. It could,
therefore, be a major instrument for accumulating and making
available to treatment personnel information about the patient.
To the patient the chart is often a repository of secret knowledge
about himself that would reveal everything the staff thinks
about him if he could only get a look at it. The less experienced
staff members, too, sometimes act as if the chart told them
everything they needed to know about the patient.

However, the chart appears more formidable than its actual
role in the information system warrants. Much information used

in making decisions about patients' treatment and about "handling" the patients is not in the charts at all, but is based on observations and conjectures passed among staff members by word of mouth and never written down by anyone. Nurses' tricks for keeping patients quiet and satisfied are often uncharted. Informal controls that nurses' aides have worked out with relation to given patients are probably never charted, although they are passed on as important information to each new aide who comes on the ward. The physician may form a definite opinion of how trustworthy a patient's pass requests are, but he is likely to store this information in his memory and pass it on orally to appropriate colleagues rather than write it in the chart.

Much of the information that *is* entered in the chart is never used except when something unexpected happens, in which case the physician may read through the entire chart in an effort to discover a cause for the unanticipated illness or other occurrence.

There is also the danger that the chart will perpetuate errors. The doctor writing the intake history may have mistakenly recorded the patient as never having had streptomycin (perhaps because he misunderstood the patient's way of expressing himself). Treatment decisions are then made in accordance with this information. If the doctor later mentions in the patient's presence that he never had streptomycin, the patient may correct him and the error will be discovered. Often this never happens. Since patients are not given access to their charts, it is likely that such errors will go uncorrected. The very fact that the information is recorded in the chart gives it the appearance of being reliable information.

INFORMATION UP THE LINE

Most nurses see relatively little of the patients. They may make formal rounds each day, sometimes not even that. They perform a few procedures—for example, dispensing medications —which bring them in contact with the patients. Nurses' aides do most of the routine work directly involving patients, including taking of temperature and pulse in most hospitals. The nurses therefore rely heavily on the aides for observational information about the patients.

Physicians rely on the nurses to report adverse symptoms, but the nurse in turn must learn much of what she knows about the patient's symptoms from the aides. Nurses are interested in patients' behavior—whether or not they appear to be ill in some way, whether or not they are following rules and procedures—but most of the observing is done by the aides.

Just what do nurses learn about patients from aides? It is difficult to give a general answer to this question because of the great variety of patterns of nursing hierarchies and functions in hospitals today. The division of labor among the different kinds of nursing personnel is in great flux, and no typical or stable relationship between the various levels of the nursing hierarchy exists. However, a few general trends may be pointed out.

Aides are most likely to tell the nurse things they believe must be known to her to protect the patients' health. They will readily report any bleeding, skin rash, or fever, even when the patient does not want it reported. Violations of rules or doctors' orders that are a clear danger to the patients' health are very likely to be reported—for example, a diabetic cheating on his diet, a severely hemorrhaging patient getting out of bed. Less obvious symptoms are less likely to be reported because the aide does not notice them. Infractions of rules and orders that are not a clear-cut danger to health are also less likely to be reported. For example, a patient who is out of bed a great deal more than he is supposed to be, or who is surreptitiously reading during the afternoon rest period, is not likely to be reported by aides, who would be thought of by the patients and perhaps even by their fellow aides as "squealers" if they told the nurse about such rule-violating behavior.

Patients frequently come to trust aides with information they do not want the nurse or doctor to have. If the aide breaks this trust, the nurse is placed in a delicate situation. Thus, the aide may tell the nurse that a patient is throwing away his PAS or that he is selling wallets he made himself though he is not supposed to be doing any leatherwork. If the nurse confronts the patient with the damning information, the patient will immediately assume that the aide squealed on him; and not only he, but other patients as well, will be suspicious of that aide thereafter. The nurse will thus not only have caused considerable conflict between an aide and the patients, but will have cut off an avenue of information that might have been useful to her in the future. The nurse may therefore avoid taking direct action, and may instead keep a closer eye on the patient with the hope of catching him at the rule violation herself. Or, she may make an effort to gain his confidence to the point where he will reveal to her what he did to the aide.

Although the physician relies heavily on information he gets from chest X-rays and other diagnostic tests, he is also interested in the day-to-day symptoms and behavior of patients, and for such information he must depend largely on the nurses. Reading each patient's chart routinely is extremely time-consuming, and therefore the physician—and also the nurse—look in the chart only when they want specific information. The physician relies on the nurses to report significant items so that he can keep up with each case without having to read everything that the nurses (and others) write. If the nurse fails to keep the doctor up on significant changes, he may not even know, for example, that a patient's medications were discontinued by another physician because of an allergic reaction, and may be placed in the embarrassing position of discussing medications with the patient and finding that the patient knows more about it than he does.

Like the aides, the nurses are most likely to pass on information that appears to be directly concerned with the patients' health. However, much more than the aide, the nurse tries to separate the important from the minor. She does not want to trouble the doctor with minor things she can handle herself. If a patient starts to hemorrhage or to show a grossly irregular pulse and chest pains, she is likely to call the physician hurriedly to get his advice and to try to get him to come to the ward to take charge of the case. However, if the patient complains of a headache, she will probably hand him a couple of aspirin, and the doctor will never even hear about the matter.

Probably the greater part of the patients' symptoms and complaints are handled in the latter manner. Such "minor things" will come to the doctor's attention only if something later "goes wrong" and if what appeared to be a minor matter turns out to be a precursor of a serious difficulty. In any event, it is the nurse who decides what is serious and what is not, and information about the patient's symptoms is filtered through her definitions of seriousness—definitions the doctor might not always agree with if he knew about them.

HANDLING THE PATIENT

The most explicit use of information about a patient by the staff is to make decisions about treating the patient's disorder. This, in fact, is the only rationale usually offered for accumulating information about a patient. A hospital staff, however, cannot concern itself solely with treating disease. It must also manage an institution, which means—among other things—exercising some control over the behavior of the inmates. For this purpose, the staff requires information about how to "handle" the patients. Even for carrying out a specific treatment procedure, staff members must know how to get the patient to agree to the procedure and to play his part in performing it.

In order to handle the patient, the hospital staff must know many things about him that are not in the chart or in the order book. The characteristics of a patient and the methods used to control his behavior are exchanged informally among staff members. Physicians who work together on the same unit or who have a patient transferred from one to the other will often tell one another how the patient may be expected to react to actions of the physicians. Nurses and aides constantly tell one another how to deal with given patients in order to elicit certain behavior.

Is a patient bluffing when he threatens to walk out of the hospital if refused a pass? How do you keep a patient from getting upset and angry when his breakfast is delayed after a blood test? How do you induce a lazy patient to get out of bed when you want to make it? How do you convince a postsurgical patient that he must sit up and cough despite the pain? How do you stall off a patient who insists on seeing the doctor? Which patient is likely to make the most trouble if you take away an extra bedside table? Which patients are most likely to sneak off to the canteen if you do not watch them? How do you deal with a patient who refuses to clear off his tray after eating? Which patients are touchy about the way they are bathed and how do you placate them?

The new nurse or new aide is told during her first day or two what the various patients are like and how she should deal with them so as to do her job successfully and not have the patients "take advantage" of her. A staff member with previous experience with a patient becomes an "expert informant" to others who have not had this experience. Thus, an aide who has recently worked on a ward from which a patient has been transferred can inform her present co-workers about the patient and tell them how to handle him without all the personnel on the ward having to find out by trial and error. In a situation like this, an aide may even become a teacher to the nurses.

Nurses must exchange information, not only on their own shifts but also between shifts, on such crucial matters as the placebos they give and what they tell the patients about them. When a patient is transferred to another ward, the nurse from the one ward tells the nurse from the new ward the details about what should be said to and done for the patient to keep him reasonably satisfied (and in what respects he is unsatisfiable and therefore should be refused or stalled off), and warns her about any aggressive or unusual behavior that might upset ward routine or place undue demands upon nursing personnel.

When Chester Carmody was on the East Ward at Shawnee Sanitarium, he was given a "pain pill"—a capsule filled with aspirin powder—when he demanded something for his chest pains. He had already rejected aspirin as not being "strong enough" to counteract his severe pain, but he accepted the white capsule when the nurses told him he could have only one every four hours to give him the impression that it was a dangerous narcotic. This gave the nurses an effective means of psychological control over him without having to get an order from the doctor (who might possibly have found their approach objectionable). This placebo was not entered in the chart. Therefore, when Carmody was transferred to the West Ward, the East Ward nurse had to get in touch with the West Ward nurse to let her know what to give Carmody when he complained of chest pains and what story he should be told about his medication. Any inconsistency in the medication given or in the story told may lead a patient to suspect that he is being given a placebo. Thus, the failure to exchange such information can lead to a loss of psychological control over the behavior of the patient.

How Patients Get and Use Information

THE OFFICIAL CHANNELS

Patients typically receive some information about themselves as a medical case through more or less official statements of the staff. Physicians tell them about the need for prolonged treatment, the slow change that takes place and the consequent long time between checkups, the seriousness of the disease, and the importance of following recommended treatment. Patients are usually informed about medical staff decisions on the medications they are to take for tuberculosis and what kind of surgery, if any, is recommended. In addition, they are usually told whether their sputum tests are positive or negative and are given at least some general notion about the appearance of their X-rays. They are advised about the kinds and amounts of activity they should take and what activity they should avoid.

For information that he cannot get from physicians, the patient often turns to the ward nurses, who are more accessible and often less frightening to the more timid patient. Nurses give patients advice and instructions about rest and activity, protective techniques intended to reduce the spread of the disease, and rules of conduct of the hospital. They will usually tell patients the names of the specific tuberculosis medications they are getting, but not the other medications. They are likely to keep patients informed on such matters of ward routine as changes in scheduling laundry pickup, linen change, and streptomycin injections. They will instruct patients on the treatment of minor ailments.

A doctor, nurse, or aide never tells a patients "everything." Though exactly what a staff member will tell a patient will vary with the individual and with the situation, there is always some information that is considered a threat to the control of treatment or hospital management if known to the patients. The staff member must always consider whether the patient may "misinterpret" what he learns about himself (or about others that can refer to his own case), or whether he will react in an undesirable way to information given him.

Thus, physicians are often reluctant to admit any uncertainty about diagnosis, treatment, or control of tuberculosis because they are afraid that patients will interpret uncertainties and disagreements to mean that the doctors do not know what they are doing, that the treatment procedures and hospital routines are mistakes, or that the patient's guess is just as good as that of the doctor. They often avoid telling a patient bad news about his case because they "just can't face" an emotionally distraught patient. They play down the subjective misery and the possible complications of the postsurgical period because they are afraid that such information might frighten the patient out of taking surgery. They frequently hide from the patient past mistakes made in his case because they are afraid that the patient may then argue that these physicians are incompetent and that therefore he does not want to be treated by them.

The treatment staff does not give all patients the same amount and kind of information. What they tell or do not tell a patient depends on the reaction they expect from him. This expectation in turn is created by their past experience with him as an individual or their experience with other patients whom they believe to be like him. The more a staff person considers patients to be alike in their reactions, the more standardized his pattern of giving, modifying, and withholding information will be.

Obviously, then, the image a patient creates of himself influences what he is told. The patient who convinces the staff that he can "take it" is more likely to be told bad news than one who has a reputation for anxiety and emotional upset. Doctors' and nurses' stereotypes (often merely the reflections of stereotypes found generally in our society) of how patients will react may determine what they will tell different groups of patients. Thus, men are more likely to be told bad news than are women.

The doling out of information to hospital patients by staff members, then, is not simply a matter of a group of specialists striving to fill the needs of consumers of information. In giving information (and in withholding it) the staff members are trying to create an effect. The effect, if successful, should be one that causes the patients to make the right decisions and to conduct themselves in the proper manner. What is right and proper in this case is defined by the staff. The patient, if he were fully informed, would not always agree. This does not necessarily mean that the staff is trying "to put something over" on the patients. It is precisely because of their concern for the welfare of the individual patient (or for patients as a group, which is not always the same thing) that they often manipulate information to the patient to get him to do what is best for him. Thus, if the physician is convinced that a patient's health will be protected by staying an additional period in the hospital under drug therapy, and if he also believes that the patient will insist on being discharged when he learns that his condition has markedly improved, the physician may feel justified in telling the patient time after time that his progress is very slow until such time that the physician considers him ready for discharge.[8]

THE DEVIOUS CHANNELS

Official information, although always welcome, is often suspect and never sufficient. Patients are, therefore, engaged in a constant hunt for information. This hunt consists in part of squeezing information out of the staff by devious means.

Sometimes a patient acquires information about himself merely as a by-product of a staff function. He may overhear two or more doctors or a doctor and nurse in a conversation about his own case or another patient's case. When there is a change of resident physicians or when a new physician joins the staff, a supervising physician may make rounds and present each of the cases to the new doctor. This is always a good opportunity for patients to learn a great deal about themselves that they were not told before.

The patient may have someone from the outside—a family member or a private physician—call the hospital doctor to get information about his case. The hospital doctors will often talk more freely about certain aspects of the case to outsiders than they will to the patient himself, and these outsiders in turn may pass this information on to the patient.

Quite often, a patient finds that when he threatens to leave against advice, the physician will show him his X-rays, and give him detailed information about his sputum status and the medical staff's judgment about his condition and prognosis and further treatment that the patient had not been able to learn about before. Patients sometimes have physicians fill out papers about social security payments, pensions, or reports required by employers that force the doctor to commit himself on the patient's condition and probable length of treatment. A patient may ask for a pass, not simply because he wants to go out on pass, but also as a way of learning more about the doctor's judgment of his present condition. He thinks: If he turned down my pass request last month, but gives me one this month, I must be getting better. If I ask the doctor directly whether I'm getting better, he'll probably give me a noncommittal or meaningless answer. But if I ask him for a pass, he *has to* say Yes or No.

Patients sometimes play the medical-status system in an effort to get more information. They may talk a new resident into giving information about test results and treatment decisions that the staff physician did not yet want to reveal. On the other hand, if a surgical resident refuses to give information about the pathologist's report on a patient's excised lung tissue, the patient may question the chief surgeon, who does not have to worry about anyone criticizing him for talking too much.

Nurses vary in what they are willing to tell patients, and

the patients learn to make use of these variations. If one nurse will not tell a patient the name of the medication he is receiving, he will try another. The patients learn from each other which nurses are most likely to give such information, and tend to save their questions for them. With three shifts each day and with relief nurses on each shift on the regular nurses' days off, a patient will have at least six different charge nurses each week to work on to get information. With the rotation of nurses that takes place in most hospitals, he will have many more over a period of time. With all these nurses, he can often find one who will give him some of the contraband information he wants.

Nurses' aides are less likely to know the details of the patient's condition and treatment. Also, they usually play safe by dodging requests for contraband information. Sometimes, however, where a friendly and trustful relationship exists (or where the patient has bribed the aide), an aide may be willing to do the patient a favor by obtaining for him information about test results, medical-conference reports, medical orders, and so on. On the whole, however, aides are likely to be more useful as purveyors of information on the minutiae of daily ward routines—information that sometimes helps patients anticipate changes in procedures or rules of conduct and their enforcement.

Social workers, psychologists, occupational therapists, ward clerks, and laboratory technicians are all likely to find themselves being pumped for information when they work with patients. In fact, patients will try to get information out of anyone who might possibly know anything relevant to their case at least once before they give up.

Since the patients are ready to take advantage of leaks in the staff information dam, those in authority must often decide whom they can trust with certain information about the patients. Thus, in one hospital nurses were no longer permitted to attend treatment conferences when it appeared that they were passing conference decisions on to some patients before the physician made rounds. Nurses' aides are frequently suspected of leaking information to patients, and in many hospitals they are prohibited from reading charts and staying in a patient's room when a physician is present, and in at least one hospital are even discouraged from listening to the nurses' report. But the medical residents and ward personnel must obviously be given much information about the patient in order to carry out their treatment tasks and to protect themselves against infection and against the demands and tricks of the patients. The control of information to patients, therefore, must rely largely on adherence to professional ethics and/or loyalty to the correct institutional viewpoint. With the involvement of many people, together with their differences in loyalties, occupational commitments, and corruptibility, and with some differences in their conceptions of what the "correct" viewpoint is, there are bound to be many loopholes in the control system.

NON-STAFF CHANNELS

Doctors are constantly warning patients not to listen to other patients on matters concerning their disease and its treatment, but this advice is almost universally ignored in a tuberculosis hospital. One of the most popular subjects of talk between patients is their own disease condition and treatment and that of other patients. Much of this talk is an effort on the part of each patient to find out where he stands and what he can look forward to in the future.

What condition am I in? How much good will the drugs do me? How safe is it for me to be up a lot, or to play cards? How often should I try to get a pass? Do I really need surgery and how safe is it? How long should I stay in the hospital? When should I go back to work and what kind of work can I do? These questions and others like them, which the physicians maintain can only be answered on the basis of expert medical opinion, are often answered in large part on the basis of information from fellow patients.

Patients often do not want to "bother" physicians and nurses, or they find that they cannot get the information that they want from the staff, or do not trust it when they get it. They feel easier about discussing their case with others who are in the same boat. They need not be afraid to ask questions. They can count on getting answers—much more definite and detailed answers than staff members are likely to give.

The "expert informant" among the patients plays an especially important role. For the new patient, any patient who has been there longer is an expert informant. A patient who has had surgery is an expert to one who is going to get surgery in the future. A patient who has been in the same hospital before or who has been in other hospitals serves as an expert to those who are in for the first time.[9]

Physicians in tuberculosis hospitals often assume that a patient who is being treated for the first time is getting his first definitive information about his condition from them. Often this is not true. Many patients have seen outside private or clinic physicians or nurses who have discussed their case with them and have even told them what treatment they might expect and how long they would have to stay in the hospital.

Patients avidly read newspaper stories about new tuberculosis drugs and other advances in treatment. Occasional television programs, books, and magazine articles about tuberculosis also provide information that is an extension of, and sometimes a contradiction of, the information they get from the hospital staff. The patient may have family members or acquaintances who have had the disease, or have worked for physicians, or have some other inside knowledge of the medical world or tuberculosis hospitals. From such people they will glean whatever information they can, and pass it on to their fellow patients.

The patient can gain information by just keeping his eyes and ears open, even when not receiving information explicitly from anyone. He can discover what rules are really enforced by observing what happens when other patients violate the rules. He can develop an estimate of how often he can get a pass by noting how often his fellows who seem to be in the same condition or stage of treatment succeed in getting a pass. His decision about how much bed rest to take depends largely on how much time the patients around him stay in bed.

HOW THE PATIENT USES HIS INFORMATION

What Does the Future Hold in Store? When the newly admitted patient anxiously asks his fellow inmates how long they have been there, what kind of treatment they are getting, how competent the physicians are, or what hospital life is like, he is simply trying to find out what he can expect in his own future as a tuberculosis patient. When he observes and questions those who are some steps ahead of him in treatment, he is seeing himself in the coming weeks and months. When he sees what happens to patients following surgery, he is gaining an idea of what to expect when *he* gets surgery. When he notes that his medical conferences are routinely preceded by a chest X-ray and a series of three daily sputum specimens, or that patients are frequently switched from streptomycin to PAS shortly before discharge, he has a better idea of what to expect in the coming days and weeks. In the same way he can pick up clues on his own future state and learn to predict the action of the staff with regard to himself on many matters large and small.

Judging Treatment. Patients are never completely satisfied with what they learn through official hospital sources of information. If the news is good, they wonder if the doctor is just trying to make them feel better. If the news is bad, they wonder if he is just establishing an excuse for holding them in the hospital longer or for refusing them privileges. They always suspect that important details are being held back. An important reason for seeking other sources of information is, therefore, to enable the patient to judge the treatment he is receiving more accurately and to help him decide to what extent he should adhere to that treatment program.

The information from fellow patients may influence patients to stay in the hospital or to go AMA,[10] to take or to refuse surgery, to take PAS or to throw it away, to take or not to take their rest. Physicians usually notice only those instances where patients have been influenced by their fellows to refuse treatment, and they universally condemn such influence. However, there are frequent cases of patients talking their buddies out of going AMA, of convincing them to accept surgery if the doctors offer it, of urging them to take their medicine, and of warning them about being overactive.

When patients accumulate information about other tuberculosis hospitals, they may use this information to decide what other hospital they might transfer to or which hospital they should go to if they need treatment again in the future. Most commonly, however, knowledge about other hospitals is used to raise questions about whether the patient is getting the best possible treatment in the hospital he is in now. Patients point to other hospitals that have less bed rest, shorter periods of treatment, more passes, less surgery, no protective techniques, and different drug regimen. They then wonder whether the doctors in their present hospital know how to treat them properly. Perhaps I should be getting different drugs. Perhaps all the surgery they do here isn't necessary. If patients can get discharged earlier at the National Jewish Hospital, why can't the same thing happen here?

Information from outside physicians and clinics is often used by patients in the same way. If the outside doctor's view is more favorable to the patient's way of seeing things, the patient may wonder if the hospital doctors have made a reasonable decision. Hospital physicians, in fact, often feel that their efforts are being sabotaged by outside physicians who minimize the seriousness of the disease and the length of necessary treatment (perhaps as a strategy to convince the patient to accept hospitalization in the first place) and thus make it more difficult for the hospital staff to get patients to accept their treatment program.

A patient's own observations can provide him with information that will help him judge the treatment. When patients see that another patient who has never taken much bed rest is promoted quickly, it makes them wonder whether a great deal of bed rest is really necessary, and they may find this a good reason for reducing the amount of bed rest they themselves take. When patients observe poor results of surgery—for example, other surgical patients being held in the hospital for a long period for treatment of postsurgical complications—they may argue that they do not want this to happen to them. In one hospital the patients noted that the postsurgical cases were not closely attended by physicians and nurses, and this made some of them hesitate to put their own lives in the hands of the hospital staff.

Bargaining for Concessions. When patients point to other hospitals that have less bed rest, shorter periods of treatment, more passes, or fewer restrictions on activity, they often do so with the hope of getting their own doctors to change in the same direction. Patients will frequently cite such variations in treatment when arguing with physicians for concessions in their own case, and the physician is placed in the position of having to defend his methods against those of other specialists (or at least the patients' conceptions of those methods).

When the *Reader's Digest* printed an article describing a treatment program at another institution that greatly reduced the ▮ of hospitalization, that institution had already abandoned its accelerated treatment [11] and had reverted to more conservative methods. The patients did not know this, and it probably would not have made any difference if they had. It was still good ammunition to use against the hospital staff in the patients' fight to reduce their period of hospitalization.

Information about variations in practice in the patient's own hospital is often used in bargaining for concessions. "Webb got a whole week at home for Christmas. How come you give me only three days?" "Harvey got discharged only four months after his surgery; I had the same kind of operation, so why should I have to stay longer?" The physician may be unable to convince a patient that such variations are justified by subtle differences in the patients' conditions. He may yield to such arguments in order to appear "fair" to all.

Political Information. Perhaps more important than the influence on treatment decisions as such is the fellow patient's influence on the "politics" of the treatment situation. It is not simply a matter of "What activity is safe?" but "What activities can I get away with?" and "What doctors and nurses do I have to watch out most for?" It is not so much "How often can I safely go on pass?" but "How can I finagle a pass from the doctor when he doesn't think I should have one?" It is not "How long should I stay in the hospital?" but "How can I talk the doctor

into giving me a discharge earlier?" or "When is the best time
to go AMA?" The question is not "When is it safe to go back
to work?" but "How can I pick up some extra money without
having the Welfare Department find out about it?" It is not
"What are the rules?" but "What rules are really enforced and
what ones are not?" On such matters, of course, the patients
must rely on their own buddies (with occasional limited assistance from the lower echelons of hospital personnel) because the
very nature of the questions precludes communication with the
doctors and other persons in authority.[12]

Summary

Although I have made an effort to outline, at least, the to[lengtl]
of the information-control system in tuberculosis hospitals, the
stress was placed—as noted in the introduction—on the staff's
difficulties in obtaining information about the patient and on
the way in which the patients obtain and use information about
themselves and their situation despite staff efforts to control this
information. The emphasis has been placed on those aspects of
information control that are commonly regarded as wrong or
unfortunate. I have tried to show that these aspects may rather
be considered an inevitable part of the situation—as "normal"
as the successful accumulation of medical information about a
patient or the acceptance by a patient of a diagnostic result
reported to him by a physician.

A normative approach is likely to miss what is intrinsic to the
situation. Labeling staff members incompetent or lazy when they
fail to obtain information that is useful in making treatment
decisions and in managing the behavior of patients over-
looks the built-in effects of the organization of the treatment setting. Thus, the manner in which hospital staff work is organized
forces the staff to use a sampling approach to obtain information about the patients—a sampling into which bias may be
introduced at many points. It also requires a process of reporting information that further selects and reduces the information
available to any given staff member. A preordained normative

approach stands in the way of an examination of the manner in which such sampling and reporting takes place and the effects these processes have on the procurement and use of information.

A normative approach also tends to ignore the differing goals of the interacting groups in an institutional setting in favor of a supposed over-all ideal. Patients' efforts to obtain more information about themselves and to use that information to make their own judgments of treatment and at times to escape institutional controls have been regarded—even by social scientists —as evidence of psychopathology. A psychiatrist, Eli Lane, expresses this typical bias when he says:

Patients tend to identify themselves with each other and it is difficult for them to understand the specificity of each person's case. In their lack of understanding, they attempt magically to divine what will happen to them through finding out what happened to others.[13]

There is nothing magical, or even futile, about the patient's efforts to get information. Contraband information that the patient can get from his own observations, from other patients, from outside sources, and from leaks among the staff serve to fill important gaps in his state of knowledge about himself and his situation. Such information, although sometimes misleading, enables the patient to make predictions about his future that are much more detailed, usually more directly useful in guiding his behavior, and sometimes more accurate, than what he would be able to make from information received from official sources only. His use of information serves his goals in the same way that the use of information by physicians and nurses serves *their* goals. The social scientist might better concentrate on explaining how the patients develop and try to reach their goals than on showing what is "wrong" with patients who are not willing to be content with the testimony of experts.

NOTES

1. Eliot Freidson, *Patients' Views of Medical Practice* (New York, Russell Sage Foundation, 1961), p. 84.

2. In most hospitals this can be easily done because the thermometers are either at the patient's bedside or else they are passed out in advance and a nurse or aide comes around to collect or to look at the thermometer at a later time.

3. Para-aminosalicylic acid, one of the three most commonly used antituberculosis drugs and the one most often causing unpleasant toxic effects.

4. Occasionally, when staff suspicions have been aroused, a physician or nurse will stand by while the correct patient spits into the specimen cup, which is then removed from the patient's possession.

5. The most commonly used and probably most effective antituberculosis drug.

6. William Caudill, *The Psychiatric Hospital as a Small Society* (Cambridge: Harvard University Press, 1958), pp. 164, 167, 171.

7. Though even here laboratory specimens can be faked or modified by patients if they are not closely watched, as noted above.

8. Quite often, such decisions are quasi-statistical rather than individual. Thus, the physician may argue that patients kept in the hospital at least three months after their lesions appear to be stabilized suffer proportionately fewer relapses in the future than those who are released as soon as they appear stabilized. Therefore, the information given to all patients may justifiably be tailored so as to convince them that they should stay in the hospital the additional period of time. Part of the tailoring would be intended to keep the patients from thinking of this as "an additional period."

9. Readmission rates are usually high enough to provide a substantial number of patients with previous hospital experience, including experience in other hospitals, to feed into the patients' information mill. During my year-and-a-half period of observation at Dover Sanatorium, 40 per cent of all the admissions had been in a tuberculosis hospital previously, and of these about one-third had been in hospitals other than Dover. During this same period, the readmission rate at Valentine Hospital was 37 per cent, most of whom had previously been in other hospitals for tuberculosis.

10. To leave the hospital against medical advice.

11. Which had been instituted as a temporary expedient to reduce the waiting list.

12. The way in which "political information" is used by institutional inmates has probably been most thoroughly studied in prisons and mental hospitals. See, for example, Donald Clemmer, *The Prison Community* (New York: Holt, Rinehart, and Winston, 1958), Chaps. 4, 8, and Alfred H. Stanton and Morris S. Schwartz, *The Mental Hospital* (New York: Basic Books, 1954), Chap. 11.

13. "The Tuberculosis Patient's Private World," from *Personality, Stress and Tuberculosis*, Phineas J. Sparer, ed. (New York: International Universities Press, 1956), p. 327.

11

The Physical Environment
of the Ward

ROBERT SOMMER
ROBERT DEWAR

Architects and others who are concerned with hospital building still proceed largely by intuition and enlightened guesswork. The least likely group to be asked for its opinions is the one that will spend the longest concentrated periods of time in the hospital—the patients. It is true that the total time spent in the hospital by the physicians and nurses will exceed that spent by individual patients, but the staff is able to leave after finishing an eight-hour shift, and is constantly on the move throughout the day. The patient is more anxious and thus more receptive to new and old sources of stimulation and hence more readily disturbed by his physical environment. His reactions may be like those of any person or animal who is forced to remain outside its territory, or those observed by zoo keepers who have worked with animals in captivity. Ellenberger [1] lists these symptoms of captivity: the initial trauma, the nesting process, syndromes produced by social competition and frustrations, and emotional deterioration.

Most research dealing with hospital patients has stressed the patient's relations with other people, especially nurses, doctors, other patients, and visitors. Much less has been written about his reactions to the physical environment. This field has been regarded as almost exclusively the province of the architect and the interior designer. When a psychiatrist or social scientist addresses a meeting of architects or administrators, he usually speaks about "the human needs of hospitals." He may wax eloquent about the need for warmth, the human touch, or effective human relations. Most of this involves the extrapolation of needs from other situations and their application to the hospital setting.

When an architect writes an article about hospital design, he is likely to deal with such matters as cost, efficiency, and types of building material. He seems largely unaware of the social research in this field. His concept of "relevant social research" consists largely of experiments showing the psychological connotations of colours and the old Gestalt demonstrations of optical illusions. Furthermore, social scientists tend to misunderstand the function and values of the architect. They see him as concerned primarily with a physical structure such as a building or other enclosure. On the contrary, the architect considers his main interest the enclosed space rather than the enclosure, and the internal dimensions of the structure rather than its external appearance. Lao-tze put it this way: "Clay is moulded into a vessel; the utility of the vessel depends upon its hollow interior. Doors and windows are cut in order to make a house; the utility of the house depends upon the empty spaces." In drawing up the plans for a house or other building, architects prefer to speak in terms of space and area to describe the place where certain things are expected to happen, instead of the term "room," which has too much of the connotation of a tightly enclosed and partitioned cubicle.[2]

When architects and social scientists talk together, they are likely to use certain key words in different ways. For example, it may be unclear whether space refers to the floor or air space and how its boundaries are defined. Roth [3] illustrates this nicely in his research in a tuberculosis hospital. He found that the lines of demarcation between "clean areas" and "dirty areas" were defined by lines on the floor rather than with respect to air space. Patients from the clean area would stand a few feet away from the dirty area even though it was generally agreed among experts that tuberculosis is usually transmitted through the air. In common speech "space" refers to the absence of something, while in architecture it refers to something very tangible such as floor space or ground area. Architects are trained to an aesthetic appreciation of space per se, and discuss the proportions and scale of their air-filled volumes that may overlap, intersect, interweave, and so forth.

Territory and Personal Space

Ecologists and social scientists generally use space in the geographic sense of area, and more commonly with reference to an animal's territory or home, for example, Eliot Howard [4] and his work with birds. He emphasized the functional aspects of territory in the processes of mating and rearing offspring. He observed that male finches quickly isolated themselves from one another and reigned supreme in small areas. Territorial boundaries vary considerably from season to season; and for the majority of woodland birds, territory is confined to the spring and summer.

Social scientists have also used the concept of territory in studying human behavior, as William Whyte [5] and Thrasher [6] in studying the territories of adolescent gangs. The idea of territoriality has figured prominently in discussion of home versus hospital treatment for various classes of ill people. It has frequently been observed that there is a marked difference in behavior and attitude between a person at home and the same person in hospital. Carse, who pioneered the Worthing experiment in home treatment of the mentally ill, observed:

At home, even though he was a sick man the patient retained his identity and the sense of belonging; he was with his family and he felt secure because he was still in the community which he knew and which he understood. In hospital, the patient is an enforced member of a group living in an entirely artificial environment bearing no relation to anything approaching ordinary home life, but where everything is strange and often frightening.[7]

Territoriality is only one connotation that the term "space" has acquired. A second meaning can best be termed the "personal space" of the organism. Like territoriality it has roots in the work of zoologists and ethologists, but it is an entirely different concept. Personal space refers to the distance that the organism customarily places between itself and other organisms. This distance may vary from species to species and from individual to individual. A person may feel comfortable when his child stands near him but be uncomfortable when an adult male occupies the same place. A chicken would not be disturbed at the approach of a robin, but a hawk would upset her. Hediger [8] speaks of "flight distance," and has measured this for hundreds of animals. Other terms that have roughly the same meaning have also been used. David Katz [9] first used the term "personal space," and compared it with the shell of a snail. Von Uexküll [10] describes people as being surrounded by "soap bubble worlds," and maintained there is no space independent of subjects. Stern [11] developed the concept of personal world. He noted that the physical world was without a center but that the personal world had the body as a natural center from which and toward which everything pertaining to it extended. Stern's analogy to the snail shell of Katz and the soap bubble of von Uexküll was to describe "personally near" as an aura surrounding the person. He contrasted this with the "personally distant," which either lay below the threshold of personal relevance or was split off from the present region. Richard Neutra,[12] an architect, uses the concept of "physiological space," which he describes as emotionally egotistic—three steps taken toward a person are quite different from three steps taken away from him, and three steps almost within arm's reach have a different significance than the same distance a mile away. Accordingly, nearness, if undesired, connotes oppression or infringement on privacy. Yet if a king or superior personage chooses to step near an ordinary mortal, it means honor and flattering familiarity.

The concept of personal space can be distinguished from territory in several ways. The most important difference is that personal space is carried around, while territory is relatively stationary. An animal or man will usually mark the boundaries of his territory so that they are visible to others, but the boundaries of personal space are invisible. Personal space has the body as the center, while territory does not. Often the center of territory is the home of animal or man. Animals will usually fight to maintain dominion over their territory but will withdraw if others intrude into their personal space. The individual's concept of his personal space can be drastically altered by confinement in hospital. His complaints about lack of privacy refer more to the feeling that personal space is violated than to an invasion of territory. Often he must lie in bed and permit a host of strangers to observe, move, and even operate upon his body. The nurses and physicians appear to have no reluctance about intruding into his personal space. They tend to view his body as an object lacking any kind of aura or sanctity. This kind of perception seems an essential ingredient of the medical role. The physician or nurse who can view a limb or body as an object often feels that his efficiency is unimpaired by consideration of how the patient feels at the particular moment. However, the apparent indifference with which a nurse or physician is able to intrude into a patient's personal space does not extend to all parts of the body. We may observe the reluctance of many nurses and physicians to use mouth-to-mouth rescue breathing as an example. Linden [13] does an excellent job in cataloguing some of the reactions of nurses to mouth-to-mouth breathing. He feels that the use of the procedure demands the overcoming of "that traditional objectivity which may be termed *professional distance.*"

Those patients who must wear plaster casts or heavy bandages often experience a restriction of personal space. Some patients feel protected and secure under such conditions, while others feel isolated and afraid. Ruff and Levy,[14] who have studied the effects of space travel, discuss the differences between the restriction of sensory input produced by bandages, goggles, and even earplugs and the effects of confinement in a small area. They use the concept of "perceptual space" to refer to the distance between the person and the point at which barriers to sensory input are placed. They have found that blocking light and sound by goggles and earplugs often produces more anxiety than blocking input by the walls of a chamber several feet from the head. Their explanation is that ego boundaries are more easily maintained when a sense of physical boundaries is preserved.

Hebb and his co-workers [15] have shown that hallucinations and thought disorder can be produced when a person is placed in a restricted environment. An almost universal symptom among his subjects, most of whom were normal, healthy college students, was an inability to concentrate or focus attention on a subject for any length of time. In our own work [16] we found that in the autobiographies of fifty former mental patients, almost all the hallucinations that the patients experienced occurred under conditions of reduced stimulation, for example, when the patient was alone in a dimly lighted room, when he was in a strait jacket, and so on. However, it would seem extreme to compare this kind of environment with that found in most general hospitals. In most cases the patient's complaint is not with the monotony of his environment but with the intensity of the stimuli around him. The comparison may be more reasonable in the case of those patients who are confined to bed or are heavily bandaged.

Effects of the Hospital Milieu

In the field of hospital design, the architect not only has a captive audience; that audience is also sick and to a certain extent helpless. Aspects of the physical environment that are relatively unimportant to a well person may loom large upon the horizon of a person confined to a hospital bed. The healthy person is able to adjust his environment to suit his own needs; he can move the furniture in his home when it displeases him or if he should become bored with the arrangement, and he can go out of his way to avoid unpleasant aspects of his environment, such as loud noises, unpleasant odors, or harsh lights. Essentially, he is able to minimize the effects of unpleasant aspects of his environment either by changing or avoiding them. A patient in hospital may be in a position to do neither of these, being physically unable to change the position or height of his bed or the color scheme of his room. He has no way of avoiding the reverberating echoes from the corridors or the odor of the hospital dispensary. One ingredient of the patient-role is the acceptance of the hospital environment as given, and this is one major difference between the home and the hospital as a locus for treatment. Returning to our discussion of territoriality, we found numerous reports of the change in the person's demeanor when he enters a hospital. His responses are not so different from those of animals removed from their territories.[17]

A review of the articles on the effects of the hospital milieu shows that almost all the work is based on surveys concerning how the patient feels about his room, the service he has received, the nurses, and so on. Few, if any, investigators have made the leap and tried to find the effects of different hospital milieus on the patients' mental and physical condition. The research into patients' preferences is a logical successor to the investigations of the ingredients of a pleasing environment. This research, which provided a meeting ground for psychology and aesthetics, has been going on for a very long time. There are innumerable studies of the affective value of colors, tones, odors, and tastes. From the standpoint of the architect, the most useful of these were concerned with color preferences. However, there is still a dearth of controlled studies of the way that people are actually affected by pleasant and unpleasant surroundings. One notable exception is the classic investigation by Mintz [18, 19] into the effects of pleasant and unpleasant surroundings on the behavior of university students. For his study, Mintz used three rooms in one building on the campus of Brandeis University. One room was generally considered attractive and pleasant; another was considered average or unostentatious; and the third was described by most people as "horrible," "disgusting," and ugly. This last room was 7 by 12 by 10 feet and had two half-windows, battleship-gray walls, an overhead bulb with a dirty, torn, ill-fitting lampshade, and was furnished to give the impression of a janitor's storeroom in disheveled condition. It contained two straight-backed chairs, a small table, tin cans for ash trays, and dirty torn window shades. Mintz was interested in how these surroundings would affect people's judgment of various pictures. He found that the ratings that were done in the attractive room put more energy and well-being into the pictures than the ratings done in either the average or the ugly room. Furthermore, Mintz kept a record of the time that each one of his student assistants spent in each of the rooms. The experiment had been so designed that there were two student assistants who undertook the testing sessions in each of the various rooms on successive days. They were instructed to alternate the rooms during each testing session.

When he checked the records of how long each testing session had taken, Mintz found that the student assistants, unaware of being "subjects" for the study, usually finished their testing more quickly in the ugly room than in the attractive room. His notes showed that in the ugly room the examiners displayed such reactions as monotony, fatigue, headaches, sleep, discontent, and irritability, while in the attractive room they displayed feelings of comfort, pleasure, enjoyment, importance, and energy. Mintz questioned all the students after the experiment. He asked them, "Did you like the experiment?" "Suppose you were a psychologist doing a study of this type, could you suggest anything that you would do differently?" He categorized the answers into those students who were aware of the room differences and mentioned that they did not like the ugly room, and those students who felt that something was amiss about the room but did not know what it was, and those people for whom everything was fine and who apparently were not aware of the differences between the rooms. He found that only 29 per cent of the 48 students mentioned the differences between the rooms. However, 46 per cent had some vague feeling that something was not right about the experiment, but they did not mention that it was the difference in rooms. This underscores the importance of architecture as a background factor, influencing interaction and behavior from beyond the focus of awareness. Huxtable [20] in an incisive article, "The Art We Cannot Afford to Ignore (But Do)," cautioned that architecture is not only essential; it is inescapable.

In any building the location of partitions and walls between rooms or wards will affect the amount and kind of interaction that takes place between people. Although this is not an important consideration in planning hospital facilities for acute patients, since we do not ordinarily expect that these patients will be wandering up and down the corridors meeting people, it does become important when the patient is convalescing. Often the patient's physician and nurse will want him to be on his feet as soon as possible after an operation, and socializing with other patients is distinctly encouraged so that "invalidism" will be minimized. Fortunately, there are many studies on the effects of enclosed areas on interaction and friendship patterns. A hospital administrator should be able to regulate the amount of interaction that takes place by a suitable design of rooms and corridor area. The relevant research comes from a variety of settings where the interaction of people in open spaces was compared with that of people in smaller enclosed areas. In an office situation Gullahorn [21] found that interaction among office workers is significantly decreased by the presence of filing cabinets separating rows or subgroups but that interaction within subunits is increased. Robert Blake [22] and his co-workers compared the friendships of Army recruits living in open and closed barracks. They found that recruits in the open barracks had more acquaintances and knew the names of more of their fellows but had fewer buddies than the recruits living in the partitioned barracks. Their interview also disclosed that it was more difficult for an outsider to enter the social system of the partitioned barracks than of the open barracks. Smaller enclosed areas also tend to produce more cliques and stronger ingroup loyalties than larger undifferentiated areas.

Contrary to popular belief, it was found in the Montefiore Hospital that patients are happier in multibed accommodation.[23] The hospital expected pressure from patients and relatives to get single rooms, but found that patients tended to resist being moved into a single room because of the lonesomeness and boredom. They concluded that a person must be fairly self-sufficient in order to occupy himself fourteen to sixteen hours a day, even with the help of radio and television. These results parallel our work in a mental hospital, where most patients did not desire a single room.

When there are several people occupying the same room, the question of crowding inevitably arises. Experimental work on this problem is very scarce, but there are observations by clinicians as to what happens when a ward becomes "crowded." Linn,[24] for example, has noted that overcrowding increases disturbed behavior among mental patients. He feels that the number of outbursts varies inversely with the amount of floor space available per patient. Pace [25] observed that when he intruded on the living space of mental patients, their psychotic behavior increased. Eventually he found that his comfortable living space was restricted to that of the nurses and aides on the ward. However, this sort of crowding seems different from that described by legislators and superintendents who speak of hospitals, schools, and jails as "overcrowded," and it seems useful to distinguish between overcrowding and overconcentration. Overcrowding is measured in terms of absolute amount of space available per patient (dividing the area of the room by the number of occupants). Overconcentration refers to the total number of people congregated in any single location. The distinction is important if one compares the situation of six people occupying a room of 150 square feet with that of sixty people occupying a room with 1,500 square feet of space. The amount of floor area available per person is identical in the two cases, the only difference being the concentration of people in each of the rooms. It seems likely that the second room has an overconcentration of people, while the degree of crowding is similar in both rooms. There is probably a point where hospital patients feel uncomfortable because of an overconcentration of people in a room regardless of the amount of space that is available per patient. The distinction between overconcentration and overcrowding bears on the staff-patient ratio within hospital. Psychiatrists are generally agreed that it is preferable to have one nurse attempting to relate to eight patients than five nurses attempting to relate to forty patients.

The Ecology of a Mental Hospital

The authors of this article first became interested in the effect of the hospital milieu while working in a psychiatric setting. While it is hazardous to apply directly the findings from a psychiatric hospital to a general medical hospital, undoubtedly some generalization from the psychiatric settings can be made to other hospitals, especially those where patients will spend long periods. The authors' research took place during the period 1957–1961 in a 1,500-bed mental hospital in western Canada. This work was supplemented by observations and surveys in other hospitals and settings.

In the light of the studies of the last decade,[26, 27] few people believe that mental patients are oblivious of their surroundings. It is assumed that even very regressed and discultured patients are aware of what is going on around them. In fact many writers state that a patient's condition is in part produced by his surroundings. This means that a great deal of attention should be directed to the physical environments in which the mentally ill are placed. If society removes a person from his home and puts him in an institution, it becomes responsible for ensuring that the environment of the institution furthers rather than retards his recovery. Many well-intentioned people speak about the needs of patients without making any systematic effort to learn what patients say about the wards on which they live. A number of our colleagues believe that patients are offended by large dormitories, and desire the privacy of single rooms. The same belief exists about large dining halls and long tables. Sometimes it appears that these ideas reflect the needs of the speaker more than the needs of patients. One reason is that many patients come from vastly different social backgrounds than their physicians or nurses.

It is also true that accommodation that is comfortable and attractive to staff can be distressing to inmates. The Report of the Royal Commission on Lunacy in Scotland, which was published in 1857, illustrates this well.[28] There was much praise of the construction and accommodation at Gartnavel Asylum, but this was tempered by criticism of the internal utilization of space. Those inmates who came from poor surroundings felt overwhelmed and oppressed by the spacious galleries. The commissioners commented, "In plain domestic buildings a more contented frame of mind is likely to arise." John Sutton, an interior designer, feels that the contemporary décor of many of the new general hospitals is disturbing to the patients. He states that "the overdone, sleek contemporary look can be an insult and an affront to fear and worry and grief. To the older age group now entering hospital in increasing numbers, it must be alien and disturbing." [29]

There is very little information, apart from autobiographical accounts of former patients, as to how the patient's status as patient affects his perception of the hospital. William Deane, a sociologist who lived as a patient for a week in a mental hospital, stated that many parts of the hospital appeared different to him when he was inside. He added: "This is in no sense a perceptual distortion. It is rather a condition of seeing things through a different set of eyes, which has the effect of making the familiar appear unfamiliar." [30] Deane also describes how his speech and actions became much slower during his stay on the ward.

Wingfield, a former patient, contrasted the pace of life in a prison with that of a mental hospital. She felt that in prison "Everyone moved at a brisk pace, as though at any moment he any patient so much as walked at a brisk pace, without the would break out into a double, while in a mental hospital, if typical institutional crawl, she was liable to be classed as paranoiac." [31]

There is also a good deal of evidence that perception of all kinds is affected by continued viewing. Extended viewing makes a bright color appear duller and an unusual color pattern appear less startling. Since some patients are likely to spend long periods on a ward, it is vital to learn how this affects their perception. Perhaps illumination that seems bright upon admission appears too dull to a patient some weeks later. It may also be that long-stay patients become accustomed to the crowding of wards, and do not mind it so much as newly admitted patients. We should therefore try to learn how the length of time a patient remains in a ward affects his perception of it. Another aspect of hospital stay concerns the passivity and docility found among long-term inmates of any type of total institution. This is a salient feature of the syndrome known as "institutional neurosis," "prisonization," and "hospitalitis." Ellenberger,[32] Goffman,[33] Sommer and Osmond,[34] and other writers have observed that long-term inmates of any kind of institution are less likely than short-term inmates to complain about their often grossly inadequate living conditions. Since these observations have seldom been subjected to a systematic investigation, we were interested in whether long-stay mental patients would make fewer complaints about their physical environment than short-stay patients.

These are several of the questions we have investigated in our research. Impetus was provided by the need to increase the amount of interaction among long-stay patients. Osmond [35] and other writers have maintained that the architecture and furniture arrangement of a hospital often reduce the amount of interaction among patients.

One of our studies [36] was done on a ward for older women that had recently been renovated. The walls had been painted in cheerful colors; a spacious day room had been created out of a series of small rooms and corridors; incandescent lighting was installed; new chairs were brought in; a television and several air-conditioning units were installed, and so on. Many visitors considered this a model ward. In fact, when the hospital submitted its application for an American Psychiatric Association Achievement Award, photographs of this ward were included in the packet. However, there was one salient feature in the pictures of this ward that was not noticed at the time. *There was no sign of human interaction.* Somehow we had given these women a model ward that effectively discouraged social relationships. Each woman could sit on her new chair and look straight ahead at the freshly painted walls or look downward at the new rubber-tiled floor. When we called this to the attention of visitors, they were quite surprised, and their opinions of the ward changed accordingly. They supplemented their compliments for the cheerful interior with remarks that it looked "like a train station" or "like a waiting room."

The dominant trend in the arrangement of furniture had been shoulder-to-shoulder seating along the walls of the room, in addition to three islands of chairs back-to-back. The unnaturalness of this arrangement was apparent when we began observing how people arranged furniture in their own homes. There we found the furniture arranged in small semicircles with people facing one another. We found that when we tried to sit and converse shoulder to shoulder, it soon became physically and psychologically uncomfortable. It seemed we had made strangers of our patients.

In retrospect, the reasons behind the ward arrangement are not difficult to understand. First, we know very little about the way in which furniture arrangement helps social interaction. The American Psychiatric Association devotes a section of its magazine *Mental Hospitals* to architecture and ward design, but the plans shown reveal only bare walls and rooms. The arrangement of furniture is left to the ward staff. Nurses and aides do not often realize the therapeutic value of certain arrangements of furniture. Ward geography is taken for granted. A chair becomes something to sweep around rather than a tool for facilitating social interaction.

The inadequacy of our ward arrangement was most apparent when we contrasted it with the furniture arrangement in the corridor outside the ward. This corridor is used by relatives and friends for visiting with the patients. Every morning at eight the chairs are placed in straight rows (shoulder to shoulder) against the walls. None the less, if one walked through the corridor later in the day he would find the furniture rearranged. The relatives had moved the chairs into small groups so that they could face one another and converse comfortably. This typically happened in the corridor but *never* happened in the ward. The moral was clear that the friends and relatives were arranging the geography to suit their needs, while the patients were *being arranged* by the geography.

This is typical of institutions of all kinds, including general hospitals. Patients, dispossessed from their homes and familiar landmarks, keep aloof from their physical surrounding by remaining in bed or sitting in the corner of a room, afraid to tamper with the physical environment. Removed from their territories and defined as sick or helpless by those around them, the patients adapt to the hospital instead of changing it to suit their needs.

Certain arrangements of furniture are most satisfactory from the standpoint of doing ward chores. In institutional settings it is common to find arrangements such as that shown in Figure 10-1 (top) with the chairs in neat rows along the walls. This makes it easier to sweep and survey the ward at a glance. Also desired are wide pathways where food carts and cleaning wagons can pass freely. All these factors join in producing a ward with rows of chairs against the walls and wide straight pathways between the rows. Food-service personnel and maintenance employees often come through this particular ward because of the ease of transit. Unfortunately, this took valuable living space from the patients and turned it into corridor space.

One must also take into account the effects of institutional sanctity. People who are confined in one environment for any length of time eventually come to accept this environment as fixed and "natural." This applies both to patients and staff, and things are done in a prescribed manner largely because of habit and ward tradition. After cleaning time on a ward, a chair is quickly returned to its specified place "because that is where it belongs." The customary geographic arrangement becomes sacred, and any deviation from it causes a disturbance among the patients and staff.

This particular attitude reinforces the antitherapeutic furniture arrangement that dominates many hospital wards. The patients come to accept the customary arrangement as good and right. In fact, they will be the first to oppose any attempt to rearrange the furniture. Various rituals will develop around keeping things in place. On most wards one will observe several patients who feel that it is their duty to move out-of-place chairs back to

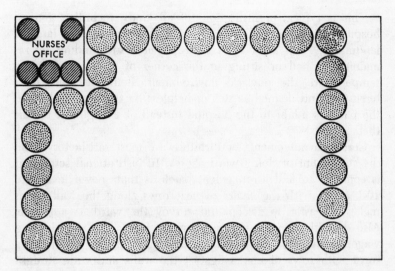

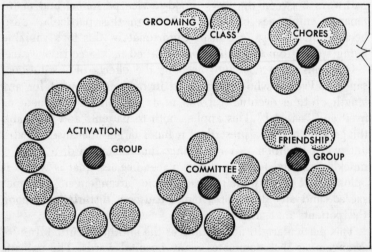

Figure 10-1. Representation of a ward for long-term female psychiatric patients. Above, a custodial pattern with the patients lining the walls of the day room and with the staff in the office. Below, a group activities.[37]

their customary positions. This makes it extremely difficult to effect any changes in ward geography. The patients prefer a stable ward environment, while the nurses admire the neat appearance of a ward with rows of chairs arranged shoulder to shoulder. It is usually true that if function does not determine structure, then structure will inevitably determine function. If the staff do not arrange the furniture to facilitate social inter-action, they may find that the chairs will arrange the patients to minimize social interaction.

In one study [38] we attempted to replace the rows of chairs along the walls with small clusters of chairs grouped around tables. (See Figure 10-1, bottom.) Our goal was to see if this would increase the amount of conversation among patients. Our observations made one month later showed that conversation and other indices of social interaction, such as magazine reading, showed an appreciable increase. However, it was not always easy to keep the chairs away from the walls. Many of the patients would replace them in their former positions when given the opportunity.

The preference of the patients for a seat next to the wall brings up a number of absorbing questions. We have observed this preference in a number of settings outside mental hospitals. When faced with a room full of strangers, people select a position next to the wall. The student of Western movies knows that the hero always sits with his back to the wall so he cannot be hit from behind. Here is an account by a London prostitute describing her life in Soho:

This is my favorite table, and here I can sit with my back against the wall, facing the door. Here is a vantage point from which entries and exits can be observed without too much effort. Nobody can get behind me, and there is safety in this. If there is any trouble, if fighting breaks out for any reason, a wall position is the best to be in. In anger or fear, I have noticed that men seek the nearest open space for maximum freedom of movement or chance of flight. . . . In the centre of a room, however alert you are, you can be knocked out of your chair by scuffling men before the first blow has landed, and if you are lucky enough to get back on your feet unharmed you will probably find yourself in the heart of the battle. . . .[39]

There has been little experimental investigation of the preference of people for a wall position. Biologists use the term "thigmotaxis" to describe the tendency of some lower organisms to congregate against a solid surface. At one time we conducted a small experiment on this, and ushered pairs of university students and nurses into a dormitory containing eight beds. When asked to express a preference of a sleeping position, almost every student favored a bed next to a wall rather than in the center of the room. One would expect this preference to be strongest when a person is in a strange or frightening situation. We have already mentioned our difficulty in getting patients to sit around tables that were placed in the center of a large room. We had suspected that patients would be unwilling to sit on single chairs in the "large ocean" of the room, and this is why we placed "islands" of chairs there. Perhaps the most feasible solution would be to use columns or partitions to provide the feeling of physical security that the patients' apparently require.

In another study [40] in this same hospital, we were interested in the characteristics of those mental patients who inhabited the corridors of their wards. Often standing or sitting silently in the dimly lighted corridor, these patients represented an enigma and a challenge to the nurses and psychiatrists. Although the corridor dwellers rarely could be induced to participate in games or activities, a few nurses maintained that the patients displayed a keen interest in their surroundings. In fact, some nurses assumed that the patients remained in the corridors so that they could see the people passing through the ward.

Our investigation involved a sociometric interview with the patients on four different types of mental-hospital wards. We were interested in whether the number of friends the patient had was related to where he customarily stood or sat on the ward. The results showed that on the three long-stay wards the corridor dwellers were the most isolated group. They had fewer friends than the patients who were found in the day room. The situation on the admission ward was complicated by the variety of patients living there, especially since the alcoholics were exceedingly clannish, remaining together and rarely associating with other patients.[41]

Later we enlisted the aid of fifteen student nurses who interviewed 117 patients on a variety of wards as to whether the patients had favorite places to sit or stand. Of those patients who answered affirmatively, twenty had favorite places in the corridor, eighteen in the day room, and ten in other areas such as verandas or small sitting rooms. The reason most frequently given for preferring the day room was the television or some other amenity such as furniture, clock, or books. Patients who preferred a corridor location could be divided into those who said that they went there for quiet and privacy and those who went there to watch people come and go. Those patients who preferred the smaller areas were mainly attracted by the quiet and privacy.

Following this, a more intensive survey was done regarding the patients' opinions of the ward milieu. A forty-four-item questionnaire was constructed that dealt with various aspects of ward milieu. Each patient was asked about the size of the ward, temperature, ventilation, lighting, furniture, noise, privacy, and crowding. Two different wards were chosen for the study, and at least half the patients on each ward were interviewed. Although both wards contained many long-stay patients, each received direct transfers from the admission wards.

Of the questions asked during each interview, thirty-eight gave the respondent the opportunity to register a complaint. Since we were also interested in the relationship between the length of a patient's stay in hospital and the number of complaints he made, we divided the sample into short, medium, and long-stay patients. Since a considerable body of research has shown that there is a low discharge rate for patients who have been in hospital for two years or longer, it seemed wise to use the two-year mark as the outside limit for short-stay patients. We also considered patients who had been in the hospital from two to ten years as "medium-stay patients," and those who had been ten years or longer as "long-stay patients."

Of the 3,610 answers of the patients, 26 per cent were com-

plaints of various kinds. Long-stay patients were found to make
fewer complaints than medium- or short-stay patients. Of the
responses of long-stay patients, 23 per cent were complaints,
compared with 28 per cent for the medium-stay patients and 30
per cent for the short-stay patients. A statistically significant
difference is found when the responses of medium- and short-
stay patients are combined and compared with those of
responses of long-stay patients. This seems in line with Ellenberger's [42] concept of the nesting of inmates in a total institution.

The vast majority of patients felt that the furniture and beds
on the ward were comfortable. More of the long-stay than short-
or medium-stay patients favored large dormitories or expressed
no preferences. The dining hall was felt to be crowded by 21
per cent of the patients, the day room by 21 per cent, the corridor by 30 per cent, the dormitory by 42 per cent, and the
total ward by 41 per cent. On each item the short- and medium-
stay patients were more sensitive to overcrowding than long-
stay patients.

Each patient was asked if there was a place he could go if
he wanted to be away from people. Approximately half the
patients answered in the affirmative, and there was a slight
trend for more long-stay patients than short- or medium-stay
patients to have private places. Those patients who gave affirmative answers were asked to describe their private places.
There was a striking difference between the wards, largely due
to the fact that one ward was locked all the time while the other
was unlocked during the day. On the locked ward the most common private places were the visiting room, toilet, veranda, or
sitting room. On the unlocked ward the most frequent single
response, given by one-third of the patients who mentioned
specific places, was that the patient would go outside if she
wanted to be alone. On the locked ward none of the patients
gave this response. This shows an important advantage of unlocked wards that is not always realized.

In interpreting these results, it should be made explicit that
what a patient wants is not necessarily what is best for him.
This is not undemocratic or antitherapeutic, but simply a realization of the fact that the patient is ill and may not know the

most effective treatment for his illness. For example, in observing the way patients on psychiatric wards sit and stand, we have seen how they use space so as to withdraw from other people. Often they prefer dimly lit corridors or soft easy chairs where they can sleep during the day. This desire for isolation is regarded by some as a main symptom of schizophrenia. Rather than design and furnish wards that further the patient's desire to retreat from people, most psychiatrists would like to establish sociopetal wards in which patients are oriented *toward* other people. None the less, wards should be designed and furnished with full knowledge of the patients' preferences even though these preferences are not always heeded.

Another problem of concern to social scientists is the change in sense perception during a stay in a total institution. There have been many allusions to sensory blunting during prolonged hospitalization or imprisonment. There is no information available as to whether this is due to the drabness of the institution or to habituation as to one's surroundings. Katz,[43] for example, found that short-stay mental patients prefer colors from the short-wave end of the spectrum, while long-stay patients prefer colors from the upper end of the spectrum. The environments of many total institutions do not seem too different from the conditions used by Hebb [44] to produce hallucinations in normal people.

The decline in complaints and lessened sensitivity to overcrowding with length of stay that we found are in line with the idea of sensory blunting. This suggests that a long-term inmate "settles into" his environment, or "nests," to use Ellenberger's [45] term. Consequently, any change in the patient's environment threatens him. Support for this idea appeared when we tried to rearrange furniture, and found that many patients and staff became upset and moved it back against the wall.

Summary

We will close this paper by again emphasizing the lack of studies showing how the physical environment of the hospital affects the condition of the patient. There is no shortage of surveys that show the patient's likes and dislikes. However, if these results are to be of any value to hospital administrators, the gap must be bridged between the patient's expressed attitudes and his physical and mental condition. More is known about the spatial needs of animals in zoos and circuses than about the spatial needs of people. As Hediger and his co-workers have shown, if an animal is given too much or too little space, it becomes sick and dies. Since it is quite expensive to replace a zoo animal, much research has gone into learning the conditions most suitable for their growth, development, and reproduction.

In this paper the concepts of personal space and territory were developed at some length. Intrusions into the patient's personal space are reflected in complaints of a lack of privacy, while the patient's inability to stake out a territory within the hospital is seen as the "impersonality" and "coldness" of the institution. In order to put the patient at his ease, the administrator of the hospital will probably want to take steps to ensure that the patient's personal space is respected, but will be somewhat ambivalent about the patient's quest for a territory within the hospital. Such a condition, often described as hospitalism, invalidism, or "nesting," is seen as a danger sign and an impediment to the patient's full recovery. We have discussed the research dealing with the way that patients in a mental hospital use space, as well as the obverse of this problem, the ways that the distribution of space within the hospital arranges the patients. It was seen that one major difference between a hospital and other settings is that the patient has very little control over his immediate physical surroundings, which increases the need for a therapeutic rather than a hurtful hospital milieu.

NOTES

1. Henri F. Ellenberger, "Zoological Gardens and Mental Hospital," *Canadian Psychiatric Association Journal*, 5 (July, 1960), pp. 136-149.

2. Katherine M. Ford and Thomas H. Creighton, *The American House Today* (New York: Reinhold, 1954), p. 109.

3. Julius A. Roth, "The Control of Contagion," unpub. MS, 1959, p. 23.

4. Eliot Howard, *Territory in Bird Life* (London: John Murray, 1920).

5. William F. Whyte, *Street Corner Society* (Chicago: University of Chicago Press, 1943).

6. F. M. Thrasher, *The Gang* (Chicago: University of Chicago Press, 1927).

7. J. Carse, "Care of Patients Outside of Hospital," *Canada's Mental Health,* 7 (June, 1959), pp. 33-37.

8. Heini Hediger, *Study of the Psychology and Behaviour of Captive Animals in Zoos and Circuses* (New York: Criterion Books, 1955).

9. David Katz, *Animals and Men* (New York: Longmans, Green, 1937).

10. J. von Uexküll, "A Stroll through the Worlds of Animals and Men," in Claire Schiller, ed., *Instinctive Behavior* (New York: International Universities Press, 1957).

11. William Stern, *General Psychology from the Personalistic Standpoint,* M. M. Spoerl, trans. (New York: Macmillan, 1938).

12. Richard Neutra, *Survival Through Design* (New York: Oxford University Press, 1954).

13. Maurice E. Linden, "Some Psychological Aspects of Rescue Breathing," *American Journal of Nursing* (July, 1960), pp. 971-974.

14. George E. Ruff and Edwin Z. Levy, "Psychiatric Research in Space Medicine," *American Journal of Psychiatry,* 115 (1959), pp. 793-797.

15. David O. Hebb, *Organization of Behavior* (New York: John Wiley, 1949).

16. Robert Sommer and Humphrey Osmond, "Autobiographies of Former Mental Patients," *Journal of Mental Science,* 106 (April, 1960), pp. 648-662.

17. The corollary situation, the change in the demeanor of the physician or nurse who treats the patient in his own home, has rarely been studied. The physician does not always stop to think that some of the change in the patient's behavior in hospital may be due to a change in the patient's perception of the physician or nurse. In a private home the physician is an intruder, coming hat in hand, apologetic because he has worn his rubbers inside the hallway, and feeling that he is disturbing the routines of the household (especially when there are healthy members of the family present). The question of ownership of hospital territory deserves some study too. We have seen cases where it seemed that the nurses had staked out this territory and where even the physicians felt they were intruders. Probably there are other hospitals where the administrator and nonclinical staff feel that this is "their hospital" even though it is a work place for the clinical staff and a locus of treatment for the patients.

18. Abraham Maslow and Norbett Mintz, "Effects of Esthetic Surroundings: 1. Initial Short-Term Effects of Three Esthetic Conditions upon Perceiving 'Energy' and 'Well-Being' in Faces," *Journal of Psychology,* 41 (1956), pp. 247-254.

19. Norbett Mintz, "Effects of Esthetic Surroundings: 11. Prolonged and Repeated Experience in a 'Beautiful' and an 'Ugly' Room," *Journal of Psychology,* 41 (1956), pp. 459-466.

20. Ada L. Huxtable, "The Art We Cannot Afford to Neglect (But Do)," *New York Times Magazine,* (May 4, 1957), pp. 14-15.

21. John T. Gullahorn, "Distance and Friendship as Factors in the Gross Interaction Matrix," *Sociometry,* 15 (1952), pp. 123-124.

22. Robert R. Blake *et al.*, "Housing Architecture and Social Interaction," *Sociometry,* 19 (June, 1956), pp. 133-139.

23. John D. Thompson, "Patients Like These Four-Bed Wards," *The Modern Hospital* 85 (December, 1955), pp. 84-86.

24. Louis Linn, *Handbook of Hospital Psychiatry* (New York: International Universities Press, 1955), p. 150.

25. Robert E. Pace, "Situational Therapy," *Journal of Personality,* 25 (September, 1957), pp. 578-588.

26. Milton Greenblatt *et al., From Custodial to Therapeutic Care in Mental Hospitals* (New York: Russell Sage Foundation, 1955).

27. Milton Greenblatt *et al., The Patient and the Mental Hospital* (New York: The Free Press of Glencoe, 1957).

28. Angus MacNiven, "The First Commissioners," *Journal of Mental Science,* 106 (April, 1960), pp. 451-471.

29. John Sutton, "Hospitals Shouldn't Look Like Night Clubs," *Modern Hospital* (September, 1958), pp. 109-112.

30. William N. Deane, "The Reactions of a Non-Patient to a Stay on a Mental Hospital Ward," *Psychiatry,* 24 (1961), pp. 61-68.

31. Alysia Wingfield, *The Inside of the Club* (London: Angus and Robertson, 1958), p. 120.

32. Ellenberger, *op. cit.*

33. Erving Goffman, "On the Characteristics of Total Institutions," *Proceedings of the Symposium on Preventive and Social Psychiatry* (Washington, D.C., GPO, 1957).

34. Robert Sommer and Humphrey Osmond, "Symptoms of Institutional Care," *Social Problems,* 8 (Winter, 1961), pp. 254-263.

35. Humphrey Osmond, "Function as the Basis of Psychiatric Ward Design," *Mental Hospitals* (April, 1957), pp. 23-29.

36. Robert Sommer and Hugo Ross, "Social Interaction on a Geriatric Ward," *International Journal of Social Psychiatry,* 4 (1958), pp. 128-133.

37. Figure from William E. Powles, "An Examination of the Concept of Milieu Therapy," *Canadian Psychiatric Association Journal,* 5 (October, 1960), pp. 203-211. (Reprinted with permisson of publisher.)

38. Sommer and Ross, *op. cit.*

39. Anonymous, *Streetwalker* (New York: Dell Publishing Co., 1961), p. 40.

40. Robert Sommer and Gwyneth Witney, "Designed for Friendship," *Canadian Architect* (February, 1961), pp. 59-61.

41. Gwyneth Witney and Robert Sommer, "Friendship Patterns on an Admissions Ward," *Psychiatry,* 24 (November, 1961), pp. 367-372.

42. Ellenberger, *op. cit.*

43. S. E. Katz, "Color Preferences in the Insane," *Journal of Abnormal and Social Psychology,* 26 (1931), pp. 203-209.

44. Hebb, *op. cit.*

45. Ellenberger, *op. cit.*

Index

(343)